BOMBSHELL

SUZANNE SOMERS

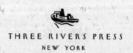

THREE RIVERS PRESS
NEW YORK

BOMBSHELL

EXPLOSIVE MEDICAL SECRETS

THAT WILL

REDEFINE AGING

Copyright © 2012 by Suzanne Somers

All rights reserved.
Published in the United States by Three Rivers Press, an imprint of the Crown Publishing Group, a division of Random House, Inc., New York.
www.crownpublishing.com

Three Rivers Press and the Tugboat design are registered trademarks of Random House, Inc.

Originally published in hardcover in the United States by Crown Archetype, an imprint of the Crown Publishing Group, a division of Random House, Inc., New York, in 2012.

Library of Congress Cataloging-in-Publication Data is available upon request.

ISBN 978-0-307-58855-5
eISBN 978-0-307-58856-2

Printed in the United States of America

Cover design by Caroline Somers and Danielle Shapero-Rudolph
Cover photograph by Cindy Gold

1 3 5 7 9 10 8 6 4 2

First Paperback Edition

To my beautiful family

who understand the importance of health:

Bruce, Caroline, Leslie, Stephen, and Olivia;

Ziane, Daisy, Camelia, Violet, Becket, and Ari.

May you all age well and live a very long time,

so we can be together always and

experience the thrill of knowing

our children's, children's, children's children!

And to Alan, the love of my life,

who will be there with me.

THE ONLY CONSTANT IS CHANGE. LEARN TO LOVE IT.

AS THE RATE OF CHANGE ACCELERATES, THE RESULT

WILL APPEAR CHAOTIC TO THE UNINITIATED.

BUT THERE IS ELEGANT ORDER IN CHAOS. FEW SO FAR

HAVE LEARNED TO RECOGNIZE AND PROFIT FROM IT.

THIS IS WHERE THE FUTURE LIES.

—*Frank Ogden, futurist*

CONTENTS

PART III
Putting It All Together

ACKNOWLEDGMENTS

Heather Jackson has been the editor of five of my books—all bestsellers—clearly it works between us. Heather is easygoing until she isn't, and I am easygoing until I am not. When the crunch is on, it's always startling that we both take such strong stands from our different perspectives. But it works for us. Heather has great respect for me as a writer, and I have great respect for her as an editor. We bounce our ideas off each other. Her choices are elegant and always with great perspective. What I'm saying is: We work together beautifully. She is my life raft. I am so fortunate to have her at the other end of my computer; and the bonus is that she is smart and such a nice, good person. The perfect editor.

Alan Hamel, my husband and partner in everything, was such a help on this one; he let me read to him each chapter as it was finished and gave me great feedback. When he said, "Wow," and asked questions, I knew that chapter was a slam dunk. When I would look over and his eyes were half closed, I knew that the chapter needed serious editing. Alan is a marketing genius, and he always has a vision beyond my own. Because of him my work has been turned into a brand. In addition, living and working with him is simply . . . fun. He shares absolute enthusiasm for all my projects and makes me feel like I am the most fabulous woman on the planet. Lucky me.

Thanks to the doctors and professionals who were my willing teachers. I loved this education and was the eager student, devouring everything all of you taught me: Ray Kurzweil, Bill Faloon, along with Dr. Steven Joyal and the scientific advisory board at Life Extension, Dr. Dip Maharaj, Noel Patton of T.A. Sciences, Dr. Bill Rea, Dr. Russell Blaylock, Dr. Garry Gordon, Dr. Jonathan Wright, Dr. Michael Galitzer, Dr. Prudence Hall, Dr. Stan Burzynski, Dr. Abraham Morgentaler, Dr. Andy Jurow, Dr. Nick Gonzalez, Dr. Joel Aronowitz, Dr. Rick Sponaugle, Dr. Ed Park, and David Schmidt of LifeWave.

I love the cover of this book. It is fresh and clean, appealing, and aspirational, thanks to my talented design team, Danielle Shapero-Rudolph with her great taste and design skills and my daughter-in-law and EVP of our company, Caroline Somers. With their impeccable taste and class they made it perfect . . . again! Thank you.

My team at Crown is always there for me, enthusiastic and respectful. I could not wish for a better publishing partner or a nicer group of professionals. Maya Mavjee is a president and publisher with faultless taste and great vision, and Tina Constable, senior vice president and publisher of Crown Archetype, has been there from my very first book, twenty books ago. Over the years, we have become very good friends, and it is always a great experience working with Tina, plus we have a ball when socializing. We have mutual admiration and trust, and I value that above all.

Christine Tanigawa, the production editor on this one as well as my last four books; Elizabeth Rendfleisch, for her always lovely design work; James Massey, for cover input; Linnea Knollmueller; Luisa Francavilla; Amy Boorstein—all these people are the unseen but crucial folks who got this book together in record time. (Sorry I was so late!) And thank you to the rest of my Crown team for your hard work and support in selling, marketing, and promoting my books: Annsley Rosner, Michael Palgon, David Drake, Jill Flaxman, Mauro DiPreta, and Meredith McGinnis.

Sandi Mendelson has been the publicist of many, many of my books, and so many of them bestsellers, which I attribute to great publicity. She's simply the best—and very sexy, too.

Cindy Gold, my talented photographer and her team, Paul Craig, John Guarente, and Bonnie Holland—all of them were my choice for the last several books. Our pictures always turn out bright and vivid, and, no small thing, you make me look so good. Great work.

David Vigilano, my agent—I love your enthusiasm for my passion about health. That's what makes the relationship work so well. You already get it. You are always thinking ahead with a vision of where this brand needs to go next. Thanks.

Marc Chamlin, my attorney who keeps the deals going book after book. I've lost count of how many we've done together; suffice it to say, a lot. But you are *the* guy. I value your literary expertise, which is a very important component for books that sell nationally and internationally. Thank you.

Thanks to my pals at SexyForever.com.

To the women who run my life on a daily basis: How could I do it without you? I love you both, Julie Turkel and Jordyn Goodman.

Marsha Yanchuck, thank you for your perfectionism, correcting my mistakes and doing the stuff I have no patience for.

Thanks to my sister, Maureen Gilmartin, who turned me on to TA-65, a great Bombshell.

I'm also grateful to Gerry Czarnecki of *The Suzanne Show* on Lifetime, who brought me a science book I devoured in two days, which got me all turned on about the possibilities of aging.

And to my cats, Betty and Gloria, who kept me company all these weeks. They walked on my keyboard, knocked over my water glass, had actual "cat fights" for my entertainment, and purred loudly while they slept in the window. Great little friends.

May you all have great health and love in your lives, and if we all follow the principles in this book, we can still be together for book number 200!

Thank you.

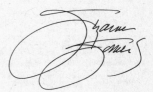

INTRODUCTION

I just turned sixty-five!

I'm excited about it. Never thought I'd feel this upbeat about an age that many keep secret.

Like so many people, a couple of decades ago, before I "saw the light," I dreaded aging. And why not? I never saw an aging person who was happy about it. My late then-ninety-year-old auntie Helen said it so well: "It sucks to get old, Sue!"

And who could blame her. Once "full of bullets" as they say—energetic, mischievous, outspoken, confident, and funny—my aunt spent her last years in a nursing home, unable to perform the simple tasks of life. "The food sucks in here," she would say. "I miss being able to cook for myself." Forgetful, with unsteady feet that couldn't feel the ground from neuropathy and bones so brittle that the wrong moves could snap them in two, she was right. It sucked.

Back when I was a kid, sixty-five was ancient. Now I see it as young. But I can remember being at family weddings looking at my old aunts (in their sixties), all of whom had their legs wrapped in support hose to hide their varicose veins and swollen ankles, their feet propped high on chairs to take some of the pressure off them. They had swollen bodies and pendulous breasts, and there was a seeming sexlessness to them. Youth was gone, bones were brittle, memories were foggy; they appeared to be living back in the "I remember whens."

Next, I noticed that the pills started, tackle boxes full—for memory, for blood pressure, for cholesterol, for bones. Soon they became the ones in the wheelchairs, stooped over, shaking, confused, not quite remembering who they were and, worse, not remembering who they used to be. We patted their heads, kissed them, and told them we loved them. They responded to the affection, but it could have come from anyone, because now in a haze of drugs and loss of self, just being touched and acknowledged, by anyone, felt nice.

When I was a kid and my parents and relatives were still young and full of fun, I remember them partying till all hours of the morning. I was supposed to be in bed, but I would sit with the door cracked open, watching, listening. They had such a good time, laughing nonstop, drinking, and playing cards all night long, then stumbling out of the house hugging and kissing one another good-bye. They were in their forties then; their sixties, seventies, and eighties were coming but none of them gave it a thought. No one back then thought about making a *plan* for aging well.

We plan for nearly everything else in our lives. Think about all the energy you put into planning a vacation, or any major event. But aging is put out of our minds; we don't want to acknowledge it; we choose not to "see" the end point. Aging is just something that "happens" and is something we want to avoid. And rarely do people think the fate they see all around in others is going to happen to them.

No one sees the nursing home, hospital, or hospice center as his or her end point. Though we know aging is inevitable, we ignore it. Even the healthiest among us choose instead to think of it as something so far off in the distance that today's choices are not directly relevant.

But we know deep within, that "time" will come and how terrible it will be if we find ourselves trapped and lost in our particular confinements: wheelchairs, oxygen tanks, knees that won't hold us up, loss of eyesight and hearing, debilitating diseases. Not us! we say. That's what happened to our parents, but not to us! But, I ask you,

WHAT HAVE YOU DONE DIFFERENTLY?

Have you taken diet, lifestyle, exercise, supplementation, hormone replacement, or sleep seriously? Have you managed your stress?

Answer yourself honestly. This book is trying to change the aging paradigm.

You don't want to hear your doctor say you have things like "auto-immune disease." Huh? What's that? Or conditions like lupus, fibro-myalgia, MS, rheumatoid arthritis, and swollen, bloated guts. You don't want to have systems that don't work properly, or experience macular degeneration, which can cause blindness or near blindness; stiff joints; brittle bones; weak limbs; damaged hearts; heart disease; minds that aren't firing; and then there's cancer. That's the big one these days. Deep down, we almost expect it. Like it's some ninja war-rior out there, sitting, waiting, ready to strike when we least expect it.

Cancer will soon be the biggest killer in the world, yet we live our lives, despite our inherent fears, as though it doesn't happen and it certainly won't happen to us. Cancer isn't inevitable. You don't have to get cancer just because you are alive in this millennium. But if you keep eating all those processed, refined, and chemically sprayed foods, you can pretty much be assured you will get cancer. (Don't skip chap-ter 15 and the interview with Dr. Burzynski, where he explains the genetic switches that protect us and how you can keep these switches turned on. This is lifesaving, life-affirming information.)

You don't have to go the way of all those people like my auntie Helen. You can choose a different course. I have. I'm having such a different experience. If this quality of life and health continues, then bring on ninety, or one hundred, or more. I believe it's all possible. Long life with quality—and I mean *long* life. This book is the ticket to a vibrant, healthy life. At sixty-five, I feel great. I'm happy, healthy, I have energy, and my bones are so strong I can do a handstand in yoga. I have perfect memory, and best of all, I have a sex drive!

Who knew this would be my sexiest age?

Things have really changed.

No, I changed.

I believe in the judo effect: using forward energy to win—in other words, turning lemons into lemonade. Like everyone, I've had a lot of things thrown at me in my life: a violent alcoholic father, an abusive childhood spent in fear. I hid in a closet at night trying to survive in an unsafe environment and experienced a teenage pregnancy and a marriage not of my choosing. I divorced at nineteen when divorce was not acceptable, resulting in immense feelings of shame and the surety that I deserved to be ostracized by family and friends. Life-threatening low self-esteem resulted and an overwhelming feeling that I was not worthy of taking up space on the planet. But I was determined to carry on, to make things better for my beautiful child. I brought him into this world and he deserved a good shot in life, and at the very least he was going to know that he was loved deeply and that he was safe.

I fell in love with a married man, which added to my personal anguish, then my darling five-year-old son was run over by a car, which almost took his life. This led to therapy for both of us with an angel who healed my son's fears and stopped his nightmares, and in addition taught *me* to see myself in a different light: that I was worthy, that what had happened in my childhood was not my fault, and that I deserved to be happy and have an incredible life.

I began to *visualize* it. I saw me: happily married, successful, respected. I kept looking at that vision like it was a "picture in the sky." I eventually married him and life took an incredible turn. He was—is—the one . . . my dream husband, and now we've had forty-four years of being in love, madly and passionately. During those years, along came unexpected incredible success on television, reaching the height of fame. But when I was at the top of my game, I was fired for asking to be paid what men were being paid. I was portrayed as greedy and lost the affection of the public.

What had happened? How could I be brought down at what I thought was the height of my life? What happened to that photo I had up in the sky?

I now realize I hadn't gone far enough in my visualization. I had more to go through to learn that the goal has to be complete. I had seen blissful marriage and professional success. That's what I got. But I didn't go far enough. I didn't work my plan all the way through. I hadn't seen how far I wanted my success to go or for how long. I hadn't seen my *end point*!

My house burned down, and then on top of that I got cancer, breast cancer. Now I was blind and couldn't see any picture in the sky whatsoever. One day, lying in my bed looking at the ocean, sicker than sick from radiation treatments that had burned the inside of my esophagus, something caught my eye outside my bedroom window. A huge whale, *huge*, leaped out of the ocean very close to shore. I called my husband to be sure I wasn't hallucinating. He saw it, too, and then I saw this whale leap out of the ocean, three times, until he disappeared.

Surely this was a message if I chose to see it as one: leaping, springing forward, joyous, life going on, energy soaring. I took the actions of the whale for the message that they were. The whale was there to show me that life goes on for a purpose, and that I had purpose. I put another picture in the sky; I saw health, great health forever. I saw joy, I saw happiness, I saw us going forward. And I saw love that was endless between my husband and me, and we were old, very old, but we weren't "old." We had youthful vitality and health, and I wanted that. So I chose it. That became my new focus. How could I use breast cancer and losing all my possessions as a new and exciting starting point?

This was the pivotal moment in my life where I chose true health and wellness as a lifestyle, as my ticket to my end point. I realized I couldn't achieve my big picture unless I started the steps to great aging immediately. I realized, too, that I could change the paradigm of aging.

I WAS IN CONTROL OF HOW I AGED!

I had read about people who lived in the high mountains of Yokohama, Japan, who were alive in their early hundreds without disease. What were they doing? What were others around the world who lived the longest and were the healthiest doing?

I began to ask doctors to guide me; I took advantage of my celebrity to get to the best and the brightest to find out what was new. What was the route to successful aging? How do we age without sickness and make aging an *advantage*? How do we aspire to enjoy aging? Can we see it as a desirable state? And what new medical advances were coming that made all the effort worthwhile? What did the future of medicine have in store for all of us? What you hold in your hands contains the answers those brilliant doctors gave me.

Your body is like a Maserati, the greatest machine ever created. It's time to start recognizing the care and upkeep it takes to keep a machine of this magnitude running at top efficiency. You would never run a Maserati into the ground; you would never put inferior fuel into a Maserati. Instead, you would be constantly tweaking, fixing, or replacing parts, and checking and fine-tuning it. Age isn't a factor with this car, it's a great machine; if you take excellent care of it, a Maserati will survive forever. You are like that machine. But you can't wait until your Maserati is broken down and falling apart. Then the job is so much harder and in some, or maybe most, cases impossible.

You have to start now, before you get too many dings and scrapes!

And just as you can restore your insides, the same is true of your exterior "finish." Wrinkles and a lack of perfect elasticity are no longer inevitable. Staying beautiful is certainly achievable without surgery today, through stem cell protocols. I have already accessed some of my "banked" stem cells and had a stem cell "neck lift" under the guidance of Dr. Robin Smith of NeoStem, a stem cell banking company. The result is beautiful and natural, a smoothing out and regeneration of the skin. How nice not to have wrinkly neck skin anymore. Injections to one's lower face using banked stem cells can smooth out and regenerate the areas that are aging: the little lines above the mouth, the large pores on the chin area, smile lines. This in itself is redefining aging. We can now roll back the clock and obtain the skin we used to have, allowing us to look fresher and more vibrant.

There is also a nutraceutical available that will smooth out skin by releasing the enzyme telomerase. You'll learn more about the importance of telomeres later on in the book, as they are key to a longer, healthier, more youthful life. I truly believe that telomeres and the discovery of telomerase are nothing short of a miracle, a real Bombshell.

Listen to what the experts in this book have to say on perfecting aging and follow their wise advice. Pay careful attention to the explosive medical secrets and groundbreaking information you will learn in *Bombshell*, which include:

- Why we age.
- What the basic steps to a longer life are.
- How you can avoid a catastrophic event.
- Why toxins will kill you if you don't learn how to escape their deadly attack.
- How environmental medicine can save your life.
- How to rejuvenate your cells and balance your hormones.
- What the top Bombshell foods are for longer life.
- Why you are in control of *not* getting cancer and the steps you need to take.

- How to strengthen and rebuild your immune system.
- Where the future—and current uses—of stem cells leads, and my journey.
- How important telomeres and telomerase are for reversing aging.
- What supersupplements are available for fantastic skin and hair, and healthy, clear eyes.
- The new kind of doctor you'll want to visit.
- Future medicine and what it promises to you today.

You'll hear from my trusted doctors and experts everything you need to know to create a healthy, bigger picture for yourself today. I've interviewed some people with the most amazing minds throughout the years, and the information they are sharing here will absolutely blow you away. Here's a little bit about who you will hear from and what they will say.

Ray Kurzweil, famed futurist, discusses nanotechnology and biotechnology and its future advancements that virtually promise to eradicate disease.

Dr. Michael Galitzer drops a Bombshell about preventing bone loss, as well as other methods in the new antiaging medicine.

Dr. Joel Aronowitz performed my amazing stem cell breast regrowth; you will read all about it here.

Bill Faloon, the editor of *Life Extension* magazine, shares explosive information on preventing catastrophic medical events that strike even health-conscious individuals.

Dr. Abraham Morgentaler shares blockbuster, life-altering information on testosterone and active prostate cancer.

Dr. Prudence Hall, my gynecologist and hormone specialist, talks about the hormone that makes you want to have sex (and improves orgasms); she asserts that a healthy person is a sexual person.

Dr. Jonathan Wright, the father of bioidentical hormones, discusses how hormonal balance and cell rejuvenation can revitalize—and lengthen—your life.

Noel Thomas Patton shares information about the new nutraceutical supplement (TA-65) that may actually reverse aging.

Dr. Andy Jurow, a Renaissance man, discusses the steps to wellness and the supplement that will redefine aging.

Dr. Russell Blaylock warns of the chemical dangers killing our brains—and shows a clear path around them to keep us sharp and vital.

Dr. Garry Gordon explains the necessity of keeping the blood cleaned to eliminate disease, and how you can naturally avoid bypass surgery.

Dr. Dipnarine Maharaj shares that there may be cancer-resistant human beings and that their white blood cells may soon be able to reverse the disease in cancer patients.

David Schmidt talks about new nanotechnology patches and nondrug approaches to slowing aging.

Dr. Stanislaw Burzynski discusses the cancer-protective genetic switches and how to keep them "turned on" to avoid the killer disease.

Dr. Nicholas Gonzalez speaks of the foods and supplements you can take to avoid the diseases of today and reiterates that cancer is avoidable and even manageable.

Dr. William Rea, an environmental doctor, discusses a detoxification protocol that will allow you to stay ahead of the toxic assault, ensuring a longer, healthier life.

And I offer a new kind of patient resource for finding doctors, Forever Health; it will make it easy to find the antiaging doctor who is best for you.

But before we read what these great experts have to say, let's find out where you want to go. Then we'll learn why we age, and what can we do about it.

PART I

WHAT AGING LOOKS LIKE NOW—AND IN THE FUTURE

I don't want to achieve immortality through my work; I want to achieve immortality through not dying.

—Woody Allen

CHAPTER I

MAKING A PLAN, DEFINING YOUR END POINT

Getting old is not for sissies!

–Bette Davis

What if I told you that you were in complete control of your end point? You are.

What if you approached aging as a coach would ready a baseball team for the World Series . . . to win? What would happen then?

How do you see yourself at the end point of your life? Are you standing straight with energy, vitality, and an intact brain? Or are you stooped over in a body that cannot hold you up, in a brain fog of confusion?

One of the greatest things anyone has said to me in the last decade was at a recent *Vanity Fair* Oscar party. A beautiful young woman came up to me—I mean gorgeous, pure perfection—and she said, "I hope I am like you when I am your age." I smiled, felt very flattered, and said, "Then start now."

She wanted what I had. She was young and perfect, yet she wanted what I had. And when I thought about it, instead of wishing for her youth, I realized I liked what I had more. I had experience and knowledge, I had wisdom and perspective, and I had an innate confidence and sexuality that made me feel great about myself. I like the way I look and I feel I deserve to be comfortable and happy. That took a lot of work. Daily, I am achieving my vision of how I see my life playing out. And by never taking my eye off that "picture in the sky," my personal projection just keeps on getting better. My end point has great clarity, and I work to make it happen. You can achieve the same results for your life; you just have to choose it.

All my life, my success has come from visualizing an achievement, whatever it might be—really seeing it before me—and then doing the work to get there.

I have visualized my end point already: I am going to live a very long time, I will be in great health, I will be thinking clearly, I will be happy, I will have abundant love in my life, and I will be sexual. I will have energy. I will have strong bones and a good working brain, and I will be a productive member of society. I will be wise, I will have great perspective, and I will be sought after as the matriarch for advice. I will be satisfied with who I am.

No wonder aging is a thrilling experience for me. It has taken on the vibe of a great adventure.

Every choice you make on a daily basis brings you closer to or further away from that picture you have of your end point. Are you vibrant? Are you healthy, energetic, and happy? Do you eat right, exercise, sleep well, and manage your stress? Every time you make a positive choice you move yourself toward your projected goal. Every bad choice leads you in the other direction.

How many times have you sat in wonder when someone close to you (usually young) has just had a debilitating, massive heart attack, and you say in amazement, "But he was so healthy!"?

I write again and again of the "language of the body." My work not only relates to these symptoms of hormone imbalance, which are so "in your face" and certainly their very own language, but also to the other "noise" the body makes: the symptoms of distress that are your body's way of alerting you to *pay attention now!* These symptoms are akin to the red warning light that goes on in your car, alerting you when the oil is low and needs checking. If you experience shortness of breath or if you are easily fatigued, you need a tune-up. If you have gut problems such as bloating or constipation, yeast or bacterial infections, autoimmune disorders such as lupus, MS, or fibromyalgia, stiffness in joints, skin problems, headaches, and a lack of vitality, your body is talking—screaming—to be taken in and checked. If your car had such symptoms, you would tend to it immediately. No sane person would run a car into the ground in spite of warnings from the dashboard light; otherwise, you might face a catastrophe that could result in the engine burning up or some other devastating fatality. Of course you wouldn't do that to your car, absolutely not! As soon as you could, you would take that car to the mechanic and have the oil checked and usually tell him, "While you're at it, give the rest of the car a good 'going over.'"

It boggles the mind that we don't revere the health of our bodies in the same way. Perhaps it's because the body is so forgiving . . . until it isn't. We continue to feed it badly, we don't rest it properly or exercise it properly, and then we are startled when the "red warning light" goes off and we end up in the ER having a first heart attack or sitting in the doctor's office being diagnosed with cancer.

It's not until something devastating, that "catastrophic event," happens that we panic. Then we try our best to pull out all the stops to cure what could have been prevented, except now it's like climbing uphill. Why don't we tune in and recognize the body's language for what it is beforehand and circumvent the catastrophe? Men generally are the worst offenders; many of them minimize, thinking it's more "manly" to do so. Men don't want to appear weak or as hypochondriacs, which, sadly, results in the early deaths of so many men who leave widows behind when they could have had more enjoyable years together. The common thinking about health, or a lack of health, is that it will all be rectified with the next "miracle drug." How has that worked out for you?

We have hit the wall with pharmaceuticals. There will always be a place for them, but the reign of allopathics has clearly come to an end. The pharmaceutical companies will not go softly into the night. They will kick and scream and discredit and ridicule and violently oppose. I understand. It is their bottom line, and oh what a bottom line they have had—the greatest ride in the history of business. They even figured out a way to get the government to pay for the drugs while they continue to make the profits. In addition, they pay off some doctors with irresistible bonuses, not only monetarily but also socially—trips to Ireland, golf excursions, yachts, lavish parties—all for writing prescriptions.

Pain, infection, mental illness, and other conditions outside my understanding may always require pharmaceuticals . . . or will they? How long will antibiotics, with the tremendous overuse of them, continue to do the job? For symptoms of menopause or andropause, why would we take drugs instead of replacing lost hormones with natural bioidentical ones? Why take dangerous synthetic drugs proven to cause cancer for the symptoms of declining hormones? Then there are the drugs for cholesterol, drugs for the heart, and drugs for blood pressure, water retention, and stomach problems. Drugs to sleep, drugs to wake up, drugs to take away depression. What are we thinking? That's the issue! We are not thinking. In fact, the overuse of drugs for every ailment is robbing our brains, leading us right to our final rest stop, the nursing homes, where patients require more and more drugs to facilitate every function of their bodies. What a bonanza for the drug companies. What a perfect business template—and we are the suckers who have bought into the sinister plan.

The pharmaceutical model of approaching medicine is ingrained in our mind-sets from the constant bombardment of television ads. These ads all say, in effect, that we need not worry as there is a drug for every condition. Think, for example, of the little butterfly that flies into our bedroom to put us to sleep (Lunesta), or the happy couple holding hands and going upstairs now that they have Viagra. There are SmartMouth drugs so you don't have bad breath, dry eye drugs, nail fungus drugs, and don't forget the doctors in white coats or the celebrities hired to tell us we can't live without these drugs. Together with big government these companies create barriers to novel and even natural treatments that can cure or prevent diseases or conditions. This makes going alternative or integrative thornier and bothersome. Most people go along without thinking of the long-term effects of taking so many drugs and their inevitable premature deaths as a result.

There is hope, great hope. The enlightened minority who seek true health and longevity understand that changes must be made. To keep on doing as we have been leads to the end result we are seeing all around us. The doctors in this book are passionate and reveal alternative, natural ways to live healthy lives while advising on not only what's coming but also what is available right now that we do not know about. These new Bombshell advancements will extend life and reverse aging. These doctors and professionals also give information on how to access the new methods of healing yourself, the goal being long life with maximum brainpower, strong bones, and the vitality of youth.

With a healthy body we can live drug-free and allow for our wisdom to emerge. Being an elder of the tribe to whom the younger generation comes for advice is part of nature, and it is the big payoff for taking care of yourself . . . wisdom is what no young person can have. Imagine having superb health and energy, plus the wisdom of our years regardless of our age?

Who do you go to for wisdom? Who are the elders of your pack? Think about it; your aunts, your grandparents? Sadly, most of them are on the "old age cocktail" of drugs that unfortunately, slowly, over time, eliminates the ability to think clearly. Years of wisdom are lost, which is a tragedy for them and for us.

Our generation has an important contribution to make because we are catching on. Our vigilance will save not only ourselves but also the coming generations. We are starting to see that the drugs are not working. Each drug creates a need for yet another and another drug. It's essential for a "call to arms" to preserve our brains and the only way to do that is to change our current habits.

Many people cannot grasp the concept of living beyond our expected eighty or ninety years (or longer). However long you desire to live, I know that you'd like to eliminate the suffering that goes with being decrepit, frail, and unable to care for yourself. It's going to take some work. But it's simple work. There is no quick *fix* . . . instead there are series of things you will do daily that will change the quality of your life for the better.

Remember this point at all times. You are the driver of this car. You are in control. Focus on the work that needs to be done on a daily basis to get to your end point. It's the food you eat, the thoughts you think, the supplements you take, the sleep you get, the stress you manage, the chemicals you avoid—that's the cocktail. It only takes a simple shift in your thinking and proactive corrections to your diet and lifestyle. By doing this you will form a great picture of your life and your future.

If you were to make two columns, on one side listing the positive choices you make on a daily basis and on the other side the negative or destructive choices, you would see very quickly what you have already decided as your end point. You might want to maintain a daily journal to keep yourself honest. It will show you with clarity which direction you are choosing.

The journey toward joyous and successful aging can redefine your life experience. What's happening and/or coming? Stem cell surgeries, designer supplementation, tune-ups for the internal organs and glands, cellular rejuvenation, and nanobots to wind through your body like little detectives finding disease and genes that are overexpressing and turning them on or off depending on the need; for example, little bots that can find islet cells and turn them on to eliminate diabetes by regenerating insulin-producing cells or stop cancer cells in their tracks. Oh yes, the future is exciting.

AGING IS REALLY ABOUT CARING FOR WORN-OUT PARTS.

Now we can tune up aging organs and parts *before* they are a problem. "Before" is key; waiting until the catastrophic event makes the job much, much harder and sometimes impossible.

Redefining aging also means creating a new philosophy, one that embraces aging as the gift that it is. If you couple this new thinking with the emerging groundbreaking science and technological advances, you will be one of the ones who doesn't deteriorate, age prematurely, or become disease-ridden and decrepit. You will flourish in good health and with wisdom.

SUCCESSFUL AGING IS CHOOSING WELLNESS

To age successfully and redefine aging, you must imagine a road map you can follow to remain youthful and vital. It takes awareness to understand what you need to do to keep your brain sharp, what you need to do to live a long life of health and quality. The antiaging world, with all its advantages, is an exciting new branch of medicine. Is it expensive? Until our government officials recognize how much healthier people will be by eating right and eliminating chemicals, it will remain an out-of-pocket expense. Currently, pharmaceutical companies largely "own" the FDA, plus they financially back the reelection campaigns of most of our officials. This certainly creates a conflict of interest, and we are the losers on this one.

To age well requires a shift in thinking, being open to change, and approaching health differently; most of that doesn't cost us anything. When chemicals were introduced into our lives through common household products and pesticides, we had no idea of the harmful damaging effects. Chemicals were seen as modern-day miracles; we blindly ate them, cleaned with them, breathed them, and drank them. But now we know the seriousness of trying to live and navigate within a poisonous environment on an ongoing basis. And for optimal health, we must start now to do everything in our power to combat the assault. Those who do will live longer and be healthier. Those who don't will most likely, sadly, die prematurely. For me, it's not a choice.

A lot of the change that must take place is simply returning to a more natural way of living life. Again, food choices are crucial. Relying a little less on modern conveniences won't hurt either (that means moving your body more and living more actively in general). Going back to cleaning your house the old-fashioned way, with lemon and vinegar and mineral oil, is not expensive and can save your life. Reading product labels will also keep you conscious and heading toward toxic-free living and long life.

IT'S A LOT MORE EXPENSIVE TO BE SICK.

Perfecting aging is a new paradigm. I live it, breathe it, and love it. I think about it every day with every choice I make, with every bite I take, with every breath I breathe. The payoff is huge. I have none of the aches, pains, and complaints of my contemporaries.

I said this recently to Oprah, who stared at me and said, "Gee, I have a hard time taking my vitamin B each day." I responded by saying that I am my own living experiment. I fully plan to get to the end, very old, very healthy, and full of life. I laughed and said, "I may be alone, but I'm going to get there."

But I really don't want to get there alone. I want all of us to be there. It's not hard, truly.

Let me be your coach. I'll be with you every step of the way. It's not a lot of work; it's a series of daily choices. I promise you the food you will eat will be plentiful and delicious, better food than what you've been eating. I promise that you are going to feel great and alive. I promise you your age will not be a factor, and then like me, you will want to shout it from the rooftops. Who knew it could be so great from here! As I said, I'm sixty-five. I love it. What a view! I must say it looks more beautiful than ever. I have so much left to do, and the great news is that I have the health and energy to do it.

Redefining aging is not about denial; it's about having plenty. It's about bounty, the bounty of great health. Redefining aging is about restoration (putting back what has declined) versus deterioration. It's about understanding that the planet has changed and, therefore, so has the human experience. To live the way we always have will no longer work.

When I was a kid, sixty-five was old age. People either retired or died. I feel so far away from that scenario. I feel young and vital. And it's all because I decided to redefine the aging experience and learn what I needed to do to navigate the new uncharted waters of these millennia. What are you going to decide? Let *Bombshell* be your wake-up call to the changes you can now make that will change your life experience.

Explosive medical advances are happening moment to moment and changing exponentially how we live. It seems that new information comes out almost daily. Once you realize that sickness and disease do not have to be part of the equation, your life can be whatever you choose. Once you learn how and where to access these new advances, you will never look back.

Start today to think about your end point. What do you want? Who do you want to be around for? What are you doing now that is helping you get there? What's blocking you?

Sit with these questions awhile, then jot down your thoughts. Paint a picture for yourself of what you want.

The chapters that follow will help you get there. First up, a glimpse at what causes aging in the first place. Then we'll look at what the future promises from the viewpoint of one of the world's most respected scientists, Ray Kurzweil; his information will give you the inspiration to make the changes needed to live your longest, healthiest life possible.

CHAPTER 2

WHAT CAUSES US TO AGE?

You're never too old to become younger.
—Mae West

We think of aging as the things we lose or that grow worse with time: wrinkles and lost looks, creaking and aching bones, loss of muscle, loss of energy, chronic disease. But with *Bombshell* I'm going to flip that scenario on its head and show you that we don't have to fear these things. With the new science and future medicine in this book, we can age to perfection. But to do that we must first understand what's standing in our way.

So the big questions that must be answered before we move on to anything else are, Why do we age? Is aging inevitable? Is it a disease? What exactly happens in our bodies?

Scientists theorize that aging is a downward spiral of accumulated wear and tear from toxins, free-radical molecules, DNA-damaging radiation, disease, and stress. The thinking is that eventually your body can't fight back. But this theory has recently been challenged by Stanford University Medical School through research that suggests specific genetic instructions drive the aging process. If aging is not a cost of unavoidable chemistry but actually driven by changes in regulatory genes, then the aging process as we know it may not be inevitable. In other words, as we have suspected:

WE ARE IN CONTROL OF HOW WELL WE AGE!

The choices we make on a moment-to-moment basis regarding our thoughts, how well we oxygenate our bodies (through exercise), and the fuel we choose for nutrition all affect the aging process. The end goal then is to slow this process and promote health. Before we do that, let's understand what's driving aging in the first place.

Clearly, the more you abuse your body by bombarding it with toxic substances, the more likely one of your repair systems will undergo a breakdown. One of the most damaging processes to happen is oxidative stress due to free radicals. *Free radicals* are molecules, like toxic waste in your cells, produced in the energy center of your cells (the mitochondria), which are the tiny power plants that convert the food you eat into a usable form of energy for your cells. In the simplest of speak . . . antioxidants "eat up" these free radicals, or clear out the waste.

As we age and in times of extreme stress our antioxidant systems cannot always keep up with the amount of free radicals being imposed on the body. When this happens, a tremendous amount of damage is done to nearby tissues, glands, and organs. In addition, the immune system goes into full swing and releases these free radicals to destroy the invaders.

We all recognize inflammation when it happens to our bodies: you cut your finger and it swells; you get an infection and it gets red and inflamed. You get the picture. What is less understood is that we also get inflamed *inside* our bodies. The problem is that we can't see it. Sometimes we feel it—an ache, a pain, some discomfort—but most often it is silent: plaque in arteries, bacteria, yeast (as in candida infections), or cells dividing uncontrollably as in cancer. Some experts believe that if you reduce your bodywide inflammation, you can slash your chances of heart disease and cancer in half, which may also be the key to preventing Alzheimer's, arthritis, and diabetes.

As I briefly mentioned earlier, one of your cell's components most severely affected by free radicals is DNA, which is the material that makes up your genes. DNA is the storehouse of all the information that makes up who *you* are. In Dr. Burzynski's interview (page 254), he explains how the reaction of DNA with free radicals can change the shape of or mutate part of the DNA and possibly cause certain genes to be turned "on" or turned "off" or even destroyed completely. If these disruptions affect critical genes, often the result is a cancerous cell. So keeping free-radical damage to the very minimum in a toxic world is an important job for all of us today. Fortunately there are now potent plant compounds that suppress free radicals much more effectively than conventional vitamin supplements. This is explained in chapter 18, "Advanced Age Reversal."

Nearly everything about the way we feel and the way we age in today's world has to do with the increasing environmental assault we undergo each day. Never before have humans been attacked by chemicals, poisons, and toxins to this degree; the result is widespread cancer as well as potentially other deadly diseases from this free-radical damage. Cancer is soon to be the biggest killer in the world, and toxins are one of the key reasons why. I was stunned early in 2012 when the President's Cancer Panel report came out, written by conservative doctors and professionals, I might add, which concluded that clearly, we are getting cancer from chemicals.

THE JURY IS STILL OUT ON ELECTROMAGNETIC RADS FROM CELL PHONES AND OTHER TECHNOLOGY. SO FAR THERE IS NO DATA LINKING CANCER TO ERS, BUT THERE HAVE NOT BEEN ANY LONG-TERM STUDIES TO DETERMINE THEIR EFFECTS.

Yet major media outlets did not pick up on it. The president himself didn't mention it. Why? We know why. What happens to big business (so dependent on chemicals, pharmaceuticals, and mutated food) if the secret gets out? So this fine report got quietly and carefully tucked away. (To read the report in its entirety, go to my blog at www.suzannesomers.com and search for "President's Cancer Panel.")

Wrinkles are just part of aging, right? Do you know that free radicals are involved in skin aging? Arthritis—yep, free radicals. Cataracts? Blindness? Macular degeneration? All free radicals. These little menaces are also involved in heart disease, cancer, stroke, and diabetes.

Okay, so how do we stop these little killers?

It's no big surprise: The right diet, daily exercise, and proper supplementation can do so much to prevent their damage. The antioxidants
in food (think plant foods like pomegranates, blueberries, cabbage,
broccoli) are potent suppressors of free radicals. And then supplements such as resveratrol can do a world of good. (A unique supplement
has a resveratrol potency equivalent to seven hundred glasses of red
wine; it also contains pterostilbene, an antioxidant, equal to twenty
cups of blueberries and the amount of quercetin, another powerful
antioxidant, in nine apples.) Imagine, one little pill every day doing so
much good. (See part III, "Putting It All Together," to get a complete
list of life-giving foods and supplements available to you.)

Yet even with the best supplementation, there is no substitute for
the benefits of eating real organic, fresh food. Nutrition is the fuel of the
body, and a diet high in antioxidants can help you control free-radical
damage. Eliminating bad oils (omega-6s, found in corn, sunflower,
and safflower oils) keeps the mitochondria (the energy centers of your
cells) from working as hard and reduces the amount of excess glucose
(a culprit in diabetes and insulin resistance) in your bloodstream.

To understand the science of why we age, it is important to know
the factors that are the age promoters. This next section is technical,
but if you gain control over the causes of aging discussed, you will be
able to have health and a long life. These causes of aging are controllable, but if not kept in check, they can cause serious problems. These
aging processes often work in concert, making one another stronger,
which, in turn, accelerates aging. To get on top of these conditions
requires a nutritious diet, lifestyle changes, and regular detoxification
and supplementation.

THE AGE PROMOTERS

- Oxidation
- Inflammation
- Glycation
- Methylation

OXIDATION

You know how quickly a freshly cut apple turns brown or exposed steel becomes rusty. These processes are known as oxidation. In the living body, oxidation creates by-products called *free radicals* that inflict enormous damage on our cells. Free radicals are bad guys, and they are unstable because each has a single unpaired electron in its outermost shell; essentially it's homeless, so it keeps trying to find a partner. These free radicals roam through our bodies interfering with normal cell function. They are constantly "hungry," latching onto any nearby molecule and damaging it by changing its shape, which makes it useless or even dangerous. This process results in a cascade: Each unpaired electron passes on unpaired electrons to other victims, creating further damage.

Right now, as you are reading this you are on fire. I'm not kidding. Free radicals are fiery unstable molecules that have been implicated in most diseases associated with aging. At the molecular level, the continuous chemical reactions that keep your heart beating, your blood moving, and your brain working look like controlled infernos. The constant exchange of electrons wheeling inside the powerhouses in your cells called the *mitochondria* throws off enormous quantities of energy. Without getting into the heavy science, let's just say that without free radicals, we'd be dead. Free radicals play an important role in cell signaling and communication; however, excessive amounts of free radicals are bad.

The problem is that as we get older, the cellular structures that once kept these free-radical fires under control begin to degrade. Our mitochondria degrade too, given the onslaught of free-radical damage over time. One expert has estimated that every single one of the trillions of cells in our bodies must withstand up to ten thousand individual hits from free radicals each day. Aging causes our cells to lose control over these reactions and makes them vulnerable to destruction.

Unfortunately, free-radical damage to your DNA increases as you age. Certain areas of your DNA are especially vulnerable to this damage, and only a limited amount of DNA is available. So when the cellular situation in your body becomes unbalanced, that's when problems begin to occur. You now have what is called *oxidative stress*. Oxidative stress happens when too many free radicals exist in the body and the regenerative and repair machinery of the cell is too sick or too old to neutralize the damage. Now you are set up for diseases like atherosclerosis, Parkinson's, Alzheimer's, heart failure, and cancer. In part III, I will explain what you can do to offset oxidative stress. As you'll read next, while suppressing damaging free radicals is important, it is only one component of a program that will protect against aging in a meaningful way.

INFLAMMATION

There is *acute* inflammation and *chronic* inflammation. Acute inflammation is what happens when you get a sudden eruption, as with inflamed joints and arthritis, asthma, even acne.

Chronic inflammation is more deadly. It is mainly silent, although it can smolder in your body for twenty or thirty years until the dreaded "catastrophic event." Heart doctors used to think that the sole cause of heart disease was the buildup of cholesterol deposits inside the walls of the coronary arteries. We now know that chronic inflammation is a major reason for cholesterol being deposited in the arteries in the first place. That's why testing for inflammation is as important as testing for cholesterol.

Chronic inflammation is a key factor involved in Alzheimer's. In the brain, inflammation increases both the production of toxic waste products like soluble amyloid protein and its conversion into insoluble amyloid fibrils. These wastes interfere with normal brain functioning and kill brain cells.

Chronic inflammation is a condition of type 2 diabetes. The elevation of blood sugar and insulin levels increases inflammation in the bloodstream, which triggers a series of dramatic events in the blood vessel wall that increases the risk of heart attack and stroke.

Medically speaking, inflammation is when the immune system creates an environment that oxidizes (or burns) certain cells or tissues in the body. Inflammation can become the root of many of the disease processes of aging if it is not controlled and regulated. The best measure for inflammation is to take a "high-sensitivity C-reactive protein" test. This blood test is extremely important in measuring the amount of chronic inflammation in your blood vessels.

The human body is a wonderfully complex machine designed to repair itself in the event of damage. But more and more humans are putting themselves at risk from poor diet and lifestyle choices. As a result, as we age many of our repair systems are breaking down and we suffer damage. Up until now, you'd go to your doctor with the complaints normally attributed to aging and he'd say, "What do you expect? You are old. This is what happens with aging." It has been common thinking that we have no control over aging and that at a certain point the best years will be behind us. What we see all around us as classic aging is not enviable—or inevitable.

Here's the good news. You can reduce inflammation by eating more vegetables and more medium- and low-sugar fruits (especially berries) for their antioxidant value. You can also increase your fish oil consumption, make sure to exercise regularly, manage your stress, and learn to sleep eight hours nightly. (Again, see more on the specific steps to take to reverse aging throughout the book and in part III, "Putting It All Together.")

GLYCATION

Sadly, it is well known that most diabetics age prematurely and die about ten years earlier than nondiabetics. One reason for this is a process called *glycation*, which binds proteins and/or fats to glucose and other sugars in the body to form nonfunctioning structures. When your body is exposed to too much sugar or carbohydrates that convert to sugar when you eat them, excess glycation is triggered. The result is called *cross-linkage*, either inside or outside the cell, which impairs the cell's functions and causes damage to it. Diabetics suffer accelerated glycation. What few people realize is we all suffer from deadly glycation reactions, only at a slower rate.

The major undesired cross-linked molecule is low-density lipoprotein (LDL). We've all heard of this one. This is the bad cholesterol everyone is so worried about because these molecules oxidize (which simply means they turn rancid) and clump to the insides of arteries and other critical places. These oxidized LDL molecules are now useless and can be deadly if they are allowed to build up. If your LDL has large particles, they are harmless, but small particles can be deadly. (You can test for large or small particles by taking the Cardiac Blood Test Panel, available by calling 1-888-884-3666 or log on to www .lef.org/goodhealth. This is a very important test for those seeking to slash their risk of heart attack and stroke. This test measures much more than just LDL levels. It helps assess LDL particle size and other artery-clogging risk factors.)

Everyone is fixated on cholesterol, yet cholesterol in itself is not bad. The problem with cholesterol starts when it oxidizes. (Remember, this is free-radical damage.) In fact, a good balance of cholesterol is essential to our health. Very high or very low levels mean you are out of balance.

Our bodies make cholesterol for many important reasons: our brains need it for neural replication, testosterone is made from cholesterol, and the body requires cholesterol for many other uses. This cholesterol-testosterone connection sheds light on why many flaws lie with statin drugs such as Lipitor. Testosterone is a vital hormone; it builds bone and muscle, plus the heart has many testosterone receptor sites. This is your *pumping power*! Why eliminate the very substance that protects the brain and is required to produce needed testosterone, which feeds the heart through the receptor sites on the heart itself? And do I need to mention the other necessary reason men should want to maintain testosterone? How many men are impotent due to low testosterone or on Viagra because they are taking a statin, which is eliminating their ability to get an erection? The lack of understanding of mainstream medicine in wanting to eliminate the body's ability to manufacture cholesterol is mind-boggling. The body makes cholesterol and testosterone for a reason. The inability of Western medicine to "connect the dots" is taking its toll on our men and women. It is robbing our brains for starters. (Dr. Abraham Morgentaler's interview on testosterone will enlighten you about this very fact.) Now many doctors are urging younger men to start on Lipitor for cautionary reasons; imagine forty-year-old brains being depleted, plus men being robbed of their very man-giving substance, and then both men and women wonder why they are out of energy, not interested in sex, and having difficulty concentrating. It's truly tragic. But I digress, back to cross-linkage . . .

The most obvious damage is when this cross-linkage creates gobs of gunk called *advanced glycation end products* (AGEs) that build up (like plaque in the arteries), accelerating aging and eventually causing death. AGEs cause the blood vessels to narrow, contributing to high blood pressure, vascular disease, and heart attacks. AGEs are also linked to insulin resistance, poor blood sugar control, and the accumulation of damaging amyloid substances in the brain and in the plaques found in the brains of Alzheimer's patients. Plus, AGEs are implicated in rheumatoid arthritis, kidney disease, inflammatory bowel disorders like colitis, and inflammatory skin conditions like eczema.

If you cut back on sugars; limit carbohydrates; avoid processed foods, prepackaged foods, and fast foods; avoid microwaving food; and avoid darkly browning your food by high temperatures or overcooking, you can reduce your number of AGEs considerably.

METHYLATION

Methylation imbalances are another aging factor. The DNA within every cell of your body requires constant enzymatic reactions, called *methylation*, for maintenance and repair. Aging cripples youthful methylation metabolism. The resulting DNA damage can manifest as cancer, liver damage, and brain degeneration.

Healthy methylation patterns have been shown to repair damaged DNA, breaking down potentially life-threatening cancer-causing chemicals and keeping blood levels of homocysteine in check. High homocysteine levels caused in part by methylation defects have been linked to an increased risk of cardiovascular disease, stroke, and Alzheimer's disease.

The problem facing all maturing individuals is that methylation gradually diminishes over time, accelerating the onset of numerous age-related diseases from cancer and heart disease to cognitive impairment.

OTHER AGE PROMOTERS

In this section I briefly describe other controllable "age promoters." The good news is that chapter 18 of this book describes scientifically validated methods to circumvent every one of these age-accelerating factors.

MITOCHONDRIAL DYSFUNCTION

The little energy factories in the center of each and every one of our approximately fifty trillion cells are the mitochondria, which require a complex series of reactions in order to maintain important functions such as carrying nutrients through the cell membrane and allowing the purging of toxic debris. Mitochondrial energy depletion can result in congestive heart failure, muscle weakness, fatigue, and neurological disease.

LOSS OF MITOCHONDRIA

Not only do mitochondria lose their ability to function by putting out energy as we grow older but our existing mitochondria also become severely depleted. For instance, a ninety-year-old man may have 95 percent damaged mitochondria compared to almost none in a healthy five-year-old. This reduction of cell energy can lead to many different pathologies culminating in death.

HORMONE IMBALANCE

Hormones are a language. They all speak to one another. It's a delicate symphony keeping perfect balance. Imbalance and missing hormones are often a contributing cause to many diseases associated with aging, including depression, osteoporosis, coronary artery disease, and loss of libido. Replacing declining hormones must be done by a qualified physician. My resource section will direct you to a doctor who specializes in hormone replacement in an area nearest you.

EXCESS CALCIFICATION

Calcium ions are transported into and out of cells through calcium channels in the cell membrane. Aging disrupts calcium transport, and the result is excess calcium infiltration into the cells of the brain, heart valves, and middle arterial wall, causing arteriosclerosis.

FATTY ACID IMBALANCE

The body requires essential fatty acids to maintain cell energy output. Aging causes alterations in enzymes required to convert dietary fats into the specific essential fatty acids the body requires to sustain life. The effects of a fatty acid imbalance may manifest as an irregular heartbeat, joint degeneration, low energy, hypercoagulation (tendency for blood to clot), dry skin, or many other common ailments associated with normal aging.

DNA MUTATION

Toxins mutate cellular DNA and cause cancer cells to form. Aging cells lose their DNA gene repair mechanisms, causing these cells to grow out of control—in other words, turn into cancer cells.

IMMUNE DYSFUNCTION

As we age, the immune system loses its ability to attack bacteria, viruses, and cancer cells. Aging people have excessive levels of dangerous cytokines that cause the immune system to turn on itself and create autoimmune diseases like rheumatoid arthritis and others.

Enzyme Imbalance

Cell function inside our bodies depends on multiple enzymatic reactions to occur with precise timing. Aging causes enzyme imbalance, mainly in the brain and the liver. This can result in neurological diseases like Parkinson's, or persistent memory loss. Impaired liver function results in toxic damage to every cell in the body.

Excitotoxicity

The aging brain loses control of its release of neurotransmitters such as glutamate and dopamine, which results in brain damage and brain cell destruction.

Circulatory Deficit

Blood flow to the brain, eyes, and skin becomes impaired as we age. Disorders of the eye due to poor blood flow include cataracts, macular degeneration, and glaucoma. Major strokes and ministrokes are common with circulatory deficit to the brain. The skin of all aging people shows the lack of nutrient-rich blood to the upper layers. The prime underlying cause of circulatory deficits is endothelial dysfunction, which destroys the inner lining of blood vessels and eliminates their ability to efficiently transport blood.

Loss of Youthful Gene Expression

As we age, genes that are required to sustain youthful cell function change. Those genes that maintain cell health are slowly "turned off" while genes that make us vulnerable to degenerative pathologies get "turned on." When cells lose their youthful gene expression, we are subject to multiple diseases and eventual death.

Loss of Insulin Sensitivity

When we are young, we efficiently utilize carbohydrates for energy with a minimal amount of them getting converted to fat. As we age and we lose our sensitivity to insulin, we begin to suffer the effects: chronically high blood glucose and high insulin.

Every one of these toxic mechanisms involved in accelerated aging can be mitigated by following the simple steps outlined in chapter 18, "Advanced Age Reversal."

JUST SAY NO TO THE TWO BIGGEST AGE PROMOTERS: SMOKING AND TOO MUCH ALCOHOL

And finally, there are two other major negative influences on health and aging that you no doubt already know about: smoking and excessive alcohol consumption. These are the two biggies. The amount of harm caused to the human body from these two activities alone is a true testament to how good our repair systems actually are.

INFLUENCE OF SLEEP, STRESS MANAGEMENT, GENES, AND METABOLISM ON AGING

How much sleep you are getting nightly and how well you are managing your stress are also key components in determining how you look and feel, as well as how you age.

Don't blame your genes, though; genetics account for only 25 to 35 percent of how fast you age. The rest is determined by your metabolism, which is largely under your control.

Anabolic metabolism: refers to regeneration or restoration activity.
Catabolic metabolism: refers to breakdown and degeneration
    activity.

The rate at which your *catabolic* (breakdown) activity exceeds your *anabolic* (restoration) activity gauges how fast you age; conversely, the rate at which your restoration activity exceeds breakdown gauges how fast and how far you can *reverse* your aging process. And that's what we are looking to do here . . . once the damage is done, what can we do to "up" restoration and put our metabolic system back to healthy, optimal, even prime function?

A BETTER FUTURE

Within the next fifteen years, as described by Ray Kurzweil in the next chapter on the future of medicine, we will have tools at hand that provide the ultimate protection as well as repair ability. He talks about nanobots, blood-cell-sized injected robots that will roam through our bodies repairing and correcting conditions that at present are taking us down, namely, heart disease, cancer, and Alzheimer's. When nanobots are a reality, the present paradigm of medicine will become obsolete.

But until then, to best access these great advancements, we must keep our bodies in the best health and shape possible to continue living with great quality. And that is the goal: quality of life. A life of vitality, energy, sexuality, and great health is ours if we understand what it is that is stealing our health and how we can reverse that. That is what *Bombshell* is all about: blowing up the myths surrounding aging, as well as taking down the obstacles that are standing in our way to the healthiest end point possible.

Free-radical damage is the biggest of these culprits that steal our lives. As such, combating it is the ticket to redefining aging. Let's see what else is out there to make our ride smoother.

CHAPTER 3

WHAT THE FUTURE LOOKS LIKE

It must be remembered that there is nothing more difficult to plan, more doubtful of success, nor more dangerous to manage than a new system. For the initiator has the enmity of all who would profit by the preservation of the old institution and merely luke-warm defenders in those who gain by the new ones.

—Niccolò Machiavelli

Let's start at the end. What's coming, what's your incentive to make healthy choices today and why? In other words, why go through all this work?

Well, imagine this.

In just a short thirteen to fifteen years from now, the diseases of today will be on their way to being obsolete. Imagine, heart disease gone, cancer cured without any of the present torturous protocols inflicted on people today. Imagine Alzheimer's no longer as the final, sad exit we now somewhat expect at the end of our lives. Imagine the end to suffering from Parkinson's and autoimmune diseases; imagine being able to grow new limbs or, as I have already done, regrow a breast taken in cancer. Imagine brains being regenerated. Imagine so much more.

I believe when you know the great strides being made, you will take your daily choices very seriously. You think you don't want to live to 100, 110, or some even say 120 years—or more—but what if you could do so in perfect health? What if, aside from this great exponential growth in science and medicine, we could even *reverse aging*?

Imagine knowing your great-great-great-grandchildren. Imagine the acquired knowledge you would have if you were able to live that long. Imagine your incredible perspective. Imagine how valuable we would be if we were the greatest wisdom pool that ever existed in humanity. As true elders of the tribe, we would be the ones the younger generations would access, not put out to pasture the way our seniors are today.

At present, just when we are at the top of our games, just when we are really good at "who we are" and "what we do," our health betrays us due to a lifetime of poor lifestyle and dietary choices. Then suddenly it's too late. You are now on a downward spiral leading to hospitals, pills, more pills, brain fog, lack of energy, bones that won't hold you up, and eventually the nursing home. That's how it goes with everyone, right? We're living longer. Can't escape it, right? Happens to everyone.

Wrong. There is another way, a new way.

This book is giving you the tools, and each one of them will be discussed in depth.

If it seems overwhelming, remember that making the choice to be healthy to live longer requires a shift in your thinking. And many of you have stuck around with me through my personal journey to these answers. In my series of Somersize books, I asked you to make the first shift: to understand that the way you had been eating was not serving you well and that to be thin and healthy, you had to completely change your thought processes about food. It wasn't about dieting; it was about eating the right foods, foods that build you up and enhance your health, weight, and energy. It worked, obviously, because ten million of you told me so by reading the books and writing to me of your tremendous successes. The letters all mentioned greater health, weight loss, renewed energy and vitality—and that you didn't think you could do it but you did.

My next set of books on health and hormones required another shift in your thinking: doing away with the preconceived notion that with aging came hormone loss and there was nothing you could do about it except accept the pharmaceutical protocol of sleeping pills, antidepressants, antianxiety pills, blood pressure medicine, cholesterol-lowering drugs, and much more. But hormone loss led to the devastating symptoms that stole your quality of life. You gained weight again, you lost your sex drive, and you felt left out of life both sexually and emotionally. You felt vacant. The pills put you in a fog. Or they numbed you but did nothing really about your symptoms. You learned to accept it, the sentence of invisibility described by so many, sexless and lonely. I asked you to assume another shift in your thinking: understanding that if the aging you were experiencing was due to declining hormones, then to feel good again it was necessary to restore yourself to perfect hormonal balance with youthful, optimal, healthy levels. I explained that you didn't have a Prozac deficiency, you had a hormonal deficiency.

You had never heard of bioidentical hormones, the natural non-drug ones, yet you took a leap of faith with me and the doctors I presented—Western doctors who had the courage to step outside of the standard-of-care box to use common sense in medicine—and you went to them in droves. These were the same Western doctors who the orthodox medical practitioners and the media tried to pass off as practicing junk science, yet you went. After all, you had been doing it their way and you weren't doing so well.

You adopted a "shift in your thinking," and millions of you around the world found "restoration" to be glorious, that reaching middle age wasn't the terrible dreaded state of "deterioration" we had been watching before us, but that your middle to later years were a glamorous, sexy, vital, intellectual time of life. You understood restoration versus deterioration and got to feel good again. You threw away the notion that the orthodox community had all the answers. You started to think for yourself. You became the contractor of your body and your good health. You began to realize that doctors were not gods but merely well-educated, well-intentioned people you hired to help you take care of your body.

You realized your body was your very own personal Maserati, the greatest piece of machinery of all time, and realizing this, you wanted to finely tune this machine: fuel it perfectly, listen to its language, and fix and repair it before it broke down. This was a new concept: true health care instead of the disease care we had all been practicing.

How different you felt taking this first step and you wanted more. You wanted perfect health, but then the environment started catching up with you. Why was there so much cancer? Why were there autoimmune diseases? Why so much heart disease? Why so much Alzheimer's?

What else could you/we do?

Plenty. Plenty now and plenty in the future.

Here's where it's going to get exciting.

You want the life you have to be of ultimate quality. That would be a wonderful thing, being happy, healthy, energetic, and vital.

Well, here's the thing . . .

That wonderful life is yours, depending on the choices you make from this moment forward. Do you realize that most people make choices on a daily basis that unconsciously constitute a slow suicide? What do you think consuming, using, eating, breathing, and drinking chemicals does to us on a daily basis? What do you think unmanaged stress on a regular basis does to us? What do you think consuming junk food; nonfood; genetically modified, nutritionally void food; and packaged, chemically treated, lab-produced food will do to you? A body requires fuel, the best fuel (remember the Maserati?), to operate.

NUTRITION IS THE BODY'S FUEL.

Feeding your body chemicals is like putting sugar in the gas tank of your Maserati; that's the end of the car. It permanently destroys the functionality of the automobile; it's ready for the trash heap, that beautiful piece of machinery, done in by the wrong fuel.

That's what we have been doing and continue to do to our bodies. Tragic, isn't it? Why can't we see the slow death we are choosing? But we do it, over and over—the cigarette that is so soothing, the extra helpings, the rich desserts, never knowing which bite is the tipping point, the one that activates the heart attack or stroke. Or the sugar that diabetes and cancer so love and thrive on.

Choices . . .

We make choices every day that move us either forward to our desired end point (the grandest vision of who we end up to be and for how long) or away from it. Aside from an unforeseen accident, we are in total charge of our health. We are in charge of our end point, whatever that means to us.

Healthy choices can become a way of life. Healthy choices can become who you are. Exercise can be who you are. These activities become enjoyable when you know they are extending your life and health. There are days when I go to the farmers' market, or to my vegetable garden, and glow with excitement at the bounty we enjoy in this country: organic, fresh, in season, beautifully colored, delectable foods and produce that inspire me to prepare delicious, life-sustaining meals, perfectly cooked or raw, drizzled with heart-healthy olive oil or sautéed in coconut oil. I seek out organic protein, grass-fed beef and lamb, organic chickens, wild salmon—life-enhancing food for all in my family. This gives me a profound sense of satisfaction that I am providing high-octane fuel for all of us.

No unpronounceable ingredients for me. Not worth it. Even though chemicals are designed to taste scrumptious, they are the worst thing that ever happened to us. They do not sustain; instead, they rob us of our health, and they rob us of our brains. Dr. Russell Blaylock will describe later our "dumbing down" through the use of aspartame and other killer chemicals most people ingest every day.

If you choose to live a healthy life, then what is awaiting you is the most exciting science of our lifetime. You can jump on this fast-moving train, but you have to start now and commit to choosing "life" and not the present paradigm of "death" by disease.

To get you excited, turned on, and give you all the reasons you need to want to live longer and healthier, I am going to start at the end. Hang on to your hats; Ray Kurzweil is the Edison of our time. What he will teach you will make you want to start right now to take perfect care of yourself and your family because the rewards in the future are so incredible.

RAY KURZWEIL

Ray Kurzweil *is the futurist of the century. He is a man whose vision of the future is clear and that includes living longer—radically longer—than humans have ever entertained. His work is based on the premise that we now have the knowledge to identify and correct the problems caused by most unhealthy predispositions as well as by environmental assaults.*

He is a highly recognized authority on biotechnology, medical applications, and the implications of molecular nanotechnology, or nanomedicine. He is also a computer scientist, a software developer, an inventor, an entrepreneur, a philosopher, and the leading proponent of radical life extension. He has a twenty-seven-year track record as a futurist. Many of the predictions in his 1990 bestseller, The Age of Intelligent Machines, *such as the rise of the Internet, have tracked accurately. He has received numerous awards, including nineteen honorary Ph.D.s and the 1999 National Medal of Technology, which he accepted from President Bill Clinton.* Forbes *has called him "the ultimate thinking machine," and* Inc. *has said he is "Edison's rightful heir." He is the subject of the widely acclaimed documentary* The Transcendent Man.

Kurzweil's theory of the law of accelerating returns is one of the reasons there will be dramatic interventions in the aging process in the near future and why you have a chance to benefit from them. Things are going to happen so much faster and so much more dramatically in biology that most humans will benefit from these advances if they are alive.

And he's a cool guy. . . .

SS: Hello, Ray. It certainly is an honor to have this conversation with you. The first time I became aware of you was in 2005, when

I picked up your book *Fantastic Voyage*, which blew my mind and inspired me to expand my thinking as to what healthy living really was. Since then I have enjoyed your other works, *Transcend*, *The Singularity Is Near*, *The Age of Spiritual Machines*, and have screened the documentary film by Barry Ptolemy, *Transcendent Man*, several times. Mind-blowing . . . I guess you could say I have been "Kurzweil"ed!

Your concepts of man merging with machines, artificial intelligence, and virtual reality are fascinating, if at times difficult to grasp. Your predictions for the future have been right on and in thinking about it, the "exponential" growth you describe regarding technology is right in front of our faces every day. For instance, recently, I went nuts when I dropped my iPhone in the toilet and felt absolutely lost without it for a day, whereas just a few years ago I had never heard of an iPhone! So for those who think man is not merging with machines, they should throw away their cell phones and try a shutdown of the Internet for a day. We'd all be lost. Your theories and predictions relevant to longer living and improved health benefits are of great interest because they are so uplifting and positive.

So let's begin with what you describe as biotechnology. What is it and how will it apply to our health now and in the near future?

RK: Thank you, Suzanne. Biotechnology is basically staying within biology, but reprogramming it. For example, when the fat insulin receptor gene was turned off in lab rats, they were able to eat all they wanted, yet they remained slim and got all the health benefits of being slim. They didn't get heart disease or diabetes and lived 20 percent longer. There are now more than a thousand drugs in the pipeline to turn off the genes that promote obesity, heart disease, cancer, and other diseases. Think of it as updating the software on your cell phone. We're updating the software in our body: turning off genes that promote disease, that promote aging; adding new genes that extend our longevity; using stem cells and reprogramming them to regrow organs or rejuvenate our tissues; and turning off cancer stem cells. So basically, we are changing the software of life using these different methods.

We can model, simulate, and reprogram biology just like we can a computer. It will be subject to the law of accelerating returns, a doubling of capability each year, a billion times more capable in twenty-five years.

SS: And this applies to all parts and conditions of the entire body?

RK: Yes. For instance, I'm working with some MIT scientists on the bad stem cells, which are cancer stem cells. We believe that cancer stem cells are the ultimate cause of cancer. Chemotherapy and radiation do kill cancer cells, but they don't kill the cancer stem cells. In fact, in many cases these methods provide ideal conditions for cancer stem cells because they are anaerobic.

SS: Anaerobic means the cancer cells don't require oxygen for life?

RK: Yes. We've actually identified and are culturing cancer stem cells. If we take a culture that has many cancer cells and cancer stem cells and radiate it, all the cancer cells are dead, but the cancer stem cells are happy and thriving.

SS: Then clearly the present protocol of cut, burn, and poison is pretty useless.

RK: You could say that the protocol is part of the solution, but of course, part of the solution is not enough. If you can't kill the cancer stem cells, you haven't gotten rid of the cancer, and these stem cells are ultimately responsible for metastasis. There is a whole field of scientists who agree with this theory, but they've never actually seen a cancer stem cell. They identified it based on certain chemicals on the surface called *antigens*. One is called: CD-44. Turns out these antigens are an unreliable method of identification. We can actually identify cancer stem cells based on their shape and their unique form for reproduction. Our work is to identify the substances that destroy them but don't harm normal human cells.

SS: Could this be accomplished with your nanobots?

RK: Yes. Nanobots will be blood-sized cells injected into the body to carry out a mission.

SS: Like a blood-cell-sized robot?

RK: Yes. They might be inserted to destroy the ultimate source of cancer, or to turn off a gene that promotes Alzheimer's. These profound diseases like Parkinson's or Alzheimer's are caused by an information flaw in the software. There's some genetic switch that gets thrown, and the answer to it can be fairly simple.

SS: Providing you know which switch.

RK: Yes, and there is probably a fairly simple trigger to diabetes, which is actually a group of diseases. We can learn to reprogram these things with technology that will not have serious side effects, because we will be very sharply focused on exactly the cause of these diseases as opposed to complex drugs used today, which are blunt instruments. These "blunt hammers" may have a positive effect, but they are not sharply focused on accomplishing their task because they are not based on a real understanding of how these disease processes work.

SS: When will we be able to access these new technologies like nanobots?

RK: I believe the full flowering of biotechnology is only about fifteen years away. That doesn't mean we're going to have nothing for fifteen years, and then suddenly we'll have it. It's already rolling out there with benefits like stem cell advancements. It's at the edge, but it's not approved in the United States. You have to go to Thailand.

Nanotech is to go beyond biology and even go beyond a reprogrammed biology by introducing nonbiological systems. But these systems are as intricate as biology and at the same level, so the quintessential application will be nanobots that are blood-cell-sized devices that have intelligence because they have little computers in them. They can have robotic capabilities.

SS: And how do we use them? Are they injected or are they a capsule?

RK: You would inject them into the bloodstream. It's a concept that's been around for some time. They were first discussed by Eric Drexler, and there have already been experiments with animals. One scientist has a little nanobot that has eight nanometer pores so it's really at the molecular level, because one nanometer is like five carbon atoms. This little device lets insulin out in a controlled fashion and has actually cured type 1 diabetes in rats as an experiment. Early experimentation in rats has shown therapeutic value. Ultimately, they can be very sophisticated. So one type of nanobot could replace a portion of your red blood cells, but they would be a thousand times more powerful. You'd have much more ability to oxygenate your tissues. You'd be protected from a heart attack if you had one.

SS: Making heart attacks a medical rarity?

RK: Yes, these nanobots will keep you going for many hours. But their uses are very varied; for instance, you could do things humans have not been able to accomplish, like doing an Olympic sprint without taking a breath for fifteen minutes, and that's just with a fairly simple form of nanobot. I believe the really useful one will be a robotic white blood cell.

SS: Why are white blood cells useful?

RK: They are very intelligent little creatures. I've actually watched my own white blood cells in a microscope outside my body and I saw two of them trap a bacterium and then ultimately destroy it. They are very slow, lumbering little creatures. I observed them doing this and it took about two hours.

SS: What are the limitations of white blood cells?

RK: They don't respond well to all pathogens. They don't recognize cancer because they think it's "you." They can attack you accidentally, as in autoimmune disorders.

SS: Why, because it thinks you are a foreign object?

RK: Exactly. We will ultimately develop a robotic white blood cell that first of all could download new software from the Internet for new pathogens, so it could work on things never seen before. With this technology, the body would not be subject to autoimmune disorders anymore. The technology could also attack cancer and ultimately protect you from virtually every type of pathogen-based disease, including cancer. I used to call it the "killer app" but that's probably not a good idea.

SS: [Laughs.] Probably not! And eliminating autoimmune disease would be life enhancing. I hear from so many on a regular basis about their lupus, MS, or fibromyalgia—debilitating, painful, degrading conditions that are treated with even more debilitating drugs, creating a vicious cycle. What else will these nanobots be able to do?

RK: Many things, and we are constantly creating new usages. They will be able to go into the brain and noninvasively interact with your biological neurons as a kind of brain extender. At present, we have computers we put into the brain or at least connect to the brain to give commands. In fact, there are dozens of different neural implants being experimented with for different kinds of neurological conditions.

Right now there's a neural implant for Parkinson's disease, and the latest version actually allows you to download new software inside the body from outside the patient. These implants require surgery because they are not blood-cell-sized, although they are pretty small, the size of a pea, but still too big to send through the bloodstream.

We will also have an artificial retina that will attach right to the optic nerve.

SS: Wiping out Parkinson's, having increased brainpower, restoring vision. This is wild stuff, and you are saying this is what we can expect in the near future?

RK: Absolutely.

SS: I read in your incredible book *Transcend* that nanobots would be able to vaporize arterial plaque and turn on islet cells, thereby curing diabetes. These are huge advancements. Is there a catch? I mean, what will keep us from being able to access this incredible technology?

RK: Poor health. That's why taking care of you today is so important. I mentioned that the quintessential application, the killer app, will be nanobots that augment your immune system. They will roam through your body and destroy disease cell by cell, actually working at the molecular level. It would be beyond what our immune system does at present, which is to destroy germs, bacteria, and viruses. These nanobots could also do little repairs, sort of like surgical repairs. They could repopulate cells that are needed, like the islet cells. We are already doing those sorts of things with stem cell therapies, but the nanobots could carry a stem cell to exactly the right place. Like a little army of machines to do maintenance in order to keep your body young and healthy while destroying disease at the level of individual cells before it becomes life threatening to an organ.

SS: So you are doing the impossible, outthinking nature. That in itself is spectacular if used correctly.

What about the hormone-making glands? I mean, rather than replacing what you are missing due to aging and stress with bioidentical hormones, which involves rubbing on the individualized, prescribed amount of cream every day, could you, in essence, "restart" the internal hormone-making machinery again?

RK: Yes, that's easy; we can already define what optimal hormone balance is. In fact, there are all kinds of trace nutrients, hormones, and other substances we'd like to see in the blood; plus, of course, there are things we'd rather not see in the blood.

These nanobots can access and process the blood. They can add substances that are needed to bring them to optimal levels. They can remove toxins and other potentially destructive chemicals, so, yes, the whole endocrine system is ultimately relatively easy to re-create in a "version two" approach, while keeping people at their optimal, youthful levels. I'm not just talking about the classical hormones but many things in the blood that are critical. The bloodstream is a whole communication system, sending all these chemical signals, which is basically what hormones do.

SS: Imagine the uses for blood cancers, like multiple myeloma. This is a thrilling concept. Will the nanobots have an intelligence to understand the rhythms of each person, that each person is a hormonal individual and some need more, some need less? Because at present, replacement, as it stands, is such a new specialty that there is a lot of discrepancy among doctors as to how much, how often.

RK: I agree. At present it is a complicated issue to correct levels. Hormones, as you write about so eloquently—frankly, Suzanne, your books have changed the quality of millions of lives—have, like you say, got to be individualized.

But what I'm talking about is intelligence within the nanobot to "know" the individual needs of that person. This will be the new method, the new technology to optimize and perfect the levels of each person.

SS: So you are saying, fifteen, twenty years from now, nanotechnology in the form of nanobots will be the answer to the diseases and conditions that have got present orthodox medicine stumped? If so, this is very, very exciting. It offers not only hope but also incentive. If you know today that you can beat the "big three" in the future, you are more likely to want to make the right choices now.

I asked before, what's the catch? In order to access this fantastic new voyage, as you say, what do we have to do to arrive there in good health?

RK: Grasp the concept . . . take the idea of good health today seriously; be proactive about it. The idea that "I don't have to take care of myself now because no matter how I abuse myself I can repair anything that's gone wrong" is just not correct. You have to make your health a priority.

SS: So help drive this home for both myself and my readers. Taking care of yourself, staying as healthy as possible, and doing the work, as in hormone replacement, getting proper sleep, managing stress, eating healthy and correctly, exercise and supplementation, good thoughts, avoiding toxins. Are these the crucial and necessary steps to take to access the coming technology?

RK: Correct. It's simpler than most people think. It will be a very exciting period fifteen years from now, but the goal of "Bridge One" (my steps to health in *Fantastic Voyage*) is what you and I both write about and practice, and that is to get to "Bridge Two" in as good shape as possible. There will be certain types of damages that are hard to repair. Let's take an extreme example, like Alzheimer's. At present, when the brain dies, it is not repairable . . . but in fifteen, twenty years, we will have the ability to turn off Alzheimer's and we will understand the genetic triggers for that. But this doesn't mean we can regrow someone's whole brain that's been ravaged by Alzheimer's. Unfortunately, that is a destructive process, a form of death, and it will not be repairable.

SS: In this book, Drs. Rea, Blaylock, Wright, Gordon, Galitzer, and others are stressing the need to eliminate toxins, to do regular detoxification, and to understand the devastating effects of toxicity to the brain and body. I see it all the time, people who are not able to connect the dots between brain damage and poor health and the every-day choices we make, such as choosing diet soda, and the chemicals in our food, homes, cosmetics, and the water and air we breathe.

I have a friend who is very health conscious, won't eat any fat or carbohydrates, yet I watch her put twelve packets of Sweet'N Low in her coffee, which is all chemicals. And then, of course, you have to ask how many cups of coffee does she consume daily? Due to lack of knowledge, she has not made the connection; chemicals are here, there, and everywhere . . . it adds up. It's a new, dangerous world, a different planet, and most of those who ignore the information, I fear won't be able to partake in your advances.

Will it ever be possible to reverse a damaged brain?

RK: I never say never. But that's not something we think we can do in fifteen or twenty years, because it would essentially mean cre-ating a new person. Basically that kind of brain destruction is very, very hard to reverse because the information, the memories, and the skills are gone. Ultimately, you will be able to re-create a new person, like I talk about creating an avatar of my father, but it's not the same as reversing the damage that's been done to an existing person.

SS: And like you say, the memories and skills will be gone. But, exponentially (your word), with so many working on this goal at the same time, it seems to me that what you don't think is possible right now may be very possible in the future. See, you are training me . . .

RK: Thank you! We are making progress faster, better, and cheaper and at a continually accelerating rate. Whereas science used to pro-ceed at a snail's pace, that is not the case anymore. We don't want to limp into Bridge Two brain damaged and debilitated. That might be hard to reverse. Why chance it?

SS: The big picture I get from you is the sure possibility of ending the conditions that are bringing us down. This is amazing stuff. Like a dream. Would we do this proactively and automatically or wait till the catastrophic event?

RK: It would be a proactive defense. Health is one application, but the quintessential future application is basically an artificial immune system that overcomes the limitations of our current immune system and would also be much faster and much more intelligent. Our immune systems are intelligent but have limitations that we will be able to overcome. Ultimately, we will send these corrected signals into the brain.

SS: Give me examples.

RK: Well, for instance, I'm talking about creating virtual reality avatars like our Ramona we introduced in my movie, *Transcendent Man*. In the future, we will have full-immersion virtual-reality environments and you will feel like you are there, and it wouldn't be just by yourself.

For instance, I have a lot of information about my father, so I believe ultimately, say thirty to forty years from now, I can create an avatar of my father.

SS: Will other people be able to see him?

RK: Yes, you will be able to go into virtual reality and it will be just like interacting with another real person.

SS: What about people who have been cryonically preserved like the famous baseball player Ted Williams, and now I hear Larry King wants to be frozen after death? I mean, frankly, at present it sounds a little creepy to me, but maybe they are ahead of the game.

RK: Well, in a way they might be. Because there is more than their DNA; you have their bodies and brains, and even though they are not functioning, future technologies will be able to map out all their brain connections and probably see the neurotransmitter concentrations. They would basically reverse the damage that the freezing process has done, as well as then curing the diseases and even reversing the early effects of death. I think that will all be feasible.

SS: [Laughs.] Yes and then they can wake up and see my Thigh-Master commercial and wonder what that's all about! [I'm referring here to a scene in a Mel Gibson movie where he was cryogenically preserved and woke up to see me. It was one of the high points of my movie career!]

RK: That's funny, and I hope you're still selling them at that time. . . . But you and I are more than DNA. We have memories, skills, and personality in our brains. It's not just the DNA that reflects our lifetime of experience. We have connections that we've grown in our brains which reflect our experiences. Every time we experience something or remember something, there are connections made in our brains that reflect that, and those connections are still intact. So you create a person who is basically a replica of the person who died.

SS: Is the human desire to live forever to preserve brain intelligence? I mean, for instance, it would be a tragedy to lose *your* brain. And tragic to lose my sunny personality (that's a joke). But the planet needs your gained intelligence, your brain's ability to understand the complexities of the universe and your amazing inventions, as well as those to come. They're all invaluable to human existence. If you were to live indefinitely, your brain would only grow and intensify if you were (and most likely will be) utilizing the technology you are telling me about. You are a valuable human asset. Your knowledge enhances life for all of us, and it would be a shame for that to die off in this generation.

RK: Definitely. And it's based on the idea that I do want to live to tomorrow and that is never going to change for me. When people say, "I only want to live to a hundred," that's not to be believed. Let's hear them say that when they are a hundred!

SS: Particularly if they are in good health.

RK: Exactly. In fact, studies have shown that the only time people take their own lives is when they're deeply suffering physically or emotionally. There are a few exceptions to that. If somebody has deep devotion to some concepts that they live by, religious or otherwise, then they would choose to follow those dictates. Or if people are suffering, they most likely would not want to live. You see, I don't have this vision of future life as being repetitive, doing the same things over and over again. My life hasn't been that way so far, and with these new advances in technology I see the opportunity to radically expand our lives, not just extend them. I'm very much looking forward to living and participating in life. But that's not something that is just reserved for me. Everyone has a lot to contribute and can continue to contribute, particularly as we unlock human potential with these new technologies.

SS: But if we extend life indefinitely, what are we going to do with all these people?

RK: That's not a problem at all. A hundred years ago there were predictions that with the population explosion we'd run out of food, and as you can see we've more than kept up with that. In fact, I have graphs that show continual progress in human wealth, health, education, and many other different resources. We have ten thousand times more energy than we need for the entire population just from sunlight. Now, for sure, we can't plug our refrigerators into the sun without converting it into electricity, but that is exactly what nanotechnology will provide. In fact, new nanotechnology-based solar panels are providing much more cost-effective solar energy and are on an exponential rise. It's been doubling every two years and has been for the last twenty-five years, and we're only eight doublings away from meeting 100 percent of our energy needs.

SS: You explain "exponential" in your law of accelerating returns, meaning, as I understand it in its simplest form, starting slow, then growing faster and faster. The rate of change is accelerating, the best example being with knowledge and technology. We hardly notice the growth at first, for example, as in cancer research so far, and then suddenly it seems to explode, particularly as I see it, outside the standard-of-care box.

RK: I wrote an energy plan for the National Academy of Engineering articulating that view. Well, within twenty years we can meet all our energy needs many times over with sunlight. We have an enormous amount of water even though right now most of it is salinized or polluted, but if we have cheap energy, we know how to clean it up. There are food technologies that are emerging.

SS: What do you mean?

RK: There will be vertical agriculture where we can grow high-quality plants in air-controlled buildings that will be very nutritious and low cost. We will have in vitro cloned meats where we can feed millions of pounds of meat from one animal basically by cloning the muscle tissue with no animal suffering. PETA is a strong supporter of this idea. There are many ideas like this that we are exploring at Singularity University. One of the projects is pursuing this new field of three-dimensional printing to print out models that can be put together into very-low-cost, high-quality housing. It goes further with nanotechnology; one of its promises is to have a desktop device where you can print out any physical object from an information file.

SS: You mean like I could print out a new blouse?

RK: Right, or a solar panel or a module to build housing. We'll have all the physical things we need. We can meet the material needs of a growing population. People say to me, "But there's going to be a 'have, have-not' divide." I respond with, Look at cell phones. Five billion of our six billion people have them. A kid in Africa with a smartphone has access to more information today than the president of the United States did fifteen years ago.

SS: Powerful stuff.

RK: Yes, and ultimately these technologies become very inexpensive and very powerful, so even if the population expands somewhat, the power of these technologies doubles every year. Even if we substantially reduce the death rate, we'd still have a doubling time of advances of like fifteen years, compared to a doubling time of the power of these technologies of only about one year.

SS: Ahh, there it is again, "exponential."

RK: Right, but the rate of growth and the power of technology's abilities to meet the needs of the population are doubling much faster. We will see advances in the next ten years or so that would have taken over two hundred years before.

SS: What do you see as your end point? What's it like? How long will it last?

RK: Well, I am sixty-three. I come out much younger on biological aging tests. In fact, I am healthier than I was twenty years ago. I don't feel I am any slower physically or mentally than I was when I was forty. So I plan to basically not age from this point on, or age so slowly that by the time I get to fifteen years from now, I'll be about the same age or less. Biologically, I am already much less than my chronological age, so I want to stay ahead of the power curve. I think our generation (you and I) can do this but not without effort put forth.

It doesn't go without saying; it takes a concerted effort, the kind of effort that overwhelms most people because they don't yet understand the benefits.

SS: I hadn't really thought about this in terms of "reverse aging," but I had a complete medical workup at the Chaum Center in South Korea last year, and my biological age came out to be thirty-four. At sixty-five, I thought that was kind of impressive, but I do put forth effort, case in point the many supplements I take daily (as I notice you do also). In fact, I enjoy when we have dined together, because you don't think I'm a quack taking supplements throughout the meal. I also noticed you take more than I do!

RK: Yes, it is great. So, clearly, your books and my books are a wake-up call to our baby boomer peers that you can make it through. Unfortunately, most people are oblivious to this perspective. So, instead, they shrug and say, "Ah well, if I try hard, maybe I'll add a few months here and there. It's not really worth it."

SS: As they take another deep puff of that Marlboro . . .

RK: Right. No one wants to be the first person in line not to make it into the theater, but when it comes to baby boomers, you have to work really hard to make it through. Our kids are going to have a much easier time. They'll probably be in good shape fifteen years from now barring an accident. But we baby boomers can make it also. Fifteen years is not that long of a time. You now see many people in their seventies (your husband, Alan, being one of them) who are still very vital. So that's my plan . . . stay healthy in order to get to Bridge Two and then ride to Bridge Three and see the Singularity [what Ray defines as a time in the future when we multiply the intelligence of the "human-machine civilization a billion-fold through merging with the intelligence we are creating"].

SS: And I'm coming with you.

RK: Great. Can't wait.

SS: Thanks so much, Ray. It has been an honor.

CHAPTER 4

ADVANCED MEDICINE—THE NEW DOCTOR YOU'LL WANT TO VISIT

Man. Because he sacrifices his health in order to make money. Then he sacrifices money to recuperate his health. And then he is so anxious about the future that he does not enjoy the present; the result being that he does not live in the present or the future; he lives as if he is never going to die, and then he dies having never really lived.

—The Dalai Lama, when asked what surprised him most about humanity

The planet has changed drastically. To live longer and healthier our approach to medicine must also change. A new type of doctor has emerged because more and more people are expressing dissatisfaction with the limitations of our present orthodox medicine and its "allopathic only" approach, meaning "a pill for every ailment." Allopathic medicine evolved at the turn of the twentieth century when a man by the name of Abraham Flexner was hired by the two richest families in the country at that time—the Carnegies and the Rockefellers, who by the way *owned* pharmaceutical companies (connect those dots). They sent him to the institutes of higher learning to promise funding in *perpetuity* to our medical schools and teaching hospitals if they would teach *only* allopathic medicine, meaning "Here's my symptom; here's your drug."

From that time on, all the other "pathics" were eliminated from medical school agendas—homeopathic, chiropractic, naturopathic, and so on—and then later these "pathics" were vilified and dismissed as "quackery." So recommendations like "Go home, drink plenty of liquids, and get some rest" and that kind of natural advice were replaced by our beloved GP saying, "Here's a prescription for an antibiotic." How many antibiotics have we taken for viruses when we didn't have an infection? (Antibiotics do nothing for viruses.) How many antibiotics have been the culprit that have disrupted our delicate gut balance and promoted a lifetime of stomach and GI issues? Allopathic medicine is a brilliant business model, I must say, but the overuse and the overprescribing of drugs when there might have been a natural solution were the beginning of the end for us!

Today, we find ourselves in a quandary. We have become a society that is "overpilled" and overtreated, resulting in our brains being robbed of their ability to think, with side effects often worse than the original ailment itself.

At first, taking a drug for every infection, flu, virus, gut problem, headache, stomachache, and so on was seen to be a miracle. Acid reflux? No problem, take the purple pill. Anxiety? No problem, take an antianxiety pill. Pain? No problem, take a mind-numbing narcotic to chase it away. But then something started to go awry . . . the sleeping pills stopped working, the water pills set up a vicious cycle, the pain pills caused addiction, the antidepressants numbed the feelings away, allowing the patient to be there, but not really . . . "there." These people got lost somewhere in a fog, their minds in a far-off place that took them out of their reality, in some cases forever.

As a result of concern on the part of not only many Western-trained doctors but also the patients themselves, alternative medicine has emerged. It's called *antiaging medicine,* or *regenerative medicine,* or *age management;* I call it *advanced medicine.* This is the best of both worlds, taking advantage, as Dr. Jonathan Wright has so eloquently coined, of "using Nature's tools" and Western medicine when necessary.

Advanced medicine also allows for the "pathics" to be relevant again. Homeopaths and naturopaths are rising up, and people are flocking to them. Alternative Western doctors now have long waiting lists. The people are speaking. They want to find natural, alternative ways for the body to heal itself, and to restore what might be missing due to age, stress, or toxicity.

One of the best doctors to explain the new medicine, and his approach to antiaging medicine, is my primary antiaging doctor, Dr. Michael Galitzer. I have a coterie of doctors, each one having his or her specialty. This is my luxury. I have made health my priority and passion. Dr. Galitzer is one of several thousand qualified doctors that you can reference in my online resource section. I have been a patient of Dr. Galitzer for fifteen years. As you will read, he has a very unique way of treating and healing the body. I go to him regularly when I am "well" for what I call a "tune-up" before and after trips. I go to detoxify and to strengthen my immune system and keep my organs and glands in top working order. You will love what he has to say.

MICHAEL GALITZER, M.D.

Dr. Michael Galitzer *is my personal, Western-trained, antiaging doctor. He practices advanced medicine at its best. He understands it all: how to balance hormones, how to strengthen the weakest organs and glands, how to strengthen the body to prepare it to fight cancer or tolerate conventional therapies. He understands the toxic assault and how to detoxify the body on an ongoing basis. He advises on lifestyle, diet, and antiaging therapies, and he also knows what to do when you get the flu. He provides all this at his office in Santa Monica, California.*

Dr. Galitzer is compassionate and caring. As an emergency room doctor, he needed to be able to handle any situation with calm, resourcefulness, and thoughtfulness, and he brings those traits to his present practice. He stays on top of new medical advancements, which allows him to take the best care of his patients. He is also my friend.

SS: Hello, Michael. Thank you again for your time. I love speaking with you as you are always so eloquent. I'd like to know what is new in the antiaging world that is contrary to present orthodox belief, and if you can, please demystify antiaging medicine for my readers.

MG: Nice to talk with you, Suzanne. Let's start with antiaging medicine, which views optimal health as when a patient is physically, emotionally, mentally, and spiritually in flow, and when the organs and glands are functioning at maximum capacity. Disease is a condition precipitated by a toxin-filled, nutritionally deficient, and stress-dominated system, which will ultimately result in changes in enzyme production and hormone production.

Traditional medicine would tend to suppress these symptoms, allowing them to smolder quietly and then erupt with increased intensity later on. In antiaging medicine, we want to remove the underlying cause and allow the embers of an illness to never get an opportunity to smolder; we want patients to have lots of energy.

As you've said in the past, our bodies are like an orchestra and our organs and glands are the instruments in that orchestra; some are in tune, and some are out of tune. Some organs age faster than others; for instance, some people have hearts and brains that are working fine, yet they fall and break a bone and that is when they find that their bones are aging faster than their hearts and brains. For other people, they may have hearts and bones that are in good order, but they can't think or remember. So in this orchestra, if we [antiaging medicine] can get everything in tune, and get the music "right," meaning all organs and systems in good working order, people will feel better.

SS: Very nicely explained. What about toxicity?

MG: When I was an emergency room doctor, we were concerned about life-threatening toxins: an overdose of sleeping pills, carbon monoxide inhalation, an oil spill, or a chemical spill. Now there are toxins in the air, water, and food and then there are pesticides and heavy metals, and they all add up and stack up on one another. Consequently the organs get overloaded, and then symptoms start; the result is people feeling lousy.

SS: Yes, but they go to their orthodox doctors who are perplexed. Dealing with toxicity and longer life that requires fine-tuning and restoration was never taught in medical school.

MG: True. Medical school was more or less about diseases and pathology; we learned all about the different diseases, but we did not learn about a model for health.

SS: But the planet has changed . . . people have conditions related to toxicity and stress that never existed before and these conditions need to be dealt with in their own special way.

MG: Yes, but instead of trying to look at how bad doctors are, I think they ought to be complimented because we became doctors and concluded that the purpose of our lives was to give. Doctors want to help their patients. They need to inspire their patients.

SS: I'm not saying they don't want to help, but science is always evolving, and to stop learning once they leave medical school cer-

tainly has to leave many of them in the dust. X-rays, CAT scans, biopsies, MRIs, and chemical blood tests have their place, but they also
have their limitations. In the case of CAT scans and x-rays, we need to
give grave thought as the radiation exposure from both is damaging.
In fact, a report came out in 2011 that CAT scans give off a thousand
times *more* radiation than they thought!

MG: Yes, that's true, and it's generally felt if all these tests check
out, then the patient is healthy. Traditional medicine does utilize
electrical technology—EKG for the heart, EEG for electrical brain,
and EMG for electrical nerve muscle, but that's where it stops. My
kind of medicine looks at the electrical signals in the liver, kidneys,
pancreas, adrenals, thyroid. In an electrocardiogram, the electrical impulse of the heart precedes the physical heartbeat. My kind
of medicine says electrical changes in the organs precede physical
symptoms. So when the electrical "firing" in the liver becomes abnormal, people have symptoms such as migraine or insomnia, and
this is something you can't see on a blood test or an ultrasound of
the liver.

SS: Dr. Sherry Rogers, in her book *Detoxify or Die*, says of Western
medicine, "Every part of the body has an electrical system, but we only
measure a couple of them like the heart and the brain," so I see where
you are on to something. I've noticed, in the years I've been coming to
you, there is a calm about any diagnosis you have given me; you are
not an alarmist, even when you find something electrically that is an
indicator of a problem to come.

MG: As a doctor, the worst thing I can do is give a patient a diagnosis of a terrible disease or condition without giving him hope. Otherwise a patient will panic, which leads to helplessness, depression, and
ultimately a weakened immune system. The wise doctor must never
destroy the hope of the patient. Patients have resources, and we must
help them conquer their fears and release those resources.

SS: What do most people complain about?

MG: People come to me, and essentially say, "I don't feel well." They
complain about fatigue, lack of energy, allergies, inability to sleep, and
aching muscles and joints. They just don't feel right.

SS: Or do they really mean they don't feel like they used to feel?

MG: That too . . . They know there is a better way to feel and they
want it back. Sleeping is a big problem for so many patients. They
either can't fall asleep or when they do fall asleep, they wake up in

the middle of the night between one and three. I find when the sleep goes, ultimately people's health really begins to diminish. In Chinese medicine, the sleep issue is looked at very easily. There are twelve major meridians in Chinese medicine. Each of those meridians is two hours of the clock. The liver meridian has one to three A.M. as liver time, which is when the body's energy is concentrated in the liver. So if people wake up, or can't fall asleep between one and three, then you know their liver energy is abnormal. Did you know you should never go to sleep earlier than four hours after drinking alcohol and three hours after eating food?

SS: Why?

MG: Because the body needs to rest. The GI system needs to relax. So many people eat a huge meal late in the day, eight or nine P.M., and it stresses the liver, the key organ in getting the toxins out. The first four letters in liver are "live" for a reason.

SS: Most people don't even know where the liver is located. And because we can't see it, telling someone their liver is stressed doesn't ring a bell until it becomes liver cancer or some other terrible disease of the liver. I know a person with a diseased liver, and his quality of life is poor. He is in and out of the hospital, and each time I see him he looks older and sicker and more worn out.

MG: Right, traditional medicine only looks at the liver with ultrasound, or doctors test for elevated liver enzymes to show that the liver is already diseased. Antiaging medicine says that most livers are sluggish, and part of what we do is to increase toxin elimination from the liver, thus reducing tissue acidity.

SS: Makes sense. Detoxify it; clean it out before there is a problem. Sounds like a no-brainer to me. How do you detox the liver?

MG: Herbs, homeopathy, acupuncture, nutrition, and there are supplements that help the liver, such as N-acetylcysteine, alpha-lipoic acid, vitamin C. Basically, if you looked at nothing else in the body but went after cleaning up the liver, you could be very, very successful in helping people feel better.

SS: Let's discuss hormones and hormone levels. I am sure that most people who come to you are declining in hormones. It's happening so early to so many people now. You mainly concentrate on the major hormones initially, right?

MG: Actually, I work with all hormones because hormonal decline in the body is so important, but especially the adrenal gland, which is one of the major hormonal glands, and basically our survival organ. It helps us deal with stress and allows us to respond adequately to stress.

SS: Most people are stressed. All you ever hear is how stressed out everyone is.

MG: When the adrenals are weak, we no longer view stress as a challenge; we view it as a threat. This is why at that point we overreact to the little stressors; then we can't differentiate between big stress and little stress. Weak adrenals set the stage for a move toward illness and disease.

SS: Ah yes, reminds me of a fight I had with Alan over almonds! Ha ha ha . . . afterward, I wondered how almonds could have been so important. Little stressors! But aren't weak adrenals triggered by an inability to sleep? Isn't it a cascade . . . toxins, weakened liver, inability to sleep, and then acute stress; they trigger high cortisol output so that person can't sleep at all? Isn't it all interconnected?

MG: Yes, and everyone thinks the doctor can fix poor lifestyle and diet habits and unmanaged stress. The patient is responsible for his or her health. We've become too acidic as a culture: too much of the wrong kinds of fats, sugar, cigarettes, and alcohol, not enough exercise. The word "emotion" has *motion* within it; if we can't move our bodies, we can't feel well. We must also know our purpose in life, and have fun.

Everyone talks about heart attacks being related to high cholesterol. But when you look at it from a deeper level, the two main causes of heart attacks are not being happy and not liking our jobs. When I was in the ER, I frequently worked Sunday night through to the Monday morning shift. Monday morning is when more heart attacks happen than any other time of the day. Why? I believe it's because many people really don't want to go to work. People aren't very happy; we don't live with passion, we stop being grateful, and we get into this belief system that looks at aging being a downward spiral. We need to change our beliefs, and it's great that you are out there pushing people to change their beliefs.

SS: Making sixty-five cool?

MG: Sixty-five *is* cool. In 1954, Roger Bannister was the first person to run a four-minute mile. Before that nobody believed it was possible. Then in the next five years, thirty or forty other people ran a four-minute mile. Once the belief system begins changing on a

large level, all sorts of things start happening. So with patients I try
to change their belief systems and help them get rid of fear.

SS: What do you mean by fear?

MG: I think fear is holding everybody back. We are afraid of pov-
erty, criticism, ill health; we fear old age, we fear death, and most
importantly we fear cancer.

SS: I have to say, I am over that one, thank goodness. Writing
Knockout in 2009 did that for me. I am not afraid of cancer. I can't
tell you how liberating that is. Doesn't mean I won't or can't get it,
but if I did, I would know what to do. The more I interviewed doctors who had patients who were managing cancer, and living long
lives with serious cancer without the use of drugs, I realized it was a
mind-set, that cancer was manageable and that, as Dr. Gonzalez says,
if "you give the body what it wants, it will leave you alone. And what
it wants is a detoxed body and good nutrition." That made so much
sense to me.

MG: That is actually a triumph. Every day patients come to me,
and every ache, pain, digestive situation that they have convinces
them they have cancer. So the cancer fear is huge. Our bodies can be
in either two modes: survival mode or growth mode. If you are totally
in survival mode, there's no way you can get yourself into a growth
mode or an antiaging mode. So eliminating fears, and fear of diseases
like cancer and ill health, is crucial for all people to move into growth
mode.

SS: How important is diet?

MG: Diet is huge. So many of my patients are attracted to your
books, which has made them very conscious about what they put
into their system. The body is a Ferrari, and you have to give it high-
octane fuel. The major problem with many people is their diet is too
acidic.

SS: Funny, I give the same analogy using a Maserati . . . same visual.
Doesn't cancer love acid?

MG: Yes, it does. So I try to teach people about what foods are
acid; animal proteins are acidic. If you are going to eat red meat, be
sure it's grass fed and hormone-free. But know that red meat is very
acidic and if you have cancer, it's a good thing to avoid. Also the contaminants in red meat are dangerous; if it's not grass fed, then you are
dealing with antibiotics, hormones, and the poor-quality feed given
to the cows to fatten them up.

SS: I don't think most people realize the dangers of corn-fed beef; not only does it go against the natural evolution of cows that are supposed to eat grass (which is why they get infections like E. coli), but the corn is also most likely genetically modified, which makes it a completely valueless food and, to my thinking, a dangerous food.

MG: It's also the lack of alkaline-based foods that most people don't consume. Vegetables are your key alkalinizing food, and people should be juicing wheat grass and green juices. The only people who take alkaline food seriously are the ones who come to me who have read your books.

SS: Thank you. I feel proud of that.

MG: You should. Tissue acidity equals toxicity. If you have a perfectly functioning liver, you could probably deal with a lot of the acids we experience every day, but most people are not paying attention to their liver.

SS: What should they do?

MG: Drink alkaline water if you can get it, eat lots of vegetables, juice green vegetables, and juice wheat grass.

SS: I have had an alkaline water dispenser installed in my kitchen sink, so I can have it when I want it. Some stores sell alkaline water in glass bottles. What about powdered Paleo Greens? Are they effective?

MG: They help. But nothing is as good as the real thing. Exercise is also key . . . it is the greatest stress reducer, and increasing blood flow helps reduce acidity and reduce stress.

The other thing that's key is vitamin C. If you are traveling by air, there are massive exposures to toxins. I advise my patients to take 1,000 milligrams of vitamin C for every hour they are in the airplane because of recirculated air, and people on the plane with colds and flu. Even the fumes you inhale when waiting on the tarmac are toxic to the body.

SS: It's amazing any of us are even walking around. What kind of vitamin C do you recommend?

MG: I like Lypo-Spheric, 1,000 mg. It absorbs so well that if you had a five-hour flight, you could probably use two or three packets. Vitamin C is also a great detoxifier and neutralizer. At my office we give intravenous vitamin C, which you have had so many times, Suzanne. All the antiaging doctors are giving intravenous treatments, and there are antiaging doctors in every city you might want to visit.

Antiaging medicine is becoming bigger and bigger, and it's being driven by patients and people who read your wonderful books and want to get more out of life.

SS: Thanks. And that's the bottom line, isn't it? Wanting more out of life! Tell me, how devastating is the heavy metal assault?

MG: Heavy metals are a huge problem. It starts with mercury fillings in teeth. There is a huge correlation to illness with mercury amalgam fillings that leak over time. Mercury is the number one toxin to the body. We've seen this in breast and prostate cancers because mercury behaves as an estrogen; it is called *xenoestrogen*, and it's a serious player. It's a huge problem in China. China burns coal, and mercury is a by-product of that; the trade winds blow it over, resulting in elevated mercury levels in the air over the West Coast. There are also very high levels of mercury in people who live in New York.

SS: How do you test for mercury?

MG: We do a urine test after giving a provoking agent that pulls mercury out of the tissues and into the bloodstream. When we get the urine test results back, we see that many people have high levels of heavy metals—mercury, cadmium, lead, arsenic. We would then give chelation, either intravenous or oral, to reduce the body's load of heavy metals. We really can't avoid the toxins, but we certainly can take steps to constantly clean our bodies. We can take vitamin C; we can get colonics; we can do infrared sauna. We can skin brush, exercise more, and juice. We can eat alkaline, and strengthen our livers and hormonal system. All greatly reduce the toxic load in our bodies.

SS: Makes sense. After all, we just don't clean our houses once and then forget about it. To keep a house tidy, you have to clean it regularly. This is what you and I have been doing for my body for years; with all the people I meet and exposure to toxins from hotel food, hotel cleaning agents, and the stress of "going on," I rarely get sick and feel energized most all the time, so I know it's working for me.

MG: I often say, if you can get people better in L.A., then you can get people better everywhere.

SS: Oh, I'd say New York is running neck and neck!

MG: You could be right. Huge cities have environmental problems—traffic, noise pollution, and pollution in general—as well as mold in those old buildings. Also, you end up with people who are in traffic an hour or two every day, working twelve hours a day, not sleeping, eating on the run, and not exercising. These are all the perfect ingredients for not feeling well. In my practice, I like to see people every four weeks, and in between they take my homeopathic drops and supplements to keep them going.

SS: What about exercise—why is it so good for us?

MG: Exercise increases blood flow; the more blood that flows, the more oxygen gets delivered to the cells, and the more energy gets created. Our bodies' cells create energy from burning oxygen and glucose together.

SS: So you are talking about the cell's mitochondria?

MG: Yes. The mitochondria are the little energy center power-houses, the energy factory within the cell. Energy equals health. Anti-aging is all about increasing energy production in the body. When you do this, people feel better. The other big thing is supplementation.

SS: Yes, every single doctor and professional in this book stresses the importance of supplementation. Tell me what supplement you feel gets overlooked.

MG: Well, we need to have thin blood. People with cancer, people with heart disease, and people who've had strokes all have thick blood. People with chronic infections have thick blood. Blood should flow like wine, not like ketchup. When blood is thick, oxygen can't get to the cells.

SS: What is the antidote?

MG: Fish oil helps. Garlic, ginkgo, vitamin E, and nattokinase all thin the blood.

SS: Yes, I know. When I was in the hospital for that terrible cancer misdiagnosis, they wanted to give me Coumadin to thin my blood because my body was in an allergic shock. I kept saying no Coumadin, give me nattokinase. They laughed at me. I didn't care. I didn't take Coumadin. I took nattokinase.

MG: If you are not going to exercise and you are over fifty, then you have to take these supplements to thin your blood. If you can thin your blood, more oxygen gets to the cells and more energy gets created.

SS: Well, you must be doing right by me. I was having a manicure yesterday and my manicurist accidentally cut me and she said, "Your blood is so thin, I can't stop this from bleeding."

MG: Well, good, that will ensure that you will live another fifty or sixty years. When I ask patients how long they'd like to live, they always say ninety but "not if I'm in a wheelchair." Here's another instance where global beliefs about aging have to change. There is a Japanese doctor, Shigeaki Hinohara, who is one hundred and still practicing. He's published an enormous number of books since his seventy-fifth birthday, including one called *Living Long, Living Good*. Amazing guy.

HE SAYS THAT ALL PEOPLE WHO LIVE
LONG SHARE ONE THING IN COMMON—
NONE ARE OVERWEIGHT!

He drinks coffee, a glass of milk, and orange juice with a tablespoon of olive oil in it for breakfast. He has milk and a few cookies for lunch, and veggies and fish for dinner.

I think when we see more of these kinds of people out there, we are inspired to live longer. You have to change the belief system and give examples of people who are being very productive when they are older.

SS: Speaking of Japan, the media is keeping very quiet about radiation contamination from the tsunami. But the ocean is all one big connected body of water and what slips in at one point is bound to travel. Have we been affected by radiation contamination, and if so, how do you in antiaging medicine address it?

MG: We are all affected; we were quite affected in L.A. Radiation is one of these slow types of situations that add up, and you don't really feel anything specific. But now it's a toxin within each person's body. In my practice, I try to neutralize the radiation with all the things we've talked about. I don't believe in scaring people, but I think this exposure needs to be dealt with by dealing with the liver/lymph/kidney drainage systems. The backup is the hormonal system; namely, the thyroid and adrenals. These glands stimulate the other organs to work better. At some point, though, these glands go on overload, and this is why the entire hormonal system is so important. If we keep our hormonal systems strong with healthy adrenal glands, and give bioidentical thyroid, estrogen, progesterone, and testosterone, along with DHEA, growth hormone, and melatonin, we can optimize the liver, lymph, and kidney drainage systems that get rid of the toxins. But with a bad diet, the drainage systems get tired, and the person moves from "I don't feel well" to "I'm becoming ill."

SS: What about minerals? No fun living longer if you don't have strong bones to hold you up, and I know minerals are crucial to bone making.

MG: You are so right. Everyone is worried about osteoporosis. Women and men have bone density tests, and the doctors report osteopenia or worse, osteoporosis, so they give them calcium and vitamin D.

SS: Isn't that good advice?

MG: Yes, it is, except . . . let's go back to your original question of what is new in antiaging medicine that is contrary to orthodox beliefs. I think the way that orthodox medicine has been looking at osteopenia and osteoporosis and bone density has completely missed a very important element.

OSTEOPOROSIS IS NOT A CALCIUM DEFICIENCY DISEASE; IT'S A DISEASE OF TOO MUCH ACIDITY.

The body's way of neutralizing acidity is to take calcium and magnesium off the bone, because calcium and magnesium are alkalinizing minerals. The acidity takes the calcium and magnesium from the bone, and then the person becomes osteopenic or osteoporotic. Minerals get depleted. In my practice, to strengthen bones I frequently give mineral IVs to patients.

SS: This is new and awesome information. I've always heard it's about calcium. But Alan discovered he was horribly gluten intolerant a couple of years ago and also was diagnosed with bone loss. You gave him a series of mineral IVs last year. Between the minerals that he still takes faithfully, hormone replacement, and supplementation, his bone density is now excellent! IV treatments are easy to make fun of. I remember a couple of years ago you allowed *20/20*, the TV program, to film me getting my vitamin C IVs from you. And when it aired, they mocked the protocol, saying "Why is it necessary to go to such extremes?"

MG: Large doses of vitamin C stimulate the immune system, help the liver work better, and strengthen our adrenals. High doses of vitamins can accelerate the efficiency and effectiveness of organs in the body. This is huge because most people come to us with reduced organ function, reduced adrenal function, and sluggish livers. So if we can help stimulate these organs to work better, we've helped them immensely.

SS: Can you test for mineral depletion?

MG: Yes, you can do a blood test for mineral depletion. But here's the vicious cycle; most people do not have great digestive systems, so therefore they don't absorb minerals well. The people who are treated with acid blockers for their heartburn and GERD will not have enough hydrochloric acid in their stomachs, which will result in decreased absorption of minerals. So, most of the people out there on Nexium, Prilosec, Aciphex, and other acid blockers are ultimately going to have mineral depletion problems.

SS: What a vicious cycle. Gut problems create mineral problems, which create bone problems; the cascade again, the downward cycle we call aging. But it's really not about aging; it's about a lack of understanding that we are living longer and that the body parts have to be addressed, listened to, and corrected, just like a mechanic listens to the sounds of a car engine.

> How long does a house last? If you take care of the house diligently, and quickly address any problem that comes up, the house can last indefinitely. If you don't take care of it, it won't last very long.
>
> —Aubrey de Grey, famed gerontologist

MG: What is also important and maybe even more important are digestive enzymes, pancreatic enzymes. The pancreas is an important organ that makes enzymes to digest protein, starch, and fat. In most people, the pancreas is not working well. The pancreas is the organ most affected by pesticides.

SS: Is this the connection to the huge rise in pancreatic cancer?

MG: We believe this is a major reason. The pancreas is put through too much stress from too much sugar and pesticides.

SS: And everyone consumes too much sugar, and everyone is affected by pesticides. And we wonder why we are sick. Pancreatic cancer is the most dreaded of the cancers. Few seem to survive, other than patients of Dr. Nicholas Gonzalez who, I've learned through my interviewing, has had such great success with pancreatic cancer patients—

probably due, in no small way, to the fact that his protocol uses massive amounts of pancreatic enzymes.

MG: Again, in the Chinese medicine clock, there are twelve different organs, systems, or meridians. They have two hours of the twenty-four-hour clock. The pancreas time is between nine and eleven in the morning. That means the pancreas is working most effectively at that time, and twelve hours later these organs work least effectively. That's why most people digest their breakfasts well because they have lots of naturally occurring pancreatic enzymes. Americans eat very small breakfasts and huge dinners. Late in the evening is when your pancreas is least able to produce digestive enzymes. So consequently these people can't digest their food, and go to bed with a full stomach and wake up feeling lousy.

To keep a healthy pancreas, don't eat late and supplement with digestive enzymes, and as far as the pesticides, we can treat and detoxify them with homeopathy and herbs.

One of the first things I do with my patients is look at the energetics of their pancreas when I'm testing in my office. I find pesticides frequently, and we deal with them homeopathically; we also use an instrument called *ONDAMED*, which stimulates the healing process within the body.

SS: Yes, I have an ONDAMED machine, and I often tell my readers to encourage their doctors to purchase one. It is an amazing piece of equipment. I used it every day recently to heal faster from my stem cell breast surgery.

MG: The earth has a magnetic field and certain frequencies within it that allow us to live. By giving these kinds of frequencies to the body, it gets the body into a balanced state. ONDAMED uses pulsed electromagnetic frequencies to stimulate and balance energy flow within the body, so that is why I use it in my office. I also offer light therapies along with other therapies as well. It's also important to eat organically, especially in today's world, and to eat lightly late in the day and take pancreatic enzymes.

SS: I'm now getting it (finally) that drinking alcohol, eating late, and then flopping into bed (and we've all done it) is really, really bad for us.

MG: Correct. Diet sodas and too much alcohol will harm you. These things weaken the digestive system and ultimately the pancreas is affected, and then you are in trouble.

If you take pancreatic enzymes on an empty stomach before you go to sleep, you are basically eating up the debris and allowing the liver to more easily detoxify the blood while you are sleeping. Taking pancreatic enzymes gives a huge advantage.

IF EVERYONE WERE TO START TAKING PANCREATIC ENZYMES, THERE WOULD BE FEWER INSTANCES OF PANCREATIC CANCER.

SS: And that is at the heart of Dr. Gonzalez's program. He will love that you have said this. It's very validating.

MG: Absolutely. I think he's completely right on. All the cancer patients who come to see me have a weak pancreas, and digestive pancreatic enzymes are critical to take.

SS: And then making a serious attempt to be alkaline rather than acidic.

MG: The acidic environment is the foundation for all illness to develop. The more acidic you are and the more toxic you are, the weaker your liver is. As your hormonal system weakens, the cells wind up not being able to utilize energy and turn into cells that can only ferment sugar. Ultimately these become cancer cells. The first step to a healthy body is to be less acidic.

SS: So what you are saying is patients need to be the contractors and understand that nobody's going to care more about them than themselves. Does it help you when a patient comes in informed?

MG: The art of being a doctor is meeting patients where they are, and taking them up slowly. Thanks to your books, patients come in understanding a lot, and what's amazing is that patients come in having read your books and now they know they are going to get better. They have "a knowing." It's not even a question with them. Again, once you expect certain things are going to happen, they happen.

SS: Well, that's how I feel. I utilize alternative medicine, and rarely ever, ever, have to access traditional medicine. I think you've given me a prescription once in the last decade.

You are very hopeful about the future relative to our health, aren't you?

MG: Yes, I am. It's not about the bad guys, the toxins out there. It's not about trying to get rid of every little bad guy and trying to eat every food that's perfectly grown. You can't do it. But there's so much in our arsenal to strengthen the body, to help the body get rid of toxins, to augment our body's hormone production with natural hormones, to strengthen these glands and organs so that we can overcome just about anything. So I'm extremely hopeful. As we move into the future and start using stem cells with their ability to help regenerate cells, organs, and tissues, it becomes very exciting . . . So the future is looking great.

SS: I'm breathing a sigh of relief. Thanks, Michael.

MG: And to you, Suzanne. As Bob Dylan said, "May you stay forever young."

PART II

EXPLOSIVE MEDICAL INFORMATION TO HELP YOU REVERSE AGE

Society, including governments and corporations, are in a fog when it comes to aging and age-related diseases.

They party on, ignoring the reality of our pending demise. They dismiss the viability of building a lifeboat to cure aging. Instead, they tend to the sinking ship's maintenance, patching leaks here and there, bailing out water when it does get in, essentially just treating the symptoms.

Then, when something critical goes wrong, people panic. They pull out all stops to cure what should have been prevented. They never considered fixing aging in the first place . . . instead passively clinging to yesterday's acceptance of the inevitability of aging and resting on arrogant pride at man's capacity to manufacture the next medicine.

All this works fine for the pharmaceutical and health care industries, because that mindset supports an extremely profitable business model. So together with big government, they create barriers to novel and even natural treatments that can cure or even prevent disease.

This makes preventative medicine and lifestyle changes seem unwarranted and bothersome, so most people march in step to the beat of big government and big pharma to a premature death.

–David Kekich, *Life Extension Express*

CHAPTER 5

BOMBSHELL #1:
BREASTS LOST TO CANCER
CAN BE REGROWN

This book is meant to blow your mind with the possibilities for your future and present health—which I'm sure the last chapters just did! A lot of the information in this book is outside the box. The new stuff is not what shows up from most orthodox medical doctors, but here is presented by cutting-edge Western-trained doctors, scientists, and professionals . . . the best of the best.

Dr. Joel Aronowitz is the doctor who performed my amazing breast regrowth using my own stem cells, and because the procedure is both personal to me and so revolutionary, it is Bombshell #1. This incredible advancement is available right now for women who can qualify for this clinical trial. It is my hope that with the conclusion of this trial, it will eventually be possible to have this procedure covered by insurance and made the standard of care. It's important to note that when having breast cancer surgery, you need to retain the nipple and the skin around the breast, if possible. Otherwise, it leaves the surgeon nothing to work with for regrowth. Stem cell protocols are very exciting and in the future, potentially any person who has lost a body part due to injury or illness will be able to regrow it.

Clearly, stem cells and nanotechnology are the future. You found out how nanobots will turn the present model of medicine on its ear in my interview with Ray Kurzweil in chapter 3, but here we'll talk about stem cells. They are available now for limited use, but they will play a huge role in new medicine, which fortunately is only a little more than a decade away.

What do you do when you've lost a body part? Up until now, prosthetics have been one option. For women with breast cancer, there have been two choices: implants or a "TRAM flap" procedure, in which a surgeon removes muscle and then moves a blood vessel from the stomach (usually) up into the breast area. The results are unsatisfactory, the look is unnatural, and the recovery time is long and arduous.

I am proud to say I am the first woman to have legally regrown a breast in the United States using my own fat and stem cells.

MY JOURNEY

In 2001, I was diagnosed with breast cancer. The remedy for my tumor was lumpectomy, followed by chemotherapy (which I refused) and radiation, finishing with the after-care drug Tamoxifen (which I refused).

Lumpectomy didn't sound so bad; the doctor would just remove a little piece of my already ample breast. I didn't think I would miss it, and then hopefully the cancer would be gone. It seemed pretty cut-and-dried. My doctors mentioned nothing about making changes in nutrition, or supplementation, or stress management; no one discussed any diet or lifestyle changes needed to make sure there was not a recurrence. Information of this sort was, and sadly still is, usually not part of orthodox medical protocol. Nutrition and natural remedies, or any other therapies such as homeopathy, not only are *not* considered but also are generally dismissed as a waste of time.

Oncologists are often good people taught a protocol in medical school that is care without a cure in many cases. The war on cancer has been a dismal failure with the exception of three kinds of cancer that respond to the approved medical standard of care: surgery, radiation, chemotherapy, and harsh after-care drugs. The cancers that do respond to chemotherapy are childhood leukemia, testicular cancer, and lymphoma.

Surgeons are taught to cut and repair, and we have the best doctors in the world in this country to do this. And to give credit where credit is due, our medical schools know their stuff when it comes to surgery. When you need surgery, you want to be in the United States. But when it comes to cancer treatment, almost always alternative options are not accepted by orthodox medicine; instead they are ridiculed and violently opposed as so eloquently stated in this famous quote (often attributed to Arthur Schopenhauer):

THE THREE STAGES OF TRUTH
First, it is ridiculed.
Second, it is violently opposed.
Third, it is accepted as self-evident.

Yet when the standard of care cannot offer a cure, it is hard to understand with life hanging in the balance why alternative options are frequently not even considered. Surely a body bolstered by great nutrition and detoxification can benefit. A weakened immune system cannot fight cancer, so it takes patients willing to go beyond what traditional medicine offers to fight their own war on cancer their own way.

In my case, the first thing my doctor told me was to stop taking my hormones, that they were probably responsible for my cancer. "Based on what?" I asked. My doctors were lovely people whom I liked very much; they were caring and had great bedside manners, and I felt I was in good hands . . . But again, "Based on what?" kept running through my mind. There was no literature proving that estrogen and progesterone caused cancer (I had looked). At that time I had already started writing about the joys and benefits of hormone restoration. I told my doctor that I had come to believe, from my research, that an environment of balanced hormones prevented disease.

My doctor then asked me, "Based on what?"

"Well, clearly," I said. "If estrogen were the problem, then why wouldn't all young women have breast cancer, because in our reproductive years we are oozing with estrogen."

"But you have an estrogen-positive tumor," my doctor said. "Yes," I answered, "but that means my body hasn't been making enough progesterone. And, if I had realized this earlier, I believe I could have restored myself to perfect balance and probably never have gotten this cancer in the first place." (At this time I did not realize I had a genetic defect, that my body did not make the anticancer component of estrogen called *estriol*, but more of an explanation about this later . . .)

We were getting nowhere.

Finally I said, "Look, I can't stop taking my hormones. It is my belief based on a lot of time and study that balanced hormones in perfect ratios are protective. For me to stop taking them would go against my beliefs."

"Well," said my oncologist, "I hope you don't die." My heart froze: I was going against him now . . . But I felt firm.

"I don't think I will," I said. "I actually believe I will die if I stop taking them."

I had thought it through. I weighed the pros and cons. I took responsibility for my life. This was my choice, and I would deal with the consequences good or bad. I also decided that I was going to change my life and eat as though my life depended on it, which I believe is true. I made my decision. End of discussion.

The day of the surgery was intense; there were a lot of unknowns. The specialists had seen the tumor, about the size of a quarter, and now we were going to cut it out. I hadn't yet mentioned to my doctor that I was not going to take the chemotherapy he had suggested.

Alan, as always, was by my side, as was my stepdaughter Leslie. But there comes a time when undergoing surgery that you have to let go of your loved ones' hands and let the doctors take you away. I looked back at Alan as I was being pushed down the hall in my wheelchair toward the operating room . . . and our eyes said it all. I was going to be okay, but . . .

Two hours later, I awakened in intensive care. Alan was there. He said softly, "They got it all . . . and nothing is in the lymphs."

This was good news. Now I only needed to heal and get on with my life.

Not so fast, my doctor told me; he said that even though I did not want chemotherapy, "radiation was a must." At the time, everyone was automatically having radiation post breast surgery. "Really," he said, "it's a walk in the park, and it is essential to kill off any rogue cells." We went back and forth on the necessity. I talked with several doctors on both sides of medicine, and all agreed that it was unsafe not to take the radiation. Finally, I agreed without much of a fight, but I didn't like this idea at all. At the time not much information was available about radiation damage.

For six long weeks every day I would lie on the radiation table and think, *Isn't it radiation that gives you cancer?*

I vomited daily; my energy was zapped as though a plug had been pulled out of me. No energy, no sense of triumph, just sickness and exhaustion.

There should be a book written on the realities of radiation and all the things that are never mentioned beforehand. I experienced horrible side effects: burned skin, burned insides of my esophagus, the killing off of my body's ability to produce hydrochloric acid (essential for digestion), injury to my gut, vomiting, exhaustion. This was a walk in the park?

There is also yet another side effect for most women that is not discussed: with radiation, the breast gradually gets flatter and flatter until it looks as though there has been a complete mastectomy. In addition, the asymmetry causes severe pain, because in order to look "even" in clothing, one side of the bra has to be pulled up so high that it injures the noncancerous breast, and taking off the bra can be excruciating.

Two days following surgery they removed the bandages. The lumpectomy breast was at first quite swollen and didn't look too radical. The treated breast was smaller than the other one, but nothing that would make you feel horrified to look at yourself. But as time went by, when the swelling subsided, it was *considerably* smaller than I had at first realized and then it began to degrade, gradually losing more and more volume from the radiation damage until it became nonexistent. Getting dressed became a challenge, and frankly, as a woman with a sexy image in the public arena, it was rather demoralizing.

Then the pain began . . . constant pain. As I said, in order to wear a bra, the full undamaged breast needed to be worn high enough to look even. This constant pulling and pressing injured the breast, making bra removal each night an excruciating experience. Also, as someone who enjoys sex, I didn't find having painful breasts conducive to that activity. In time, I was always in pain. Something had to be done.

As an avid participant in antiaging and alternative medicine, the idea of a foreign object in my body was unacceptable. As I mentioned previously, at the time of my cancer surgery, I was offered only two options. When I refused the first choice, implants in *both* breasts to assure evenness and symmetry, the other option offered was the TRAM flap procedure, which was also unacceptable to me.

I had first learned about the use of stem cells in growing new breast tissue from Dr. Robin Smith of NeoStem, a stem cell banking company. I was fascinated by the notion that we could bank our stem cells while we are healthy and store them cryogenically for later use. I also learned that stem cells could be used for a complete breast regrowth from reading literature about a doctor named Kotaro Yoshimura who was working out of the University of Tokyo. He had successfully re-grown breasts on over four hundred women in Japan. Although Dr. Smith made it clear there were no FDA-approved therapies for breast reconstruction, as an optimist I banked my stem cells with NeoStem in 2009, hoping one day to be able to use them for this procedure. I feel that banking your own stem cells is "bioinsurance." I believe that in the near future, our country will loosen up and allow stem cell protocols and therapies due to high demand. Those who bank their stem cells when they are healthy will be ahead of the game, particu-larly if facing a catastrophic event.

The official name of my breast regrowth is "cell-assisted lipotransfer." The procedure is not FDA approved, so for Hollywood Presbyterian Hospital to agree to participate in this groundbreaking procedure, the hospital administrators insisted I obtain an IRB (Institutional Review Board) approval qualifying me for a clinical trial. It took me three years to get this permission. I was disappointed that under this bu-reaucratic restraint, the FDA would not let me use my banked stem cells as I had wanted, only stem cells taken from my fat during the procedure. (But as you read on, you will see how I was able to use my banked stem cells for other aesthetic procedures.)

I met with Dr. Joel Aronowitz in Los Angeles, and together we went to Korea to learn more about stem cell procedures. I also asked Dr. Yoshimura to come to L.A. to examine me, and he agreed to work with Dr. Aronowitz who already had some expertise in adult stem cell technology and breast rejuvenation. Dr. Aronowitz worked with Dr. Yoshimura to learn this new groundbreaking procedure, and I felt secure that he was properly equipped to do his "virgin" surgery on me. He was successfully able to perform this advanced procedure using my enriched adipose-derived stem cells. Other doctors around the country are doing autologous fat transplantation for cosmetic breast surgery, but I am the first to have Dr. Yoshimura's advanced technique utilized, legally, using only my fat enriched with adipose-derived stem cells. Because of Dr. Yoshimura's pioneering work in Asia, this ad-vanced technique has now proven successful here in the United States. This is a great advancement, the best use of a scientific breakthrough. It is a modern approach to beauty, which in my opinion is safer and much less invasive than surgery.

The procedure is really quite simple. In layperson's terms, the sur-gical team removed the fat from my stomach by liposuction (boo hoo, hated to see that go!), then they took that fat and spun it at supersonic speed, separating it into three layers (like a mousse). The first layer was fat, the second layer was blood, and the third layer was stem cells. They took the stem cells, cleaned them, separated them, discarded the weak ones, then converged the strongest stem cells, which were now in high concentrations, and put them into a small concentration of fat so that the fat was supercharged with stem cells. With a "turkey baster" (my term), the surgeon injected the stem-cell-laden fat into my breast until it was of the correct volume. Poof! There it was.

Like a miracle, fat was removed from my abdomen to provide the stem cells that were then sorted in a high-technology procedure to extract the strongest and largest amounts of stem cells to be reinjected into my breast. Here's the thing: fat can be taken from any part of the body. I would imagine each individual woman would have her favorite places for removal: love handles, thighs, inner thighs. So the whole procedure is a win-win-win; you get a new, real breast, full feeling is restored, plus you get rid of unwanted fat! The whole process took about ninety minutes.

The most painful part of the procedure is the liposuction; it's not for sissies!

What women do need to know if they are having a mastectomy or a lumpectomy and want to consider this procedure afterward is that it is crucial to maintain the skin around the breast and the nipple. The mastectomies of yesteryear took away everything, the skin and nipple included, making this regrowth procedure impossible. Today doctors approach it differently, and if there is no concern of cancer in those places, the skin and nipple are left intact, which makes regrowth possible.

Now I look down where once there had been no breast and it is beautiful . . . high and real and firm, soft and unscarred. Talk about reversing aging! My breasts now look like they are those of a young woman. I can't tell you how this has positively affected me psychologically.

The thrill about this procedure for me is the medical advancement. There is an aesthetic component, of course, but the real joy comes from knowing what this means for all women. It's a huge advancement for breast cancer.

I researched and persevered, and I never gave up. As I mentioned, it took me three years to obtain legal permission. I did everything right to establish a legal precedent, so other women could qualify for a clinical trial and thereby allow for insurance to cover it. This is a real merger, truly *integrative*, of the best of Western and the best of alternative medicine.

I could have gone to Japan to do this three years earlier than I did, but instead I spent a considerable amount of time persuading an American doctor to learn this methodology. I allowed him to use me as his first patient because I wanted this to be an American achievement, by an American doctor on an American woman. At present, Americans who want to utilize stem cells mostly have to go to Japan, or the Dominican Republic or Germany, to name a few countries using stem cell procedures. We have been behind on this one. We have the best doctors on the planet in the United States, yet in so many cases our doctors have their hands tied, the laws prohibiting them from being all that they can be. I hope my surgery will open up this progressive and cutting-edge procedure to more people.

With the success of my regrowth, all women who are choosing to have implants now have a *real* option. Personally, I can't imagine why any woman would ever want to have a foreign object put in her body when she could have this procedure instead. Implants are laden with side effects, such as leaking, infections, and rejections, all of which simultaneously degrade health. A woman can now utilize a safe procedure of taking fat from her own body to regrow her breast and do a better job. Maybe the simplicity of the procedure is why there was such resistance and difficulty to my getting permission to do it. My procedure required less surgery, fewer drugs, no foreign objects, and less money; sometimes you have to sit back and think about who might have a vested interest in this procedure not being available. Whatever the reason, what could have been an easy stroll was made a long and difficult road for me instead.

No matter. It was worth it to help move the dial forward and bring this type of change to all who need or want it. All I know is that every time I look down at what hadn't been there for eleven years and is now replaced by a beautiful real breast that is a part of me, I smile.

Now, as for my banked stem cells . . . After the breast procedure, I asked my doctor to request that NeoStem send out *some* of my banked cells (I still have enough left cryogenically preserved to last me a lifetime) that originated in my bone marrow but were obtained through my blood. He injected these cells to improve the appearance of the skin on my neck, giving me, in essence, a stem cell neck lift using my banked stem cells. These mixes of cells contain something called *VSEL* (very small embryonic-like) cells, which have many regenerative properties. The result of the injection? Natural smooth skin, without any surgery. The wrinkles on my sixty-five-year-old neck are greatly improved, all without surgery. (For detailed information on stem cell banking and an accompanying video, go to my website, www.suzannesomers.com, and find the episode on my Internet talk show called *Suzanne Somers' Breaking Through*, which features Dr. Robin Smith discussing banking your stem cells.)

Using banked stem cells as a beauty enhancement is a huge medical advancement, showing off the skills of our doctors when working at their best.

CHAPTER 6

BOMBSHELL #2:
YOU CAN AVOID CATASTROPHIC EVENTS—
LIKE HEART ATTACKS!

Great spirits have always encountered violent opposition from mediocre minds.

—Albert Einstein

Everyone is afraid of catastrophic events! These are the unforeseen health incidents that occur: crippling autoimmune diseases, cancer, and the big one, the one that scares people the most, a heart attack! We think we have no control over any of these things, but this is a book about aging well and avoiding the conditions that are killing others. So, how do we control this fear and avoid the "catastrophic event" that brings down so many?

There is a way!

My family has been plagued by heart disease; it killed my mother and father and so many of my relatives. My sister has already had heart surgery for her coronary arteries. Thankfully, she caught it in time and now is on a regimen that will prevent heart problems for her in the future. I am grateful she has adopted these protocols because I cannot imagine living in a world without my sister.

The answer is not in pharmaceutical drugs! If it were, then heart disease would not be the number one killer in the country.

Yet what goes wrong, particularly with people who *are* health conscious but are brought down by the "big event," for instance, like Jack LaLanne? With his aim to live well past a hundred, what did this famous health pioneer miss? With his diet and exercise regimen he should have lived even longer. What causes people who take exceptionally good care of themselves to die of age-related diseases? What else could he have done?

And how is it that people who do make good choices and avoid bad habits—eating healthy, exercising, and taking supplements—still develop a serious illness?

This chapter will answer these questions. There is a nice reward for making healthy lifestyle choices: It will add years to your life, free of the afflictions you see in others who may be younger than you. Yet there are other things you can do that you might not realize exist. Read on.

BILL FALOON

Bill Faloon *is a cofounder of the Life Extension Foundation, the largest longevity organization in the world. Life Extension members take extraordinary measures to slow their rate of biological aging with the objective of forestalling the onset of degenerative disease.*

I wanted to find out from Bill what prevents people from living as long as they should, even when they make major efforts to remain young and vigorous.

Bill Faloon is also the publisher of Life Extension *magazine, which reports on cutting-edge health and science issues. It is printed monthly and is, I believe, the most impressive gathering of the newest medical information in the country. It is jam-packed with information to improve life quality and teaches readers how to save their lives.*

Bill Faloon is passionate about eradicating age-related disease; both he and his scientific advisory board have a remarkable grasp of the latest lifesaving therapies. This interview about avoiding the "catastrophic event" that robs so many of us of life is eye-opening.

SS: Hello, Bill. First, tell my readers how the Life Extension Foundation started.

BF: Thank you, Suzanne. Back in 1980, I helped assemble a group of people who wanted to slow our rate of aging. None of us liked the odds we faced of contracting degenerative disease, so our group developed what were some aggressive interventions at the time aimed at slowing our biological clocks.

SS: What were people doing back then to remain younger longer?

BF: The biggest handicap was that most of us lived in the United

States. That meant we would be the *last* to access medical advances because of the FDA's obstructionist policy toward scientific innovation. We had to import coenzyme Q_{10} from Japan for personal use because the FDA claimed it was a drug and not a dietary supplement. The vital hormone DHEA was approved in Europe, but of course not in the United States. Potencies of vitamins were so low that people had to swallow a lot of pills to obtain a meaningful dose. The challenge back then was gaining access to therapies that had demonstrated antiaging potential in scientific studies but were banned by the FDA.

SS: Amazing that a supplement as important to life as coQ_{10}, particularly for those people on statins, could be prevented from being sold in this country for so long. How many of you were there initially?

BF: There were only about three hundred of us back then. We worked together in a loose-netted confederation, talking on the phone and corresponding by mail to exchange information. We had doctors, research scientists, and dedicated laypeople who didn't like their odds of contracting cancer, stroke, heart disease, or senility. None of us accepted these inevitabilities, so we wanted to see how far we could go to prevent age-related illnesses.

SS: What motivated you to form the Life Extension Foundation?

BF: Our group knew there was an abundance of information that was being ignored by the medical establishment. We didn't believe that mainstream doctors had all the answers. For instance, when we would go into a hospital and look at the charts of members in our network, we would often see that the patients were not getting optimal care. In some cases, they were ill because of anemia and obvious malnourishment. Simple problems like this, if corrected, could result in the patients getting *out* of the hospital, as opposed to continuing a downward spiral until they died. It was our ability to *reverse* disease states related to aging that motivated us to form the Life Extension Foundation as a nonprofit organization.

SS: So . . . how has medical practice changed today?

BF: There's a lot more we can do today because consumer rebellions have stripped the FDA of some of its oppressive powers. Over the past thirty-two years, there has been an astounding increase in knowledge about what can be done to prevent and treat disease. The problem remains that much of this knowledge is not being utilized in the clinical setting. It's shocking that we've got all this good science and so little of it is being translated into medical practice.

Our mission is to bridge that gap so that Life Extension members gain access to the fruits of research findings that are published in the scientific literature.

SS: Okay, let's get to the meat of this interview. I believe we all worry about the unknown. What are the things lurking in the body that could take us by surprise and bring us down? I ask because there are many people who take good health seriously yet succumb to a catastrophic event. It doesn't feel fair. So what are they missing?

BF: The greatest impediment is that many people who think they are living healthy are missing just a few critical components. The result is they die needlessly. There are eighteen known mechanisms of aging. They are chronic inflammation, glycation, methylation deficit, mitochondrial dysfunction, hormone imbalance, excess calcification, digestive enzyme deficit, fatty acid imbalance, DNA mutation, immune dysfunction, enzyme imbalance, loss of mitochondria, excitotoxicity, circulatory deficit, loss of youthful gene expression, loss of insulin sensitivity, loss of bone density, and oxidative stress.

The reason health-conscious people die prematurely is they leave themselves vulnerable to just a few of these age-*accelerating* factors that are easily containable with today's technologies. [See chapter 18, "Advanced Age Reversal," for a list of supplements that address each factor.]

SS: Yes, these age factors are very important to understand. That's why I put them at the front of the book in chapter 2, so people would realize they need to know what the terms mean to be able to get a handle on reversing damage already done to their bodies. But let's talk about those who do follow a comprehensive program and still die early. What are these people missing?

BF: Sometimes they overlook just one important factor. Think of all those who seem to be aging well but succumb to pneumonia. What some people accept as "normal aging" in reality involves a hideous decline in healthy immune function. Scientists refer to it as "immune senescence," and aging people have to be particularly vigilant in maintaining youthful immune surveillance. They also need to immediately and aggressively treat any kind of infectious agent that could cascade into pneumonia.

SS: What should we do to maintain immune function?

BF: You need to restore your natural hormones to youthful ranges. A deficiency in the hormone DHEA, for instance, can result in a horrific disruption of immune responses. Conventional medicine has frightened a lot of people away from the proper use of natural hormones. The fatal result is that elderly people succumb to infectious diseases they may never have contracted had they maintained a youthful hormone profile. But there is a lot more that aging people need than any single hormone to guard against pneumonia.

SS: Makes me happy that your organization feels so strongly about natural hormone replacement, but Jack LaLanne seemed to be doing everything right. He restricted his calorie intake, exercised vigorously, and took a ton of supplements (never heard if he replaced hormones), yet he died in 2011 at the age of ninety-six. Now that's a long time and a long life, but could he have lived even longer with the current science?

BF: We aggressively sought out reasons why Jack LaLanne died at ninety-six considering his objectives of living well beyond one hundred years. From what we can gather, his first major event occurred in 2009 when at the age of ninety-five he underwent aortic valve replacement surgery. A little over thirteen months later, he died at age ninety-six of respiratory failure due to pneumonia. Even in healthy elderly individuals, the impact of aortic valve surgery can be what we call the "catastrophic pathological event" that leads to a downward spiral culminating in death.

SS: So give me the Bombshell! What should have Jack LaLanne done to prevent it?

BF: Jack LaLanne was ahead of his time in so many ways, yet he appears to have missed out on one key nutrient—vitamin K_2—that may have prevented *calcification* of his aortic valve. When a valve or other tissue in the body calcifies, it hardens like a rock and becomes nonfunctional. In reading Jack LaLanne's last book published in 2003, he mentioned the importance of vitamin K only in the context of normal blood clotting, and he recommended green leafy vegetables as the main source. We now know that almost everyone obtains enough vitamin K for their blood to clot, but not nearly enough vitamin K_2 to protect against deadly soft tissue calcification.

SS: So you are saying that he might be alive today had he taken vitamin K supplements?

BF: It's hard to say since we only started recommending vitamin K supplements in 1999, but a compelling volume of data published since then substantiates the role of vitamin K_2 in protecting against tissue calcification throughout the body, so people who have not yet developed aortic stenosis can benefit enormously by taking it.

SS: So with everything Jack LaLanne did, the simple omission of vitamin K_2 may have led to his dying whereas he could have lived even longer had he supplemented K_2?

BF: I'm afraid so. At the same time, we pay tribute to Jack La-Lanne's foresight in promoting healthy lifestyle practices decades before others, but we must acknowledge the lethal consequence of omission. New information is published daily that provides *clues* as to what aging individuals can do to prevent the lethal catastrophic event that initiates a downward spiral of terminal degenerative disease. We fear Jack LaLanne's *omission* of vitamin K_2, and perhaps certain hormones, may have created his catastrophic event, that is, the aortic stenosis that predisposed him to pneumonia.

SS: It's amazing that one simple supplement can be so important to living longer. Vitamin K_2 will come up several times in this book. Clearly it is very important. How much vitamin K do most people need each day?

BF: There are two forms of vitamin K_2 and everyone needs both. So one should look at vitamin K supplements to ensure they contain MK-4 and MK-7.

> **Read labels; your supplement should contain: 1,000 mcg of MK-4 and 100 mcg of MK-7. The reason MK-7 is important is that it produces sustained levels of vitamin K over a twenty-four-hour period, whereas MK-4 has been shown to be particularly effective in protecting against osteoporosis.**

SS: What are other countries doing to treat aortic stenosis?

BF: Since 2007 Europeans have had an option to avoid the horrific surgical trauma associated with aortic valve replacement. Instead of open-heart surgery, a balloon catheter carrying a highly compressed bovine tissue replacement valve is inserted into an artery in the leg and threaded to the heart. Once the catheter reaches the beating heart, the balloon inflates and secures the new valve in place to replace the calcified aortic valve. Patients are functional within days as opposed to sometimes months of recuperation required for conventional open-heart procedures. In addition to improved survival, patients experienced substantially better quality of life afterward.

SS: Why aren't we doing this procedure here?

BF: This method is being used around the world, but the *FDA* may not approve it in the United States until after *2014*. This is unfortunate as many elderly Americans are so sick that they cannot qualify for open-heart surgery, and if they do, they may die from surgical complications.

By way of real-world example, an eighty-eight-year-old aunt of our magazine editor was told by her cardiologist that she had only a short time to live if she did not have her aortic valve replaced. She was taken to four different surgeons in New York City who all wanted to do conventional open-heart surgery. There are many concerns with a person this age, including cognitive deficits that occur in many patients placed on heart-lung machines and heightened risk of pneumonia and other infections during the long recovery phase.

Now here's another Bombshell, Suzanne . . .

Dr. Michael Ozner, a member of our scientific advisory board, informed us of a clinical trial in which surgeons were inserting the bovine tissue valve with cobalt-chromium frame via catheter *without* open-heart surgery. None of the top-rated surgeons in New York City who were initially visited were aware of this new procedure.

The eighty-eight-year-old patient enrolled in a trial location in New York at Columbia-Presbyterian Hospital not knowing if she would be randomized for open-heart surgery or this new procedure. Fortunately, she was chosen to be a part of the experimental group and was spared open-heart surgery. The procedure was done on Thursday, she was up and walking on Friday, and she went home on Monday. Two years after the procedure and now approaching ninety, she continues to work out with her trainer and takes her supplements. Equally as impressive, she does not need to take the anticoagulation drugs that mechanical valve patients require that carry a host of side effects, including increased stroke risk.

SS: I am an Irish woman, and my family dies of heart attack and stroke. I learned early on that the Irish tend to have high homocysteine, which is probably a genetic factor and why most of my family has had heart problems. Knowing this, I have kept my vitamin B levels at optimum. What are your feelings about this?

BF: Some cases of elevated homocysteine are genetic and require aggressive supplementation with an activated form of folic acid called *L-methylfolate* along with vitamins B_6 and B_{12}, and other nutrients. This genetic predisposition has been reported in some Irish population studies. As far as the Irish or anyone else is concerned, high homocysteine may reflect diets rich in methionine-containing foods, which include virtually all protein foods, meaning they are hard to avoid. Methionine is found in beef, pork, chicken, nuts, and even fish, so taking B vitamins is very important for most people to suppress the formation of homocysteine from methionine in food. As we age, our natural detoxification mechanisms become impaired and homocysteine levels tend to creep up, thus making proper B vitamin supplementation even more critical.

SS: Yes, I have been aggressively taking vitamin B_6 and B_{12} for years. Early on I injected it because we found my homocysteine was so high. I believe as a result of aggressively taking vitamin B, I have skirted my genetic predisposition and may have avoided a heart attack or stroke.

Explain the role homocysteine plays in heart disease and stroke.

BF: We know that very high homocysteine levels can cause premature atherosclerosis that manifests as coronary heart disease in very young people. A debate has been raging between Life Extension and mainstream medicine as to how low homocysteine needs to be to not be a heart disease or stroke risk factor. By way of example, a group of doctors at the Cleveland Clinic assessed the association between homocysteine levels and various degrees of aortic valve disease in seventy-six surgical patients.

- In patients with normal aortic valves, mean homocysteine level was 10.9 (umol/L).
- Patients with early-stage stenosis had homocysteine mean levels of 11.4.
- Those with the more severe *aortic stenosis* had a significantly higher mean homocysteine level of *15.4*!

While the small size of this study limited its predictive value, the doctors stated, "It is conceivable that the elevated homocysteine levels seen in patients with renal impairment and older age could contribute to more rapid progression of aortic stenosis seen in these patients."

SS: How come so many relatively healthy aging women and men who suffer just one bone fracture never recover? They don't always die right away, but they seem to develop endless complications that wind up killing them.

BF: Sadly, bone fracture is a classic catastrophic event. It creates a deadly downward spiral in the elderly. It first causes immobility that makes aging individuals vulnerable to pneumonia. But bone fractures also create systemic inflammation that can thrust an otherwise healthy person into a degenerative state that can manifest as dementia, stroke, or other age-related pathology. Had these people been able to prevent the initial bone fracture, they would have lived much longer in good health.

SS: People don't realize they can avoid bone fractures and that it's not just a bad stroke of luck. Everyone should be taking calcium and vitamin D to prevent bone fractures, right?

BF: This helps, but it is not enough to maintain optimal bone density in the later years. The public and most doctors are unaware of the magnitude of bone loss suffered by women and men as they age. The sad result is that people who take calcium supplements still suffer fractures that cripple and create ancillary pathological conditions.

SS: What else should people take to protect their bones?

BF: Strong bones require the minerals boron, magnesium, zinc, and manganese in addition to calcium. Vitamin D should be in far higher doses than found in typical multivitamin formulas, along with sufficient potencies of vitamin K_2. Men need to maintain their testosterone in youthful ranges, while women should achieve a youthful balance of estrogen and progesterone.

SS: Well, I've been writing in my last several books about the optimal, joyous quality of life that results when you replace the missing hormones due to aging, but I've also written about the protective nature of hormones in particular for strengthening bones. Would you explain why taking hormones strengthens the bones, even though one is taking supplements with enough minerals and vitamins?

BF: Because bone's skeletal-building cells, called *osteoblasts*, are directed by testosterone in men and progesterone in women to take up minerals from the blood and incorporate the minerals into the bone matrix. Adequate estrogen is needed by women and men to stimulate other skeletal cells, called *osteoclasts*, to remove older osteoporotic bone so that osteoblasts can pull in the minerals to build new stronger bone. Aging men and women lose these hormones and the result is significant loss of bone density that can culminate in osteoporosis and bone fracture.

SS: That was a wonderful explanation. The body in its wisdom never ceases to amaze me. You mentioned vitamin K again. Most doctors think the only function this vitamin has in the body is to ensure proper blood clotting. We know that without proper blood-clotting factors we would bleed to death internally. Yet as people age they develop sticky platelets that can clump together and block a vital artery in the heart or brain. How does vitamin K protect against osteoporosis and maintain healthy blood clotting?

BF: Calcium plays critical roles throughout the body that are strictly regulated by vitamin K_2. If there is not enough calcium in the blood, the body will pull it from the bones to ensure other critical functions are met, such as electrolyte balance needed to keep your heart beating. As people age, they suffer an imbalance in their calcium-regulating proteins that results in too much calcium being removed from bone and deposited in the arteries, brain cells, and heart valves. These calcium-regulating proteins are controlled by vitamin K_2. Supplementing with vitamin K_2 keeps calcium in the bone to maintain youthful density while keeping it out of our brain cells and arterial system where it causes disease. Interestingly, there is no danger for healthy people taking vitamin K as the body will only use enough of it to ensure necessary clotting. It will not cause abnormal clots to form in blood vessels of people unless they are on a medically supervised program designed to restrict vitamin K intake.

SS: Let's talk about senility. This is truly a catastrophic event.

BF: Yes, it is, especially from the standpoint that short-term memory loss is accepted by too many doctors as "normal" aging.

SS: I know. It disturbs me when I am out with a group of women and they refer to a memory lapse as a "senior moment" and laugh. I no longer find it funny because I realize it's the beginning of brain loss.

BF: You are right, and short-term memory loss can be a signal that serious underlying degenerative changes in the brain are happening. In some cases, there are circulatory disturbances that, left unchecked, result in a disabling stroke. When detected in time, relatively simple steps can be initiated to improve blood flow to the brain. In other cases, chronic inflammation is the culprit that inflicts massive damage to our brain cells. Suppressing inflammatory fires is a critical step to protecting against senility.

SS: Then how do you restore healthy blood flow to aging brains?

BF: At Life Extension, we perform blood tests to evaluate what risk factors may be causing blockages to occur in an individual's blood vessels leading to his or her brain. Once we identify the underlying factors, we advise members to aggressively correct these atherogenic factors. For example, in a peer-reviewed published study, pomegranate juice when added to conventional therapy was able to restore carotid artery blood flow by a remarkable 44 percent after only one year.

SS: I once read a report that eight ounces of pomegranate juice a day has been shown to actually reverse and flush out arterial plaque. But how do you suppress chronic inflammation?

BF: We utilize blood tests to ascertain the degree of chronic inflammation and what may be the underlying causes. Our health advisers then help customize a nutrient and natural hormone program to suppress the inflammatory factors that create so much destruction in aging brain cells. Nutrients like DHA from fish oil and extracts from green tea can exert significant inflammation-suppressing properties in the brain. Curcumin extinguishes inflammatory fires via several established pathways. A new form of magnesium has shown the remarkable ability of increasing the density of brain synapses, which enables our neurons to communicate with one another, which in lay terms means helps restore our short-term memory function. The key is attacking senility at the first sign of memory impairment instead of waiting for full-blown dementia to manifest.

SS: What is the most prevalent catastrophic event?

BF: Atherosclerosis, manifesting so often as coronary artery disease, is still the leading reason why health-conscious people don't live as long as they should. You may remember growing up, Suzanne, how men in their forties and fifties were suffering acute fatal heart attacks. The number of middle-aged people dying from acute blocked coronary arteries has plummeted over the past forty years due to better preventative measures. The burden has now shifted to people over age seventy who enjoyed healthy coronary blood flow most of their lives, but suddenly develop acute angina or heart attack that requires stenting or bypass surgery. Side effects from these invasive medical procedures plus accelerated atherosclerosis can become the catastrophic event.

SS: What causes these people's arteries to suddenly clog?

BF: The underlying cause we recognized long ago is a phenomenon called *endothelial dysfunction*. We observed people in their midseventies who had only 30 percent coronary artery blockage, yet a mere two years later, they were 90 percent blocked. What had happened is around age seventy-five, the inner linings of their arteries deteriorated so quickly that plaque rapidly accumulated in what were relatively healthy arteries just a few years prior. It was not because their LDL or triglyceride levels suddenly increased. The problem was the structure and function of their endothelium (inner arterial wall) had rapidly deteriorated and was attracting atherogenic agents from the blood.

SS: How do we protect against endothelial dysfunction?

BF: The blood test panels that Life Extension members take annually provide clues as to what blood components may be attacking the inner arterial wall. In aging people, however, a major problem is *nitric oxide* deficit. The endothelium requires nitric oxide to maintain its structure and function. As nitric oxide levels diminish with age, our arteries lose their ability to shield themselves from the many atherogenic blood compounds, cholesterol being just one of them.

SS: So how do we boost nitric oxide levels?

BF: It used to be thought that if enough of the amino acid *arginine* was taken, one could maintain adequate endothelial nitric oxide levels. The problem is that arginine is rapidly degraded in the body, so relatively little is available to create a sustainable volume of nitric oxide needed to protect the endothelium. To overcome the inability of arginine to produce sustainable nitric oxide, we looked at the problem from another direction. We knew most people produced enough nitric oxide, but the loss of natural antioxidant enzymes was causing the nitric oxide to degrade too rapidly. So we compounded several plant-derived antioxidants that targeted the free radicals that destroy nitric oxide. The results from published scientific studies show that these plant-derived antioxidants spare nitric oxide and improve blood flow to critical organs of the body such as the heart and brain. It is regrettable that conventional cardiologists have not caught on to these natural approaches that can partially reverse atherosclerosis.

SS: One of the reasons I take pomegranate along with my resveratrol, a powerful and miraculous supplement, is to decrease and hopefully eliminate inflammation and also to keep the blood in my arteries flowing perfectly. How far behind are cardiologists today when it comes to treating and preventing coronary artery disease?

BF: About twenty-five years behind. Cardiologists today recognize the dangers of elevated cholesterol, LDL, and triglycerides, but many remain in the dark about vascular disease blood markers such as fibrinogen, C-reactive protein, hormone imbalances, and other factors that contribute to atherosclerosis as people age. Cardiologists today are failing to control all the known risk factors that cause coronary artery blockages in aging people. The result is too many maturing individuals are requiring hospitalizations that only temporarily restore blood flow. Complications from hospital procedures, such as stroke, can be the catastrophic event that destroys a lifetime of healthy living. Congestive heart failure is another problem people with severely blocked coronary arteries encounter. Of course, sudden death heart attacks still kill over 156,000 Americans each year, so taking aggressive actions to maintain healthy circulation is critical to an extended healthy life.

SS: Elizabeth Taylor died in 2011 from congestive heart failure. I'm sure she had all the very best doctors. What did they miss and what does Life Extension recommend to improve cardiac output?

BF: Those suffering congestive heart failure need to restore the energy-producing capacity of their heart muscle cells. This involves taking the proper doses each day of acetyl-L-carnitine, taurine, and a special form of coenzyme Q_{10} called *ubiquinol*. A study on patients with severe congestive heart failure showed that 450 mg a day of conventional coQ_{10} did not improve the heart's ability to pump blood, but that 450 mg a day of ubiquinol improved recovery rates from congestive heart failure by 88 percent. In addition to these nutrients, Life Extension has uncovered solid data showing that restoring hormones like DHEA also improves cardiac output. I doubt Elizabeth Taylor's mainstream doctors were aware of this research showing that congestive heart failure is reversible.

SS: Okay, tell us, what steps do we need to take to prevent a catastrophic event from destroying our bodies?

BF: We have found that virtually anyone over the age of forty has markers in their blood that indicate their future disease risk. When people join the Life Extension Foundation, they gain free access to health advisers who can help identify an individual's particular vulnerability. We use blood test results and other data to customize a personalized longevity program to minimize one's odds of suffering a catastrophic health event.

SS: I think my readers will appreciate knowing they can take advantage of all your sophisticated testing and supplementation by joining Life Extension. It's one-stop shopping for lack of a better term. I don't think today's doctors are paying enough attention to people's medical issues as their patients grow older. It seems that most physicians accept age-related disease as being normal and are not recommending aggressive programs to protect against it. I've often heard it said to me by my readers that their doctors have said, "Well, what do you expect? You are old!"

BF: You're so correct, Suzanne. Few physicians are taught how to manage the multiple disorders caused by aging, and they fail to lead their patients through this period when they are susceptible to encountering a deadly catastrophic event. People join our Life Extension Foundation so they can learn to manage their own bodily issues with personalized guidance by our knowledgeable health advisory staff. Members receive a 110-page magazine every month that keeps them updated on the latest medical breakthroughs and, most important, that informs them how to utilize this information to maintain or restore their youthful vitality.

SS: Thanks again for all the great information, Bill.

BF: My pleasure, Suzanne.

You can obtain a free trial copy of *Life Extension* magazine by calling the toll-free number 1-888-884-3666 (twenty-four hours a day) or visiting www.lef.org/goodhealth.

CHAPTER 7

BOMBSHELL #3:
TESTOSTERONE SUPPLEMENTATION
DOES *NOT* CAUSE PROSTATE CANCER

After ninety, there's no need to worry about dying. Not many
people die over the age of ninety!

–George Burns

Now I'd like to introduce you to three doctors who will give you their
perspective on achieving a good quality of life and longevity. These
outstanding, highly educated Western doctors are *hormone specialists*, along with having expertise in other medical areas.

Dr. Abraham Morgentaler is an associate clinical professor of urology at Harvard Medical School and the founder of Men's Health Boston, a center focusing on sexual and reproductive health for men.

Dr. Prudence Hall is a graduate of the famed Keck School of Medicine of the University of Southern California and is the founder of
the Hall Center in Santa Monica, California.

Dr. Jonathan Wright has degrees in cultural anthropology and medicine from Harvard and the University of Michigan, is the medical
director at Meridian Valley Lab, and is the founder of the Tahoma
Clinic, both in Renton, Washington.

All these doctors, along with the other physicians and professionals
presented in this book, understand not only hormone replacement but
also the *art* of hormone replacement for both men *and* women. Replacement is an art, because it takes a doctor who is able to finesse an

individual's biochemical makeup and work with it. If your doctor has not chosen to specialize in bioidentical hormone replacement, then find one who does. It truly is a specialization, and going to a doctor who does not understand it is like going to a plumber for a heart by-pass. It's that important. These doctors also understand the daily dietary and lifestyle habits that hamper your efforts at achieving optimal hormonal balance.

Read on and let them teach you what you are unknowingly doing that is taking away from your health and also learn the benefits that come from having a balanced body.

Living longer with an efficiently working brain and robust health will keep you productive, allowing you to reinvent yourself as many times as suits you. Because I embraced antiaging medicine, my health and energy have allowed me to pursue an entirely new career. My writing endeavors are rewarding, and my age has become my asset. I am a productive member of society, and part of that is the wisdom I can bring to the table. If I were all "pilled up," if my brain was foggy from lack of hormones, and if I had been eating nonorganic food all these years, mine would be a completely different story. I cannot tell you how great it feels to be alive. I feel upbeat, healthy, energetic, and sexy. I am so busy there doesn't seem time in each day to do it all, yet I never feel worn out. There is a difference between worn out and tired, by the way. It all started with replacing my depleted hormones. Bioidentical hormone replacement keeps my brain sharp, my bones strong, my joints limber, my energy at peak, and my libido rockin'!

I set out to have these doctors answer the following: (1) How can we create a line of defense that allows our bodies to outsmart the present overwhelming environmental toxic assault? (2) How do we live with quality and optimal health in this new longer life that technology has afforded? and (3) What's new? Get ready . . . this is a fast-expanding science and what you will learn will give you the "edge" you are looking for to stay feeling young, healthy, and relevant.

THE FIRST SIGNS THAT YOU MIGHT WANT TO SEE A HORMONE DOCTOR

The first signs of deterioration are when your doctor might say something like "Your thyroid is a little off." A little off? The thyroid is a major player; it governs and regulates the minor hormones, although why they call estrogen, progesterone, and testosterone *minor*, I'll never know. Those of you who have low hormone output know that it is no minor thing.

To have a greater understanding of low hormonal output, think of your father and testosterone deficiency: out of gas, sleeping in his easy chair at all hours of the day, his big belly heaving, shoulders no longer straight but sloping, and, no small thing, notice his grumpiness. These are all indicators of testosterone deficiency.

But it's not the outward physical look of testosterone deficiency or the state of his mood (albeit not pleasant) that is alarming relative to aging successfully. Instead, it represents what is happening internally, in particular, the depletion of the pumping power of the heart, the largest muscle in the body, the muscle with more testosterone receptor sites than any other organ in the body. According to Dr. Abraham Morgentaler, whom you'll hear from next, lowered testosterone levels lead to an enlarged prostate. That is how important hormones are to our health and quality of life. It is very clear that testosterone depletion accelerates aging, and testosterone replacement in the right individualized dosages is a powerful player in aging well.

Your mother wouldn't have believed that, compared to who he once was, that same guy would end up being the guy she is married to today. The guy she fell in love with "back when" was a testosterone machine; he had energy, muscle tone, virility, sharp thinking, strong bones, a strong heart, and he was full of life, love, and passion. Where did all that go? Unfortunately, it drained out, as his testosterone drained from his body. But the good news is that now, with what we understand in antiaging medicine, he can get it back. Keep reading. It's reversible. This is the exciting aspect of new lifestyle medicine, and it's available to everyone who is interested. What an exciting notion.

ABRAHAM MORGENTALER, M.D.

I had the pleasure *of meeting Dr. Morgentaler at a dinner party outside of Salt Lake City several years ago. To my delight I was seated next to him and was so impressed with his relaxed charm. I found him to be the most unpretentious, affable, lovely man who, in spite of all his success at Harvard, still had boyish curiosity. We talked hormones all evening, and as you can imagine I was in heaven.*

Dr. Abraham Morgentaler is an associate clinical professor of urology at Harvard Medical School and is the founder of Men's Health Boston, a center focusing on sexual and reproductive health for men. He is the author of a number of popular books including The Male Body, The Viagra Myth, *and the one I devoured, the life-changing breakthrough book called* Testosterone for Life.

This book put the medical community in a quandary. For once he couldn't be called "one of those quack doctors" for stepping outside the orthodox beliefs. Here was a prestigious doctor from Harvard, on the faculty, saying the impossible: testosterone replacement was necessary for men's health!

Up until now, the inaccuracies and lack of understanding of this vital hormone have put so many men at a disadvantage. Without this vital youth-giving, bone-building substance, their lives get robbed of the very thing that gave them their male "edge." What Dr. Morgentaler has to say in this chapter is, I believe (along with many others), the greatest advancement in men's health in decades. I appreciate deeply that he called me to deliver the important news you are about to hear.

SS: Thank you for your time, Dr. Morgentaler. Harvard is an unlikely place for someone such as yourself to come out with cutting-edge information about testosterone replacement, particularly in light of the fact that most orthodox information promotes the theory that testosterone gives you cancer, or at the very least, raises the possibility. How important is it for men to replace testosterone as an antiaging ingredient?

AM: Thank you. It's nice to speak with you again, Suzanne.

Our ideas about testosterone are evolving rapidly. We now know that having a normal level of testosterone keeps men healthy. But, like many things in health, science, and medicine, we get "stuck" with very old ideas, and once they take root it's difficult to change the thinking.

SS: Why has traditional medicine been so conservative in its ideas concerning testosterone?

AM: Part of the reason is that there are so many myths and misconceptions about testosterone that are pervasive even at the highest level of academia. Early in 2012 there was a study reported in the *Wall Street Journal* about a group of young Filipino men. Testosterone levels of this group were obtained as young men, and then again several years later when some of these young men had become fathers. When they compared testosterone levels between the men who were fathers and the men with no children, the fathers had lower testosterone levels. That was kind of interesting.

But what was flabbergasting was the interpretation of this study. I gather it was done by a number of anthropologists. They concluded that there must be an evolutionary reason that fatherhood lowered testosterone, and when interviewed, the authors and other researchers made comments like "The lower testosterone levels in men with children means these men are less likely to leave the marriage and they will be better fathers."

Whereas with the higher-testosterone guys the thinking was, "If he goes out for drinks he may see some woman who interests him and he will be a worse father."

SS: Really, this is the thinking in academia?

AM: Right, this idea that men are just a function of our testosterone is misinformed. The big problem with the field of testosterone is that nearly everyone thinks they know all about it, but in this case what we think we know is often incorrect. In this study I mentioned, the authors appeared to believe that those men with lower testosterone are more domesticated and more likely to be faithful. What the authors seem to be unaware of is that testosterone levels can fluctuate widely even from morning to evening, especially in young men, yet our personalities don't change hour by hour.

To me, the likely explanation for the lower testosterone in young fathers is that they were sleep deprived! Any kind of sleep disorder drops your testosterone. The proof was the men with the very lowest testosterone were the ones whose babies had arrived within the last month.

SS: It's good to know that the men are not sleeping after the arrival of the new baby either!

So why is testosterone a good thing for long health?

AM: All men have testosterone, and our levels decline as we get older. When it gets below a certain point, men start having symptoms. However, lower levels of testosterone also affect some biological systems. For instance, studies show that men with low testosterone are at an increased risk of developing diabetes.

SS: Thank you. I've been saying this in my books . . . why do diabetic doctors not understand that testosterone replacement is so important relative to treating older diabetic male patients?

AM: I don't know why this is, but they haven't connected the dots, which is amazing. Some of them are starting to get tuned in, but not many. I work with the Joslin Diabetes Center in Boston, which is one of the premiere diabetes care centers in the world, and through our work together the physicians there have started to pay attention to the link between diabetes and low testosterone. A number of studies have now shown that between 40 and 50 percent of men with adult diabetes have low testosterone levels. It's one of the greatest risk factors for low testosterone. Other studies have shown that men in the lowest 25 percent of the group with low testosterone ended up with more than double the risk of developing new onset of diabetes. In other words, having diabetes means that a man is at high risk of having low testosterone, or "low T" as I like to call it, and low T itself is a risk for *developing* diabetes down the road.

Also, in separate studies they found men in the lowest 25 percent had two to three times the risk of getting fractures because testosterone is crucial for bone density in men.

SS: Because testosterone is an anabolic steroid?

AM: Yes. Testosterone is good for bone in men just as estrogen is good for bone in women.

SS: Because anabolic steroids build bone and muscle?

AM: Right. Furthermore, in four population studies involving a total of several thousand men, men with low testosterone died sooner than men with normal testosterone.

SS: That's quite significant . . . and I'm sure they were a lot grumpier while they were alive.

AM: You're funny! Yes, low testosterone can make men grumpy. Within the conservative medical establishment there is a way of thinking that's, "Let's wait until we see all the data as proof before we move on this." As a physician who sees patients, there are some situations where the evidence may be less than perfect, but my patient is sitting right in front of me, and I have to make the best judgments based on what I do know.

Here's what we know so far. When you give testosterone to men with diabetes, their blood sugar control gets better. Testosterone changes the body's composition from fat to muscle, which not only sounds good but also helps with blood sugar metabolism and probably atherosclerosis, too.

SS: Then it's tragic that older men are not given testosterone routinely. It just doesn't make sense not to. We're talking not only health but also quality of life.

AM: It just hasn't gotten into the mind-set of a lot of doctors; they have funny feelings about testosterone. That's part of the challenge.

SS: The medical establishment has funny feelings about hormones in general. Yet the men and women who have embraced replacement all say (myself included) that it's life altering.

AM: Why do *you* think there is resistance?

SS: Because it wasn't taught in medical school and I think doctors have been caught unprepared, and there is an embarrassment factor. So there's a tendency to brush it off as junk science. Do you agree?

AM: Yes, I do think that's part of it. There is a widespread belief in the medical establishment that testosterone causes trouble, and it's seen largely as a hormone for sex rather than for your heart, muscle, and fat and for your health in general. But sex has the biggest implication in terms of perception.

One of the areas in which I deal is sexual medicine. Doctors are supposed to be talking to people about sex but actually they are about the worst people to talk to anyone about sex, right?

SS: Well, what doctor talked to you about sex when you were a kid?

AM: Right. Nobody! I went to Harvard Medical; we were taught to be politically correct, as in when you took a sexual history you were supposed to ask without judgment in your voice, "Are your partners male, female, or both?" That's about all I learned about sexuality in med school.

SS: Luckily, many female doctors (primarily gynecologists) and antiaging doctors as well are now asking about sexuality.

Because you are a Harvard doctor you have credibility that can (excuse the term) slop over into orthodox offices making HRT [hormone replacement therapy] a viable choice. Your book *Testosterone for Life* was a true breakthrough. When you wrote about the merits of testosterone replacement, people listened. It essentially said: testosterone does not cause prostate cancer, and that a man could take testosterone if he had had prostate cancer.

Now you have new information saying that if a man has active cancer, he can take testosterone replacement. Can you elaborate?

AM: Thank you. That's essentially correct, but we have to be careful because it is not necessarily safe for *all* men with prostate cancer to take testosterone.

HOWEVER, IT HAS BECOME CLEAR TO ME
THAT THERE IS PROBABLY NO PROBLEM FOR MOST MEN
WITH PROSTATE CANCER TO TAKE
TESTOSTERONE THERAPY.

One group I do worry about is men with advanced prostate cancer, especially if they are on medicines like Lupron, which lowers the testosterone almost to zero.

SS: You mean giving testosterone to these men is a waste of time because they are taking a drug to take *away* testosterone, so what's the point of giving it to them?

AM: Right. This is not good. Another group is men who happen to naturally have extremely low levels of testosterone. Most men diagnosed with prostate cancer do not fall into those two groups.

SS: Where did the theory about testosterone causing prostate cancer originate?

AM: In 1941, a urologist named Charles Huggins of the University of Chicago was doing studies on dogs with BPH (benign enlargement of the prostate). At that time it was known that around the 1900s, castration had been used to treat men who were in urinary retention, who couldn't pee because of their big prostate. Castration caused their prostate to shrink, and some of these men were then able to urinate again.

SS: Ouch!

AM: Right. So Huggins and his colleague Clarence Hodges began performing castration on men with widely metastatic prostate cancer, hoping that the cancer would respond the same way as the enlarged prostate in dogs. They used a blood test called *acid phosphatase* to determine how these men responded, and sure enough, many of the men felt improved, and the acid phosphatase level fell, indicating that the cancer had regressed, or shrunk. Huggins went on to win the Nobel Prize in 1966 because his idea of castration helping with prostate cancer was the biggest news in oncology in the early 1940s. Everyone thought this was amazing and jumped on it, and Huggins became one of the most prominent medical doctors in the world.

SS: When you say castration, you mean prostate removal?

AM: No, it means removal of the testicles.

SS: I am speechless. That's a heavy-duty procedure.

AM: In my training between 1984 and 1988, we did a lot of these operations.

SS: Are they still castrating men today?

AM: Yes, although in the United States, we tend to now use medicines to lower testosterone. Those medicines are relatively expensive, though, so in much of the world, removal of the testicles remains the standard treatment for metastatic prostate cancer. Lowering T [testosterone] to castrate levels definitely shrinks the prostate, lowers the blood test PSA, and can reduce bone pain if there are metastases in the bone. In some men, it can also provide a long-term successful treatment outcome, but in most cases the cancer eventually comes back.

The big fear about using T in men for health and symptoms, though, comes from a misunderstanding of what Huggins and his colleagues showed. The overly simplistic idea has been that since lowering T is a good treatment for prostate cancer, then it seems logical that raising T would be dangerous. It's not that simple, though.

In my training at Harvard I had done some undergraduate work with lizards showing if you manipulate testosterone and put it back into the right parts of the brain, these male lizards acted as though they were fine even though there was nothing circulating in their body and they went after females just like they should have.

SS: Why manipulate the testosterone in the brain? Is it because there are testosterone receptors in the brain?

AM: Yes! Some of the most important actions of testosterone stem from the fact that it is a brain hormone. I had been interested in testosterone, and had researched it in animals since the 1970s, but when I did my medical training and training in urology, all at Harvard, I was taught essentially that testosterone was dangerous, particularly for prostate cancer. Harvard had taught me never to give testosterone to men with elevated PSA or any suspicion of prostate cancer, for fear of activating the cancer. I learned that giving T to a man with prostate cancer was like pouring gasoline on a fire. I was also taught that low testosterone in men was rare, and that even if it were present, treatment with T was highly unlikely to be helpful for any symptom.

I don't always listen so well, though, and I like to figure out for myself if what I've heard is really true. Because of my experience with the lizards I was curious about testosterone in men, and I started measuring testosterone in a lot of patients who came to see me with sexual symptoms, or who complained of fatigue or depressed mood. I was surprised to find quite a few with low T, since that went against my training. So I started giving testosterone to these patients and not only did their libido return, but they often said things like "I feel like myself again." That was pretty impressive for me. But I still worried that some of these men might have hidden cancer of the prostate and that testosterone might promote its growth.

SS: So you were taking a big chance.

AM: It felt risky, since I didn't know a single physician who was treating men in this way. Testosterone therapy had been primarily the province of endocrinologists, who prescribed T almost exclusively to men with severe T deficiencies, usually due to genetic problems like Klinefelter's disease, or whose pituitary glands had been removed for tumors, or men who had lost both testicles and couldn't produce any testosterone on their own. The idea of treating men who were otherwise healthy, and who had developed low T simply due to aging, was unknown to me at the time, although later I found a few sympathetic souls around the country who were doing the same thing. Nonetheless, I still worried that I might provoke a hidden prostate cancer to grow in some of these men. Around 1992, I went to our national urology conference and I ran into one of my former teachers in the hallway who said to me, "Abe, I understand you are giving testosterone to men, and I don't think you should do it." He said, "I gave testosterone to a man and within a couple of months his PSA went up. I did a biopsy and he had cancer." Well, I freaked when he said that, since that had been my biggest concern about T therapy. My treated patients were doing unusually well, but prostate cancer was the big bugaboo. This teacher of mine went on: "I don't think you should be treating men with testosterone because of the prostate cancer risk. However, if you do, I strongly recommend you do a prostate biopsy first to make sure they don't have cancer."

I was sure I wanted to continue to treat with testosterone, but I took my teacher's comments to heart, and when I returned from the meeting I went straight to my chief and told him I wanted to do prostate biopsies in men who were candidates for T therapy. He said, "Go ahead."

Almost as soon as we started doing prostate biopsies in these otherwise normal men with low T—they had normal PSA, normal prostate exams—I found a few cancers. That was a shock. The traditional teaching had two parts. One was the caution that higher T was a cause of prostate cancer, and the other was that low testosterone was supposed to be protective against prostate cancer. In fact, almost everyone who trained in the field of prostate cancer was taught that men who developed severely reduced T early in life would *never* get prostate cancer.

A year or two later I presented this information to my colleagues, again at our national meeting. These men had no known risk factors for prostate cancer, and I had performed biopsies only because they had low T and I wanted to exclude the possible presence of cancer before I started T therapy. We found six cancers in our first thirty-three men, which at that time was considered a very high rate of cancer. That wasn't supposed to happen if the T was low. At the end of the presentation, an internationally famous urologist stood up and said, "This is garbage! Everyone knows that high testosterone causes cancer, and low testosterone is protective. You guys just hit a few cancers you never should have found in the first place. I can guarantee if you do another hundred biopsies you won't find another cancer."

I thanked him for his comments and when I returned home, I continued to do biopsies and found more and more cancers in men with low testosterone. We wrote up our experience and submitted it to the *Journal of the American Medical Association* [*JAMA*], and one day the editor called me and said, "This is highly unusual information you have submitted. It's the opposite of what we've assumed for decades. We'd like you to accumulate more data, and if the numbers hold up, we will consider publishing it." When we had prostate biopsy results in seventy-seven men with low T and normal PSA, and eleven of them had cancers, they published it. That was 1996.

SS: This must have rocked the establishment.

AM: It did. But I think no one really knew what to do with the information. Clearly we proved that low testosterone was not protective against prostate cancer. These men with low T had cancer rates of 15 percent, which was as high at that time as men who were supposedly at high risk, with elevated PSAs or a prostate nodule.

SS: You know, I'm enjoying this because it's been the thinking in antiaging for years, but the movement needed your research and, as I said before, coming from Harvard carries a lot of weight. It must be difficult for the "old guard" to let go of established ideas.

AM: Right. From that research, I no longer believed low T was protective against prostate cancer. So I was curious where that idea had come from. I went back in the earlier journals and found that that theory was essentially based on *nothing*. It just fit neatly into a story line in which T was seen as the devil; high levels were bad, low levels were good. For years, urologists have seen themselves as the "protectors of the prostate." My work and the conclusions I was drawing from our results were challenging to traditional ideas, and they didn't like it. They saw me as kind of a "nut," or let's say they indulged me. Sometimes they would get angry.

But I saw firsthand how well men were doing on testosterone, not just with sex but a general all-over improvement in their health, vigor, well-being, and mood. Some years later, a training fellow and I went through all the published literature on T and prostate cancer for a review paper on the risks of testosterone for the *New England Journal of Medicine*. We looked at several hundred articles from medical journals to investigate the association between high testosterone and prostate cancer. In the end we couldn't find a single article that showed any compelling evidence that high T, or raising T with treatment, was a risk for prostate cancer. Not one.

SS: So the theory of low testosterone being protective from getting prostate cancer was totally inaccurate? That's an amazing story. Think of all the men who suffered as a result of this inaccuracy.

AM: Right. The traditional idea, taught for decades, that raising T would cause prostate cancer or would make an existing small cancer grow like wildfire was based on a misunderstanding of data that went back to Huggins in 1941. All this time the medical establishment had been relying on old outdated information, and because it seemed to make sense to people, it had never been seriously questioned or challenged.

Probably the single best thing I ever did in medicine or science was going to the basement of the Countway Library of Medicine at Harvard and pulling out the original Huggins paper. I couldn't believe my eyes when I read it. Huggins and his coauthor, Hodges, had removed the testicles in a relatively small group of men with metastatic prostate cancer and showed that a blood test called acid phosphatase dropped quickly, presumably due to lack of testosterone. This indicated that the cancer had regressed, which was very cool. This was the first successful treatment for advanced prostate cancer, and as I mentioned before, we still treat metastatic prostate cancer by lowering T, although we tend to do it now with medications rather than removing the testicles.

In addition, Huggins and Hodges wrote that they had also administered T injections to men with prostate cancer, and the acid phosphatase went up in all of them. That sounded bad when I first was reading it. But when I looked more closely, they only gave testosterone to three men. In the Results section they only gave results for two men. One of these men had already been castrated, which put him in a different category altogether. In the end, the theory that prostate cancer will grow like wildfire if an otherwise normal man receives testosterone was based on a single man! And the actual data provided for that one man was not particularly convincing. That blood test, acid phosphatase, is no longer used because it's so erratic. And in the one individual who supposedly showed a definite increase in acid phosphatase during testosterone administration, his levels were bouncing all over the place.

I found a few additional stimulating articles among the old literature. Prior to 1982, there were several studies where investigators had actually treated men with testosterone even though they had metastatic prostate cancer. At the time, the idea that the prostate was hormonally sensitive was new, and they were trying to figure out what happened when they gave T and when they took it away. Although no one really was prepared to say it at the time, it became clear to me from these various studies that if T was given to men with prostate cancer after their own T had been reduced to zero (by testosterone-lowering drugs), their cancers grew rapidly. However, when T was administered to men without any prior hormonal treatment, if they had just been left alone before receiving T, then nothing happened to them.

SS: So your conclusion is . . .

AM: Prostate cancer needs some testosterone in order to grow. But it can only use a little. Adding more doesn't seem to do anything bad.

SS: We are talking about active cancer.

AM: Yes.

SS: Well, that makes sense. Men are individualized just as women; everybody needs what they need.

AM: I like to use the analogy of a houseplant. If I go away and don't water a houseplant, when I come back it's going to be dry and shriveled up. If I come home in time and water it, the plant will grow and gain mass again. Once it's had enough water it doesn't matter if I let a garden hose run into that plant night and day, it will never grow to the size of a tree.

SS: Are you saying that excess testosterone won't make prostate cancer metastasize?

AM: That's right. In multiple research studies, there is no evidence that men with higher T are at any greater risk of metastatic or aggressive disease than men with lower T. Like the plant and water, prostate cancer can only accommodate, or use, a certain amount of its nutrient, testosterone. My colleague, Abdul Traish, Ph.D., and I have written this concept up and called this the *saturation model*. At some point that plant is saturated, like a sponge that's full of water.

On a biochemical level, the way hormones usually work is that they bind to a receptor molecule. If you don't have the receptor to recognize and bind to, the hormone doesn't do anything. Each cell has a limited number of copies of the receptor molecule. Once all the copies of the receptor are filled with androgen (testosterone), additional testosterone has nothing to bind to. It turns out that human prostates have their androgen receptors completely filled (we say the receptors are "saturated") at extremely low T concentrations, about 120 nanograms per deciliter. That's why men with advanced prostate cancer in those old studies who received T did fine if they hadn't yet been treated to lower their testosterone. And it also explains why men in those studies who had undergone castration did poorly with T administration—because the androgen receptors weren't filled yet with T, so there was still opportunity for T to bind to the receptor and thereby influence the cells to grow or divide more rapidly. We think of a normal level of testosterone to be above 350 ng/dL. If you drop a man's testosterone severely by administering medicines like Lupron, the prostate actually becomes "thirsty," if you will, for testosterone, and now the prostate is deficient and that allows the low testosterone to cause trouble, which wouldn't happen if levels were normal or even modestly reduced.

Testosterone makes men feel better. However, the fear that T will necessarily cause prostate cancer to appear, or grow if already present, has been the number one reason physicians have shied away from offering this to more men. And until very recently, it was believed that T was contraindicated in any man with a diagnosis of prostate cancer, even if he appeared to be cured of his cancer.

In the May 2011 issue of the *Journal of Urology*, my colleagues at Baylor Medical College and I published a study that seriously challenges that old taboo, in which we gave T to men with untreated prostate cancer. I got started with this project about five years ago when an eighty-four-year-old man walked into my office with some sexual complaints. He couldn't have an adequate erection, he couldn't have an orgasm, and he felt tired all the time. He was a lawyer, in great shape, with a beautiful shock of white hair on his head, and he still went to work every day. We tested his blood and he did have low T, as I suspected, but he also had a very high PSA. His value was 8.5, and anything above 4.0 ng/mL is considered abnormal and a risk for prostate cancer. I don't do a lot of biopsies in men in their eighties, but he wanted to know if he had cancer, so I did a biopsy on him. The biopsy showed he had relatively low-grade prostate cancer in both sides of his prostate. He said he really didn't want to treat the cancer, which I thought was reasonable given his age and the likelihood that this low-grade cancer wouldn't cause him any trouble for many years, if ever. But then he told me he wanted to try the testosterone treatment we'd discussed before his biopsy! I told him I had never given testosterone to a man with active prostate cancer.

SS: What did you do?

AM: I told him conventional wisdom is that his cancer will get worse. I also told him I do a lot of lecturing and research on this topic, and I wasn't sure that it was true. He asked, "If you give me testosterone and the cancer gets worse, will you be able to know?" I said, "Most likely because your PSA will go up." He's a lawyer, very smart, intelligent, and logical. He said to me, "Listen, I'm eighty-four years old. What have I got to lose?"

SS: Did you give it to him?

AM: Yes. You know what happened? Over two years, his PSA dropped from 8.5 to the sevens, into the sixes, into the fives, and then stabilized in the low sixes. After two years of testosterone treatment, I published his results as the first case of long-term T administration in a man with untreated prostate cancer, revealing no progression of disease.

SS: That's fantastic, one man, one case, two years of testosterone therapy in a man with untreated prostate cancer. How is he today?

AM: He's fine! He still comes to see me a couple times a year. He's eighty-nine, he's been on testosterone the whole time, and there's no evidence of cancer progression. His case gave me the courage to start giving T to other men in the same situation. The paper we published in May 2011 gave the results of testosterone therapy in a small group of men, thirteen of them, all with active, untreated prostate cancer. They were rigorously monitored, and all of them had follow-up biopsies—an average of two sets of follow-up biopsies per individual. The average time of T therapy was two and a half years. Amazingly, none of these men had any progression of their cancer. Their PSA did not rise, and the size of the prostate measured by ultrasound when we did the biopsies did not go up. In fact, 54 percent of all the biopsies we did in these men showed no cancer at all.

I had another patient fifty-nine years old, more money than God, flies everywhere in his private jet. He was diagnosed with prostate cancer and had his prostate removed surgically.

SS: Didn't he do any research?

AM: This guy is smart, but when you are diagnosed, even the smartest get scared. He'd been on testosterone for a year and had done very well with it. But when his cancer was diagnosed, all his doctors were telling him, "You gotta get off testosterone, it's making the cancer grow." So he did, stopped cold turkey. While recuperating from surgery in one of his homes in the Bahamas or somewhere, a place he loves, he became suicidal. He told me he was watching a show on assisted suicide and he was taking notes on how to do it. He had only been off testosterone for a few months. So he decides, screw it, I'm going back on testosterone. Within a week he felt like himself again.

But his wife was worried and said, "You can't do that or it will wake up those sleeping cells."

SS: But . . . he wanted to kill himself when he was off it.

AM: Right. So he finds me and explains how great he feels on testosterone and is it safe for him to take? He asks, "If you told me that I would live three years with testosterone versus ten years without it, I would take the three years." He went back on testosterone and his cancer numbers have gone down.

SS: The testosterone theories have never made sense. If high testosterone were the problem, then every young man would have cancer.

AM: That is absolutely correct.

SS: I believe this research deserves the Nobel Prize. When you consider all the men who have been castrated, had prostates removed, been put on useless drugs, and destroyed their quality of life, to find that it might be as simple as T replacement is revolutionary.

AM: Thank you, Suzanne. You are so good for my ego! You know, I've been doing this for twenty-plus years and it's been a serious challenge to get the message out there. There is such resistance to this information. Historically we've been depriving men of androgen and in so many cases been wrong! I hope I'm not getting too technical. Do you know the difference between androgen and testosterone?

SS: No, I don't.

AM: "Androgen" is a general term for chemicals similar to testosterone. I mentioned earlier that there are receptors that hormones bind to; anything that's in a class like testosterone and binds to the androgen receptor is called an androgen. As a rule, androgens have positive effects on muscle and bone. There are several fairly well-known androgens. The best known, and most plentiful in the body, is testosterone itself. Others include DHT (dihydrotestosterone) and androstenedione.

SS: Isn't too much DHT dangerous?

AM: No, I don't think there's any reason to believe it is. Some people have raised concerns about DHT because most testosterone is converted to DHT within the prostate cells, and DHT binds more tightly to the androgen receptor. So some have believed that higher levels of DHT are risky for prostate cancer. However, as we've discussed, whether it's T or DHT in the prostate, the theoretical evidence as well as my own research shows that excess androgen is exactly that, a mere excess.

DHT appears to be responsible for some good things for men, such as erections. DHT is involved in the signaling pathway that allows cells in the penis to release the chemical that causes erections.

Testosterone creams tend to increase DHT because there's an enzyme in the skin called 5-alpha-reductase that converts testosterone to DHT. So it's fairly common to get higher DHT levels with T gels or creams. I am not aware of any evidence that high levels of DHT are a problem, and in fact there have now been several studies in which men were treated with DHT gels. Their blood levels of DHT increased quite dramatically, but those men experienced no significant problems. I don't worry about high DHT levels at all.

SS: This is new information. I thought high DHT levels were worrisome, just like overly high estrogen levels in men.

AM: Estrogen in men comes from the conversion of testosterone to estrogen. As men age, their testosterone goes down but so does their estrogen. Higher estrogen is often found in men who are obese. If you have more fat tissue, you have more aromatase, which is an enzyme that converts testosterone to estradiol. If you have more aromatase as a man, you are going to end up with more estradiol. If those levels are excessive, you are at a higher risk of getting breast tissue (you've seen those man boobs on guys who are heavy). Actually, some studies show that when estrogen levels are too high or too low in men, there is a higher risk of atherosclerosis and stroke, and when estrogen levels are too low, a greater risk of osteoporosis.

SS: Is there danger in those scenarios?

AM: Well, if he has boobs, he's in danger of somebody thinking he's a woman.

SS: There's always somebody for everybody! [Laughs.]

AM: There may also be some rare instances when a man has extremely high estradiol levels and it interferes with his response to testosterone therapy. However, those cases are rare. It is not unusual to see a mild or modest increase in estradiol in men who are receiving T therapy, or in overweight individuals, and by and large, the elevated estradiol is unlikely to cause any trouble at all. Men with more abundant fatty tissue may have more aromatase, but I'm not aware of any problems that arise from too much aromatase. Specifically, there is no reason to think that aromatase itself is a risk for cancer.

SS: Is it true that the prostate is akin to a woman's breast?

AM: In what way?

SS: My understanding is that a woman's breast has ducts where we make the milk. Similarly, the prostate has ducts where testosterone makes food for the sperm. In connecting the dots, it seems to me that when a man stops producing or is not making very much testosterone anymore, the prostate enlarges, looking for its key ingredient, testosterone, which was always there and now is not. And that the remedy (it seems to me) is to replace the missing or deficient testosterone; it would calm the prostate down because now it has what it needs and will, therefore, return to its original size.

AM: Well, that's a brilliant conclusion, Suzanne! Of course I say so because I've wondered the same thing! Enlarged prostates happen to older men and do not happen to twenty-year-olds. When I lecture, I usually find somebody in the audience who is under thirty and I point him out and ask if he realizes that he is at his peak of production of testosterone? They are always very proud, and then I ask, "Do you feel your prostate growing right now?" People laugh because it's absurd.

But then why has the thinking been that enlargement of the prostate comes from high testosterone? If that were true, every young man would have prostate cancer or enlarged prostates and it just doesn't happen. That model for T and enlarged prostate growth, and prostate cancer, has been wrong. It makes more sense, logically, that testosterone (or DHT) may actually prevent prostate growth, since enlarged prostates occur when we age and T has declined.

SS: So the prostate is looking for testosterone? I ask because men have been given testosterone as a cancer preventative in Europe for over fifty years.

AM: What exactly causes cancer is open for debate. Could be a lot of things, particularly in this environment of toxicity and stress; but I think yours is as good a hypothesis as any that happens in the normal environment for the prostate where the hormonal environment has been disrupted. I wrote an editorial this past year for the journal *Cancer* about how low testosterone is now being seen in many studies as a risk for bad cancers. I'm talking about *low* testosterone, not *high*! I enjoyed writing that article about how the original thinking has been turned upside down.

Suzanne, perhaps I think overly simplistically about some of these things, but I believe one can make a reasonable argument that testosterone therapy may reduce the impetus for prostate cancer to grow or metastasize. It's like a bear in the woods that has lots of berries and fish around. He's happy, he has lots of food, and he doesn't have to travel very far. Suddenly you take that same bear and take away the food; no fish, no berries. That bear now has to go far afield to find food and survive. He might even need to start changing its habits to find other sources of nourishment. Similarly, think about a prostate cancer that likes testosterone; if there's not much around it's going to find other "food sources" or might find ways to travel far afield to get what it needs. There are multiple studies that show that men with low testosterone are at risk for getting not only prostate cancer but also higher-grade and more aggressive cancers. A number of studies performed in the laboratory have shown that prostate cancer cells appear to behave less aggressively when exposed to abundant levels of testosterone, and more aggressively when deprived of testosterone.

SS: It makes sense.

AM: I believe before too long the data will be strong enough so that it will be possible to say that having normal amounts of testosterone is protective from developing prostate cancer. It may well be the *key factor* to keeping those cancers well behaved.

SS: Well, it has been my belief for the last six or seven of my books that it is an environment of balanced hormones for men and women that can prevent cancer. The theories you have just stated apply to women as well as men; if high estrogen caused women to get breast cancer, then all young women, who make tons of estrogen, would have breast cancer. The environment in a young woman is of balanced hormones; it's not until menopause when the balance is "off" that the cancers and problems begin. You know, connect the dots.

AM: Having normal testosterone doesn't necessarily mean somebody's going to live forever, but I do think it's a key component for general health.

SS: You are speaking of quality of life, and for a man, maintaining his mojo?

AM: Yes, it's impossible for a man without testosterone to keep (your word) his mojo. Aging is complicated, and there are many factors that determine why one will age well and the other doesn't.

SS: So what we've said in this interview, if I may paraphrase, is: Testosterone does not cause prostate cancer, and if a man has had prostate cancer he can and should take testosterone replacement. And now the new big news from your research; if a man has active cancer, he can and should take testosterone replacement?

AM: Almost. I'm not prepared to say yet that a man *should* take testosterone if he has been diagnosed with prostate cancer. At this point, I do feel that many men who are symptomatic from low levels of testosterone will benefit from it, and the evidence so far, which is still quite limited, is that most of these men with prostate cancer who do receive T will not have any problems with it. However, there are situations where I would *not* give testosterone. And although the evidence regarding aggressive prostate cancer and *low* testosterone is intriguing, I'm also not ready to say yet that T therapy is a good treatment for prostate cancer. Right now that is just an idea—an interesting one—that may or may not turn out to be true. Hopefully we'll have a chance to explore that possibility over the next few years.

As for the use of testosterone therapy in men without prostate cancer, I do think there is more and more evidence that a normal T concentration is good for health and longevity.

However, there is a strong public and even medical sentiment that the decline in testosterone as men age is "natural," and therefore "good." It is as if God/Nature designed us this way, so why are we mucking around with the natural decline in hormones? It's a struggle to convince those with that thinking that there may be important benefits to hormone treatment in men. Sometimes, nature isn't wonderful!

Your books, Suzanne, with the message that there is a new way to age and that hormones are a key ingredient, have had a huge influence. Some of the men who come into my office tell me that their wife or girlfriend read "that Suzanne Somers book," they're now feeling great, and they want their man to feel as good as they do, so he can keep up!

SS: [Laughs.] Glad to boost your business!

AM: The present notion that whatever happens to us as we age is "supposed to happen" makes my brain hurt! There is this idea that we are supposed to age gracefully like Katharine Hepburn in *On Golden Pond*.

SS: Yes. I don't think that beautiful lady was aging gracefully. Her head was shaking; she had all sorts of problems.

AM: Yes, but it is a very romantic notion. What most people don't recognize is that aging sucks! Big time! This is how I respond when people ask, "Why can't we age gracefully, naturally?" Aging is associated with all sorts of lousy things—bad eyes, bad hearing, bad brains, bad teeth, bad joints, bad blood vessels. And cancer! All these are "natural" events that occur with aging. We treat all these to improve the quality of our lives, and in many cases to live longer and better. The testosterone deficiency that accompanies aging in men is really no different. I had perfect vision until I turned forty or so, and now I can't read anything without glasses. Should I give up my glasses because the diminished vision of aging is "natural"? That would be ridiculous!

SS: We have to help ourselves, and your work is redefining that paradigm. Hormones are the antidote for everything you just mentioned except for bad eyes and that will be taken care of by nano-bots thirteen or so years from now. For instance, it was Dr. Jonathan Wright who told me in my book *Breakthrough* that loss of hearing was a result of low aldosterone [a hormone] and by replacing aldosterone, many of his patients' hearing is coming back measurably. My own husband, who had lost 5 percent of hearing in the upper ranges, has had his hearing restored by replacing aldosterone daily.

AM: It's time science starts thinking about quality of life. We've been depriving men of testosterone for no good reason other than a fear based on a misunderstanding of a small study performed over seventy years ago. Since the time of Huggins we started depriving men with advanced prostate cancer first by castration and then with medicines like Lupron and Zoladex. Those medications can be enormously helpful in some men with very advanced prostate cancer, particularly if they have metastases and pain, and also if given for a short while prior to radiation therapy, where it seems to improve outcomes. However, these testosterone-lowering medications have been used far too frequently, and at a considerable cost to the health and lives of men. Lowering testosterone levels to zero, or close to it, causes osteoporosis, which puts men at risk for fractures; it also increases the risk of heart attacks.

When the PSA goes down with treatment, patients and their doctors tend to be pleased because that seems like a good thing. It may be good for prostate cancer, and bad for health. A huge study published last year found that "cancer-specific survival" was improved in a group of men treated with androgen deprivation, but the overall survival was the same.

SS: What does that mean?

AM: It means that fewer people who were deprived of androgen died of prostate cancer, but they still died at the same rate as men who were not androgen deprived. They died of other things, like heart attacks. And in all likelihood they were miserable—low or absent sex drive, chronic fatigue, depression and irritability, weight gain.

Lowering testosterone severely causes men to increase their fat and increases their risk of getting metabolic syndrome and diabetes. The risk of a fracture increases substantially. The medical establishment jumps for joy that we saved a man from prostate cancer, but in doing so we produced conditions that killed him anyway. That's not much of a victory.

SS: And along the way they look and feel like crap.

AM: Right. The big issue is this. If men don't live any longer with a treatment, and they have no quality of life due to the loss of testosterone, then what the heck are we doing? Is this good medicine? I don't think so. But in medicine there has been too much emphasis on statistics and pieces of data that do not tell the whole story, such as "cancer-specific survival." Not enough thought goes into the misery men experience when deprived of the very essence of what makes them a man.

SS: I believe I am not alone in thinking that I am interested in being on the planet for a long time but only with a quality of life.

AM: Same for me . . . but here's the good news: Little by little it's changing. More and more people, even within the medical community, are opening their eyes and paying attention to what makes us healthy and vital. So, with that, I am not only hopeful, but enthusiastic.

SS: This is all good news. Thanks so much for your time, Dr. Morgentaler, and keep doing your good work.

AM: Thank you, Suzanne. It's been my pleasure.

MY SON'S EXPERIENCE

I've spoken throughout this book of the need for a *plan*. Rarely do young people follow through with planning how they age. I thought it would be interesting at this stage in the book to get the point of view of a *young person* who has made a plan, who has been on supplementation, testosterone, and human growth hormone (HGH) replacement for many years, and how it has affected his quality of life. I'm not one to resort to nepotism, but I am going to do exactly that right now.

My son Bruce Somers actually was the one who got me on the

path to health. He started supplementation very early in life and the results for him have been an *ageless* experience. He looks younger than his peers, his body is athletic and strong, his outlook is always bright and sunny, and his health is pristine. I believe he offers incentive to other young people to take it all seriously. Please enjoy his description of his life *plan*!

My name is Bruce Somers Jr. and I am Suzanne's son. I'm forty-six years old. I've been taking supplements since I was thirteen years old. However, the supplements I was taking when I was thirteen are quite different from the supplements I'm taking now. These days, we know so much more. For the past twenty years I've been having my blood drawn every six months. In this way I've been able to track vital vitamins, minerals, and, most important, hormone levels in my body.

One of the most important supplemental changes that I incorporated in my life was bioidentical hormone replacement. It started when my doctor noticed that my HGH had started to decline soon after I turned thirty. At that time we started a regimen of HGH five times per week. A couple of years later, my doctor added DHEA to my regimen. Shortly after that he added HCG (human chorionic gonadotropin), which I injected three times per week. In essence, you are helping your body make its own testosterone. Of course, at a certain point, a man's body stops being a good engine for testosterone production, so around forty years old, I started using a cream-based testosterone supplementation. Again, this is bioidentical, not synthetic.

In addition to the supplementation, despite some of my bad eating habits (alcohol and cheese), I do eat a lot of raw, steamed, and sautéed vegetables. Perhaps more than anything, good nutrition makes me feel the cleanest and healthiest. However, it is the full orchestration of supplementation, hormone replacement, exercise, and nutrition that makes me feel my best.

Though I am blessed to come from a family with pretty healthy genetics, I try to listen to my body both mentally and physically in order to make the adjustments to complete my health. There isn't any one thing that is the panacea for health, but it is a continual search for the knowledge to help maintain my health and increase the efficacy of my supplementation and nutrition and exercise. Like

anything else, you must believe in your lifestyle protocols, as I believe
this perspective is perhaps the most important aspect of one's health.

Whether or not the positive effects of supplementation are psycho-
somatic or actually have a direct benefit on the health of my blood,
organs, and entire body, the one thing I know for sure is that in the
past twenty to twenty-five years I've only had two antibiotics (and
even those were required for two minor surgeries). In the past twenty
to twenty-five years, I've never had more than a common cold or the
occasional stomach infection. And by no means have I lived a pious
or strict life outside of my supplement intake. In fact, I enjoy wine,
tequila, the occasional filet mignon, nachos, and lots of cheese. I'm
fairly active, going from occasional workouts during some months
of the year to compulsive cycling for stretches of time. My point is, I
have lived and continue to live a full life.

CHAPTER 8

BOMBSHELL #4: THE HORMONE DISCOVERY THAT INCREASES ORGASMS AND MAKES YOU FEEL SEXY

If you want my body
And you think I'm sexy
Come on sugar, let me know...

–Lyrics from "Da Ya Think I'm Sexy?," sung by Rod Stewart

A HEALTHY PERSON IS A SEXUAL PERSON

Think about it. If you are not healthy, you are not going to be "in the mood." But if you are a man or a woman and you desire to have a healthy sex life, read on.

Dr. Prudence Hall is my gynecologist and also a hormone specialist. I have sent hundreds, maybe thousands, of women and men to her to help unravel the mysteries of missing hormones. Replacement, as I have said, is an *art*, and very few doctors have chosen to specialize in this art form. Our medical schools today still do not teach the intricacies of hormone replacement, instead spending approximately only *four hours* on prescribing hormones. That means by the time you finish this book, you will have had more instruction on hormones than any doctor in medical school! This is why I stress that you must ask up front whether your doctor is a hormone specialist in bioidentical hormones and if the answer is no, then this is not the right doctor to be handling your replacement.

Real bioidentical hormones offer a better quality of life. If we are talking about redefining aging, then hormones are at the top of the list. That is why I have chosen to offer a meaty section on BHRT (bioidentical hormone replacement) and the new advances that have come down the pike since I last discussed them. (For basic information on BHRT, you can read the relevant sections in my books *Ageless* and *Breakthrough*.) What is offered in this section is the advanced art of hormones, and how to truly use them for health, cancer prevention, and waking up the libido to new highs. Aging can be an enjoyable, pleasurable, wise experience . . . and hormones can help make it that way.

PRUDENCE HALL, M.D.

Dr. Prudence Hall *is youthful, smart, and sexy. She addresses the problems and pain women experience due to a lack of understanding regarding hormones and a good quality of life. She was educated at the esteemed Keck School of Medicine, of the University of Southern California. Today, she is the founder and director of medicine and gynecology at the Hall Center located in Santa Monica, California. At the center she helps her patients, both men and women alike, to rejuvenate and regain their vitality, energy, and well-being. Her approach to health is guided by the principles of functional medicine—a revolutionary, science-based practice of cutting-edge medicine. Along with her practitioners, she identifies and balances hormones and treats inflammation, adrenal stress, metabolic problems, and detoxification problems. Her work aims to rejuvenate and increase the energy of her patients, leaving them balanced and healthy. She prescribes bioidentical hormones as well as specializes in nutritional interventions, acupuncture, and physical therapies as needed. She believes her clients should be advocates for their own well-being and offers guidance to get there. She has been my gynecologist for over fifteen years. She is progressive, very sweet, and compassionate; and she's on hormones herself, which is a big advantage in treating women's hormonal issues. She's been there and knows how to fix them.*

SS: Thank you for your time, Prudence. I hear from women over and over that as they age, they lose their sex drive from loss of hormones. They refer to a sense of loneliness because they aren't getting touched as much, or not at all, and they speak of the feeling of a "sense of invisibility."

PH: Yes, that loneliness comes up with so many of my patients.

It's tragic that loss of hormones seems to suck the life out of both women and men. But, fortunately, as I sit there listening to patients, I know I am going to be able to help them; the mere fact that they are sitting in my office is an indicator that they want to do something about it. I always talk to my patients about their lives and what makes them happy. So often they express isolation and loneliness, a lack of sexual intimacy and intimacy in general. We also talk about the things that used to give them real joy but they now feel cut off from. I know by talking to them and looking at them what is wrong, but I always confirm by lab and blood work that we are dealing with an estrogen deficiency and/or an oxytocin deficiency.

SS: Oxytocin?

PH: Yes, when people have a deficiency of oxytocin, it causes them to feel cut off, and this in turn affects their health negatively.

SS: Tell me about oxytocin. Isn't this the "cuddle" hormone we associate with pregnancy?

PH: Yes. Oxytocin is actually one of the newer hormones that I've been using. I originally learned about it when I was in training as a gynecologist because we would give women in labor oxytocin to induce labor.

SS: So if I take this, my body is going to think I want to give birth?

PH: Very funny. Oxytocin is the hormone responsible for a mother being able to nurse, while at the same time helping her relax and feel loving toward her child, rather than stressed.

SS: Nature always amazes me. But I'm still not getting the connection to we women who are nonreproductive.

PH: Well, for instance, I nursed all three of my children for a total of twelve years. I loved it. It caused me to feel relaxed, loving, and bonded with the children, and that is what oxytocin does.

OXYTOCIN CAUSES PEOPLE TO FEEL NATURAL
HAPPINESS AND LOVE AND REDUCES ANXIETY. IT ALSO
CAUSES WOMEN TO FEEL MORE *ORGASMIC*!

SS: Okay, now I get it. How fantastic. You mean if we take oxytocin hormones, we have better orgasms?

PH: Yes, absolutely, and it causes better arousal. So it's one of the important sexual as well as social hormones, and we are sexual and social animals. We naturally want to bond with other people and have those relationships.

SS: So it's a relationship-bonding hormone. Again, nature never ceases to amaze me. Why did you start giving this to men?

PH: I started working with oxytocin ten years ago to help women have better orgasms. It worked, so I started wondering what it would do for men. I asked the male practitioners in my office if they would try it and see how it made them feel. Even though they said they didn't feel anything dramatic except being more relaxed, the women in the room knew differently. We all felt the men were much more talkative, touched us more, felt sweeter, more present, and, to put it frankly, were just sexier. As I worked with my male patients and gave them oxytocin, they reported better orgasms and better ejaculate. Research supports that, and lots of other benefits, as well. It decreases blood pressure, increases the amount and the intensity of ejaculations, and decreases anxiety. It is also one of the tried-and-true ways I help people lose weight. About 10 IUs of oxytocin every day helps curb appetites, resulting in weight loss and a sense of well-being. So actually there are a lot of benefits of oxytocin for men. When I first started giving women oxytocin, I gave them 10 IUs, which didn't have much effect on their orgasms, so I increased their dosages to 50 IUs, knowing that when a woman is nursing she releases a tremendous amount of oxytocin with no side effects other than perhaps wanting a lot of sex.

SS: [Laughs.] How bad could that be?

PH: I would say not bad at all. A side effect that isn't as pleasant is that occasionally oxytocin can lower cortisol levels in patients who have low adrenals. It is rare, but it might cause them to feel more tired.

SS: Why, because they are so busy having sex and orgasms?

PH: [Laughs.] Perhaps! But probably the fatigue is due to lowered cortisol levels. Actually, oxytocin also maintains a sense of peace, and it has beneficial physical effects in decreasing pain in the body; in addition, it helps with insomnia and general vitality. Also, Suzanne, it helps to increase low sperm counts.

SS: But do men know to come to the Hall Center for erection or sperm motility problems?

PH: Yes, men come to us every day, frequently because they are having problems with erections. I put them on oxytocin, and it really helps them. It's a combination of several things for them—oxytocin, testosterone, human growth hormone, and thyroid—and it all brings the men back to life.

SS: My readers are really going to react to this. First of all, who doesn't want to have better orgasms and who doesn't want to have a renewed interest in sex? We are all looking to feel good. I can confidently say, my readers are smart and they want to find the answers with natural remedies and protocols.

PH: Exactly. You are spreading the word, Suzanne! One more thing: The effects of oxytocin and estrogen are magical when replaced in balance. Unfortunately, low estrogen causes low oxytocin.

SS: So that explains why so many middle-age women have zero interest in sex. Low estrogen=low oxytocin=zero interest.

I think you are onto something, Prudence. This is a real Bombshell. The compounding pharmacists' phones are going to be ringing off the hook once this book is published. By the way, can you send me a prescription? I'm no different from any other woman. I want some of this. Woo hoo!

PH: Sure, Suzanne. I'll send you a few bottles via courier. While you're waiting for it to arrive, there are also ways to increase oxytocin naturally. You can exercise, and you know, just hugging or touching increases it. In medicine we are taught to touch our patients, and it's important to touch our loved ones because it helps to increase oxytocin. And of course, replacing estrogen and all the missing hormones are important, too.

SS: Do you have any other Bombshells, Prudence?

PH: Well, there's pregnenolone.

SS: Let's talk about that. It's kind of a forgotten hormone. Rarely do I hear about any doctor putting a patient on pregnenolone.

PH: It shouldn't be forgotten. Pregnenolone is a hormone made by the adrenals that protects our brain and keeps our memories sharp. It gives energy, vitality, and a better sex drive and is an important hormone in weight loss.

SS: How does that work?

PH: When the adrenals are low due to stress, it's very common to find that pregnenolone levels are low. Pregnenolone is a "mother hormone" because it helps to make a lot of other hormones in the body. I like pregnenolone levels to be around 100 to 150 in both men and women.

SS: Sounds great to me. And it's a hormone our own body makes, so we're just putting back what we have lost in the aging process. Another way to redefine aging and make it the pleasurable experience it should be.

So oxytocin and pregnenolone make for a serene, happy, loving, crazy sexy life. These are Bombshells!

I was speaking with a friend of mine recently; he's an entertainer, about forty-two years old. He's always on the road, has lots of stress, and goes through different time changes; I'm sure his cortisol is all off. We met through my books because he wanted to take testosterone. Nothing blunts hormones faster than stress and traveling. All the "rock and rollers," I am sure, are more of an "act" than we realize, because with the drinking, poor diets, traveling, late nights, cigarettes, et cetera, believe me they cannot be the sex machines they make themselves out to be. It's not physiologically possible, unless they are Viagra machines, too.

So anyway, this guy I'm talking about said he stopped taking testosterone because he was getting vertigo. I said to him, "I'm no doctor but you might want to have your adrenals checked as well as your cortisol levels." So many people write me about dizziness and they usually end up at the neurologist. Can you address this?

PH: What you just said about adrenals is probably one of the major causes of dizziness. With stress, sleeplessness, travel, and the like, the adrenal glands run out of hormones, just like a car running out of gas. Those hormones are cortisol, pregnenolone, DHEA, and testosterone, and part of their job is to keep our hearts beating and our blood pressure normal. Patients with low adrenals have low blood pressure and get dizzy; they can't remember things, their libidos are low, their thinking is unclear, and they can get angry, depressed, drowsy, and light-headed.

SS: So the remedy for him would be cortisol replacement?

PH: Yes, and pregnenolone, DHEA, along with his testosterone and whatever else his lab work shows as depleted. If he was only replacing testosterone and had not checked the levels of all the other hormones, then that also might have been what threw his entire balance off.

SS: It's alchemy—a little of this, a little of that until you get it just right for each individual. I wonder how many people end up at the neurologist's office with expensive testing, MRIs, and so on, when the answer is really so simple.

PH: I always want to get to the root cause of symptoms, and I agree that a lot of testing being done isn't giving us those answers. Of course, other causes, like viruses, can affect the inner ear, or heart disease, but always the first thing I think of when somebody has been experiencing extreme fatigue with these symptoms is adrenal deficiency. It's the same when women go to the cardiologist because they have heart flutters, but it's really related to menopause, estrogen imbalance, or an imbalanced thyroid. So a good place to start with this patient is to get a good test done for hormones in the most precise way possible. In the case of measuring thyroid hormones, I always use the cutting-edge Thyroflex exam, which is more accurate than blood work.

SS: To redefine aging I believe hormones are crucial and the first step in a new way to age. Do you agree?

PH: Yes, definitely. But there are many other things to do to age well . . . something as simple as taking vitamin D, which is actually a prohormone. But usually I find a number of hormones are low, such as estrogen, progesterone, testosterone, and more major ones as well, such as cortisol, thyroid, and insulin. Of course, lifestyle and diet play a crucial role. Almost 50 percent of all people in this country are gluten intolerant along with other food intolerances and allergies. These intolerances are a big impediment to health unless discovered. Dairy is not good for most people.

SS: Do you test for allergies by stool testing and when doing so are you looking for the HLA gene?

PH: Stool testing and gene testing are the most effective ways to uncover gluten intolerances, and people who carry the HLA gene are very affected. The digestive tracts of people who carry that gene become inflamed much more than those of the other patients who don't carry it. I carry this gene.

SS: Yes, I carry the gene also; so does my husband. I wrote about this sensitivity in my book *Sexy Forever*. I took the stool test and realized I was very, very "off the charts" allergic to eggs. Giving up eggs was a big one. But I lost ten pounds in two weeks and my gut calmed down and the bloating went away. I miss eggs, but they simply are not worth it. When I tell this to people, they immediately say, "I'm going to give up eggs." And I always reply, "No, this is what I am allergic to; that doesn't mean you are." That's why the stool test is so important. EnteroLab has a very comprehensive test for this.

PH: Yes. Also, food intolerances and allergies profoundly affect dementia, and cause inflammatory states, so how you absorb your food is critical in terms of how you age. People with this gene also don't absorb protein very well. And no small thing, stress and repetitively eating so much sugar and wheat are not sitting well with humans. When you look at people living in Paleolithic times, they didn't have any gluten in their diets. What we've done over the centuries is bring large quantities of processed and "unnatural" foods into a stressed intestinal environment that is not able to really process it well and it causes problems.

SS: Let's talk about men. What is the connection between low testosterone and disease?

PH: Testosterone is so important for men's health, and having the right levels decreases just about every cause of death in men. I'm sure there are some obscure diseases that are not decreased, but the data documenting the dangers of low testosterone is definitely clear.

SS: What diseases are you specifically talking about?

PH: First, prostate cancer, which is a common problem of men as they age, is a disease related to low testosterone. As men age and lose their testosterone, they are at higher risk for elevated cholesterol, heart attacks, strokes, dementia, and diabetes. Also with low testosterone they put weight on around the middle, their brains don't function as well, and they get grumpy, tired, lose their energy, and have problems with erectile dysfunction. Some men are able to revitalize erections with testosterone alone; others need Viagra in conjunction with testosterone, depending on the depletion levels.

SS: Are you talking only about older men?

PH: No, younger men also. I measured the testosterone levels of Berkeley students who were nineteen and twenty who had just finished their exams. I found that the average testosterone level was about 350 nanograms per deciliter out of these ten men. Now, nineteen-year-olds should have testosterone levels in the 800 to 1,200 ng/dL range.

SS: The levels were lowered due to stress?

PH: Yes. Stress plays a large role in decreasing testosterone production. The army looked into the testosterone levels of young men who had been in combat in Desert Storm. After two weeks of being in combat, their testosterone levels were lowered to prepubertal lev-

els. This kind of stress just wrecked their T levels. Now this is a problem because these men have to be fit and proactive and strong. They
get this way from their high testosterone levels. Without it, muscles
and bones also get affected negatively. Their overall strength gets affected. Also it sets them up for osteoporosis.

SS: What did they do about these soldiers?

PH: I hope they gave them testosterone replacement, but I don't
know for sure. Without testosterone, it's like tying one of their arms
behind their backs. And this is how loss of testosterone affects older
men, also. That is why you see them literally fade in front of you, and
they are no longer the men they used to be. They no longer have drive,
ambition, and the abilities they once had, but really all they need is
someone to understand that they need their testosterone replaced.

The thing is, men are much easier to balance. I give them testosterone, DHEA, HGH, vitamin D, thyroid, and they start to feel
amazing. Women are trickier because of their reproductive systems
and their need for multiple hormones to achieve the perfect balance.
Takes time and patience.

SS: Are young women coming to you also?

PH: Certainly by their late thirties women are experiencing peri-
menopause. The youngest patients I'm dealing with are teenagers
who have been put on the birth control pill and now they are feeling
depressed or sad. Or the very stressed young women who don't get
regular periods.

SS: I have always felt teenage girls need short-term replacement.
They have raging hormones. It would make the age so much easier
and I believe healthier.

PH: Oh, Suzanne, that has been my message for so long. Young
boys and girls are very affected by hormonal imbalances, and I am
seeing lots of thyroid disease and it causes terrible depression.

Also, teenagers can experience low cortisol. It can also affect babies, and an infant with low cortisol can end up with more ear infections, rashes, and asthma.

SS: But no doctor would think to measure the cortisol levels of an
infant!

PH: And that's too bad . . . it happens, and when corrected it saves
a lot of pain and suffering.

SS: So what you are saying is every person is a unique little scientific individual. And your job is to work like a chemist with each
patient.

PH: Yes. I look for how hormones are broken down, a person's genetics, allergies, intolerances, mercury, lead, cadmium, and the molds and bacteria that slip into our bodies. Testing something as basic as a homocysteine level and finding it elevated could mean a patient is not detoxifying properly, allowing toxins to pass through his or her liver into the body. It's important to really look at our patients, not just to look at a piece of paper with lab results on it. If a patient has puffy eyes, I know to check her thyroid. If she has tight and constricted shoulders, she probably has low human growth hormone. If she has more wrinkled skin and lax muscles, I think of estrogen, DHEA, and HGH deficiency. If she has memory loss, she's probably pregnenolone deficient and estrogen deficient. Once hormones are balanced we go from there. I start slowly so as not to overwhelm.

Then we start supplementation. I make sure patients are sleeping and add 5HTP, melatonin, and GABA if they aren't. Also amino acids and fish oils, and mineral deficiencies are important to correct, too.

I generally find that after patients have been on their hormones for about four weeks, we can begin rapid fat loss with a detox/cleanse, and start looking at their diet and exercise regimens. After they are really starting to feel good and lose weight, we attack the sugar issue. It all has to be done slowly and methodically, so they are not turned off or overwhelmed. But the patients who stay with it achieve a quality of life they never imagined. It's much the way you have chosen, Suzanne, to approach your health. You literally glow with health and vitality, and I know it's because you have dedicated yourself to wellness.

SS: I have and wouldn't have it any other way. Are you enthusiastic about the progress men and women are making relative to living longer?

PH: I believe we have the potential now to live to 120 or more. Look at those of us who have embraced this approach to health. Both you and I are halfway through our lives, and I certainly can see both of us here for another sixty years. We have the potential to stay extremely healthy, active, and vital for many, many years. We know things; for instance, we know that human growth hormone helps to prevent dementia, and so does thyroid and oxytocin. If we can maintain our brains, then living longer is very attractive.

We know so much more about living longer as vital, sexy beings. As a gynecologist, I am always talking about sex and the importance of hormones. It's our connection to joy. Another powerful way to connect to love, sex, and intimacy is through proper breathing. Check out Mark Whitwell's work at www.thepromise.com, to learn his secrets. When people age, they become isolated and are no longer in contact with their body. This is not the purpose of aging. The purpose of aging is to love and be loved.

SS: And that brings happiness.

PH: Cultivating intimacy is the greatest gift we can have and give. So I see it as a progression. We balance hormones so we can give our greatest gift back to the world. Why are we here? What is our soul's purpose? When you are sick, you can't begin to entertain those concepts.

SS: Also, without hormones you can't access the wisdom that is the gift of aging. Do you worry about the lack of wisdom because so many are not practicing this kind of medicine and instead are on drugs that rob the brain?

PH: Certainly, that is true. My hope and prayer is that this type of medicine will permeate down rapidly to everybody, so everyone can practice this style of medicine. We are an aging population, and how we age is going to affect a large community of people. I want everyone to be involved in healthy, joyful, intimate aging.

SS: You have a lucky constituency at the Hall Center. They come to you so you can guide them through this maze of confusion until they see the light.

How do you see yourself at 120 years of age?

PH: I see myself just as engaged in the mystery of life as I am now, with lots of walking—not Rollerblading because recently I had a bad fall—but walking, making love, teaching, traveling, hiking, certainly in the Himalayas, the Alps, and in the Sierras. Being in nature, doing yoga every day, and being part of a community that celebrates life. Because at a certain age what we have to offer is our wisdom, compassion, love, and understanding. So whatever expands me, I will be. It's within all of us, but it needs to be discovered and connected with; that to me is the goal of aging.

SS: Well, Prudence . . . I'd like to go on that great hike with you when we are both 120. I truly believe we'll both be doing it.

PH: Oh, Suzanne, I have no doubt! Let's go up to about twelve thousand feet!

A TESTIMONIAL:
MY HUSBAND'S PERSPECTIVE

Many may wonder if all that has been discussed in this book is really worth the effort. I started out by telling you in the beginning of this book that aging well takes a *plan*, and then the determination to follow through with this plan. I thought you might want to hear from someone near and dear to me—who has taken his life plan seriously—about how it has impacted his quality of life.

My name is Alan Hamel. Suzanne and I have been married for many years. I am seventy-five, ten years older than Suzanne. Fifteen years ago at age sixty, my body and my thinking went through a strange and unexpected metamorphosis; I gained eighteen pounds around my middle, my muscles were shrinking, and I lost my interest in things that up until then I was passionate about. I just didn't feel like doing much of anything, and I was thinking that I was entering the cocktail hour of my life. I didn't much like the direction in which I was headed.

Suzanne sent me to her endocrinologist. She did a hormone panel and told me I had lost most of my male sex hormones and she would begin the process of restoration. It took several months, but I lost the eighteen pounds, my muscles came back, and so did I. I was my old self again. I loved my work, and I looked at my wife through new eyes.

I happily gobbled down all the supplements, rubbed on testosterone and DHEA creams, injected my human growth hormone, injected vitamin B complex, ate only organic food, and followed Suzanne around the house like a dog in heat; we both laughed at that one.

Once I was back to the old Al, I became extreme. When we traveled, I always had the hotels bring in organic almond milk, Greek yogurt, organic vegetables, and gluten-free cereals. I brought a small bag of organic nuts and dates and cheeses along with organic Fuji apples and HoneyBell citrus (the greatest oranges on the face of the planet). I set up EZ gym, our door exerciser, slapped on my LifeWave energy patches, and couldn't believe the energy I had; it felt like I was in my thirties.

I suddenly knew I had many decades ahead of me of robust health, a healthy brain, and good bones. The brain thing was in-

teresting. I had been one of those guys who said "senior moment" when I couldn't grab a name or a situation. Also, in the middle of a sentence, I would forget what I was talking about and either suffer that moment of embarrassment or say "I'll get back to that in a minute" . . . which of course I never did. I would walk into a room and couldn't remember why. I would dial a phone number and experience a moment of panic because I couldn't remember who I had called and hoped I would recognize the voice that answered.

All that became a thing of the past. My memory came roaring back and I enjoyed recalling moments and dates and names with deadly accuracy; I was back big time.

One night, we dined with a famous physicist and my memory actually reached back over fifty years as I proudly recited Isaac Newton's three laws of gravity . . . perfectly.

I have several lifelong friends who are spiraling down and refuse to do anything about it. When we are together, they say, "Hey, Al, you're looking great. What are you doing?"

So I tell them what I do and they say, "I could never do all that." Or the Canadians say, "It's not covered," which means that their socialized health plan won't pay for it. So they are all suffering the fate of aging and doing nothing. However, their wives look at Suzanne and can't wait to get on bioidentical hormones and prescribed supplementation, lose that menopausal weight, and go shopping for a new wardrobe. When the wife gets it all back and is proud of her new body and sunny outlook and feels sexual and the husband is the old couch potato, nibbling on nachos and farting, grouchy, and accepting of the direction his life has taken and not interested in sex . . . this is a plan for marital disaster.

I love my wife. I love my kids. I love my grandkids. I love my work. I love my life.

If it all gets any better, I will explode.

CHAPTER 9

BOMBSHELL #5: CELL REJUVENATION THERAPY MAY EXTEND YOUR LIFE SPAN

First, you know, a new theory is attacked as absurd; then it is admitted to be true, but obvious and insignificant; finally it is seen to be so important that its adversaries claim that they themselves discovered it.

–William James

Imagine that your aging organs and glands can be rejuvenated! How would that change your rate of aging? What implications would that have on your health?

As I have said repeatedly in this book, aging is about worn-out parts. If there were a way to restart burnt-out adrenals, stimulate the pancreas to work more efficiently, or get the thyroid gland working the way it did when you were young and at optimum, wouldn't you be interested? Especially if I said none of these things required drugs?

Well, that is the bombshell Dr. Jonathan Wright is about to drop. He explains that by determining your weakest organs and glands and rejuvenating them, you can turn back the clock! The results are renewed vigor and energy. Cell rejuvenation may make you younger and healthier, and best of all, it's drug-free.

Read on.

JONATHAN WRIGHT, M.D.

Dr. Jonathan Wright *is a fearless and passionate seeker of true health care. He has coined the phrase "using Nature's tools," an anthem he lives and breathes. He is the "Father" of bioidentical hormone treatment, being the first doctor in America to prescribe bioidentical hormones as replacement therapy, twenty-five years ago. He is a sought-after lecturer and teacher, responsible for educating thousands of doctors and professionals on natural hormone replacement as well as natural and alternative methods of allowing the body to heal itself without drugs. As a result, patients flock to him in his Tahoma Clinic in Washington State. "In forty years, I've never healed a patient," says Dr. Wright. "They heal themselves." His modesty notwithstanding, over thirty-five thousand patients have come to see him, and more wait their turn. An in-demand speaker in Europe, he's also considered a hero in Japan, and thousands of professionals have temporarily put their careers on hold to attend his famous seminars.*

In my book Breakthrough, *Dr. Wright demystified the replacement of natural hormones and woke up America to alternative healing. In this book, he goes deeper into explaining the nuances of hormone replacement essential to living longer and as a key necessary element to redefining how we age. In this interview he also explains that it is now possible to cut cancer off at the pass using anticarcinogenic replacement creams, and to bypass cancers that might have become life threatening. The end result: extending life without disease.*

In addition, he drops a huge Bombshell: Cells in the body can actually be rejuvenated to, in essence, restart themselves again. This is reversing aging at its best; organs and glands rejuvenated to youthful levels, using

*once again, as he so eloquently says, "Nature's tools." He is my friend,
my doctor, and as an educator, a gift to humanity.*

SS: Hello, Jonathan. Thank you once again for allowing me to
pick your incredible brain. This is the fourth time I've had the privi-
lege of featuring you in one of my books, and I know we have only
touched the surface. You have taught me so much over the years.
Along the way we have become very good friends, and I treasure
that. You are one of the first, if not *the* first doctor to recognize there
is a better way to stay healthy and age well, and that lost or diminished hormones rob us of our youth and vitality. When they are replaced, a person starts to feel good again and thus lives longer. So to
start, how would *you* describe yourself?

JW: Thank you, Suzanne. It is indeed my honor to be featured
again in another of your important books. To describe my work—it's
actually fun, too!—half of what I do is body chemistry and the other
half is hormones.

SS: Okay, then let's begin with your Bombshell! *Cell rejuvenation!* This is body chemistry at its finest. I am fascinated about this
great breakthrough. It's underground, a true explosive "secret" that's
really not so secret, just not yet hit the mainstream.

Cell rejuvenation sounds too good to be true except for the fact
that I have been utilizing cell rejuvenation under your guidance for
six years now, and I have noticed a real slowdown of my aging process. Can you explain?

JW: Certainly. In the late 1920s, a professor named Paul Niehans
of Switzerland started using cells from fetal animals to strengthen
the parts of the human body that were weak or diseased; for instance,
"heart cells" to strengthen the heart, "kidney cells" to treat kidneys.
But even he wasn't the first to recommend something similar: The
tradition goes all the way back to Ayurvedic doctors who would recommend eating tiger testicles to treat testicles.

SS: Yuck! Makes me glad I'm a female!

JW: If you recall from your studies, even in Greek mythology,
Homer had Achilles eating bone marrow from lions to gain strength.
So the idea of using fetal animal cells for a person with, say, an organ
problem is not new.

SS: But it is not the standard of care in today's orthodox medicine . . .

JW: It got lost in the patent-medicine-oriented approach to health, but it is truly a great advantage to health. There are growth factors in those fetal animal cells that, when injected, end up in the target organ and help that organ to get healthier.

SS: So injecting the fetal cells from the same organ or gland of the animal can be used to treat a human organ or gland?

JW: Yes, but its other major use is as an antiaging factor. Cell therapy can be used to put those fetal growth factors back in all the cells and organs, and, in doing so, we find the organs literally work better. So cell therapy can be used as a targeted therapy for a specific problem, or it can be used as an overall antiaging therapy. This therapy has been used in Europe since the 1920s.

SS: Yes, and I recall in the 1950s you'd hear about Hollywood stars flying to Switzerland to have sheep's placenta injections.

JW: That's true. Placenta is kind of a wild card because it makes any cell more effective. So what they were doing was using sheep placenta with sheep heart or sheep lung or others. The reason they use fetal animals is that fetal animal cells are not antigenic. They do not set off allergic reactions. Even though they are from another species, the growth factors are mostly the same or extremely similar.

SS: Have there been any negatives associated with these injections?

JW: No, there hasn't been a single problem with fetal animal cell therapies since they were invented in the 1920s. Let me give you an example of the effectiveness of this therapy. Dr. Niehans wrote of a woman, fifty-three years old, and she was shaking, shaking, shaking. She could hardly walk because she had this giant goiter removed, but the parathyroid glands were mistakenly removed, too.

SS: Goiters are enlarged thyroids from lack of iodine?

JW: Yes, and I will explain that in a bit. When you get a goiter, like you said, it's because your thyroid is enlarged from lack of iodine and the thyroid gets big. Hers was so big it impaired her breathing. In the thyroid gland that has enlarged into a goiter are embedded parathyroid glands, which are the glands that control calcium in the bloodstream. Without the parathyroid, the calcium in the bloodstream drops very low and you get all spastic. Usually a person would die within a few weeks of that problem, but Dr. Niehans obtained fetal sheep parathyroid cells, injected them into the pectoral muscle, which is the muscle under the breast, and within two days her calcium in her bloodstream was normal, she quit shaking, and she lived to eighty-five.

SS: After one injection?

JW: Yes. Now does it always work that well? No. But it does work very, very often.

SS: My first experience with cell therapy under your guidance was when my adrenals had flatlined. I was completely out of energy, was experiencing depression, couldn't sleep, and had a host of other problems. My situation remedied when I was given bioidentical cortisol pills, which I'd have to take four times a day. You mentioned to me that I might have to do this for life because I had so damaged my adrenals from the stress of overworking, and then you asked would I be interested in another way.

That is when you gave me the adrenal cells shots, and in a very short period of time I was able to wean myself off the cortisol and all my symptoms disappeared. Then you mentioned when Alan and I were patients at your Tahoma Clinic outside of Seattle, in Renton, that we could rejuvenate *all* our cells for antiaging purposes. We had pancreas, thymus, thyroid, skin—Alan had testicle shots—and all the other organs rejuvenated. I think it was a total of about twenty-five injections over three days. (They didn't hurt by the way.) The results are subtle, but I haven't been sick or tired, or fatigued, for a few years, and people are saying to Alan and me, "I don't know what you two are doing, but you sure look great." I figure it's the effects of the cell rejuvenation. I also notice the effect on you and your wife, Holly; she looks fifty, yet you say she's seventy.

JW: Hard to believe, isn't it? She gets carded when we go to the movies and I try to buy her a senior's ticket.

The adrenal is an area where we apply the most cell therapy for two reasons. One, so many people who develop weak adrenals don't know it. It's a diagnosis that's most often missed, and second, people are so stressed and that affects the adrenals. Adrenal fatigue does cause burnout and that is what you were experiencing. We use a combination of adrenal cells, a little bit of hypothalamus, thyroid, and a little bit of ovary if it's appropriate. It takes about two to four months to start working, but then it works really well. Cell therapy is "protected" from the FDA because in 1993 the law was changed so that the government couldn't interfere with giving entirely natural substances if they did not harm people.

SS: How often do you have to reinject?

JW: About every three to five years. I think in your case, Suzanne, with all the other things that you do, and the way you eat and sleep, you probably won't need reinjection for a long, long time. To finish the cell therapy explanation: If people have a weak liver, we give liver cells, and their liver gets better; we give people with low white blood cell counts a combination of bone marrow cells and liver cells, and their white blood cell count goes up.

But antiaging rejuvenation is more than just looking better. It is about improving the overall internal health.

SS: As in, if your insides are young and rejuvenated, it resonates on the outside?

JW: Yes. My mother-in-law came up to stay with us a few years ago for the summer—she's in her nineties now. She was eighty-five and looked it. While she was here we gave her an overall antiaging cell rejuvenation program. By the end of the summer, when she went back home, everyone was asking her if she had had cosmetic surgery. She also got her energy back. Now, she didn't look thirty, but she did look at least ten years younger.

So cell rejuvenation is not going to prevent us from dying ultimately, but it is going to keep us healthier. Stem cells are certainly the future, but at present with having to go offshore, it can cost in the $25,000 to $50,000 range, and many of these offshore clinics are not using effective stem cells. A course of cell therapy runs about $4,000 to $5,000.

SS: Will it allow us to live longer?

JW: Well, definitely. If it makes you more active, more energetic, and look better, it will add years to your life; but most of all, you will be healthier.

SS: I wish this had been available for my mother when she was alive. I find it exciting that you are providing this kind of regenerative medicine at a time when doctors are at a loss. They haven't been trained in medical schools to deal with the changing planet, the longer life span, and the conditions created today from toxins, stress, chemicals in the house, outgassing, fluoride in the water, and poisons sprayed on our food. We have to take care of ourselves in a different way, and that is what you are offering and teaching other doctors. You are doing a big service to humanity.

JW: Well, thank you. And yes, we have to focus on staying healthy. In caveman days, all you really had to worry about was not getting eaten by a tiger, or getting an infectious disease, but the food was organic—there weren't any other choices—and there were no synthetic chemical toxins. People were outside a lot of the time, so most were getting plenty of vitamin D.

SS: Now let's talk about hormones. Why are bioidentical hormones crucial in order to live longer and healthier? Also, why are they the first step in achieving that goal?

JW: With the loss of hormones, people experience a great deal of bodily discomfort, which is too bad because that doesn't have to happen. In the last half of the last century, there was quite a rise in Alzheimer's disease, so let's start right there. The evidence clearly indicates that replacement of bioidentical hormones is not only vital but also needs to be sex-specific to reduce the risk of Alzheimer's disease. And the risk reduction is very significant if bioidentical hormone replacement is started as soon as your own hormones drop too low.

SS: Meaning both sexes need replacement, individualized to the needs of either the man or woman?

JW: Correct. For men, testosterone is the major hormone, along with perhaps needing some DHEA (another hormone) and thyroid, and in a few cases they might require some progesterone. The restoration of these hormones—particularly estrogens for women, testosterone for men—reduces the risk of Alzheimer's disease dramatically. Frankly, I can't think of a better reason for using bioidentical hormones than to protect our brains.

SS: Yes, and I believe the biggest fear most people have regarding their health is getting Alzheimer's.

JW: In the early part of this century—not so long ago actually—researchers at Rockefeller University made some amazing discoveries. They obtained autopsies of people who had no brain disease at all, maybe died in a car crash or something like that, and they put the neurons from these people into cell cultures and grew them, also adding in all the right nutrients, but no hormones. What they observed was pretty incredible: relatively rapid accumulation of large excesses of natural substances, beta-amyloid, tau protein, and neurofibrillary tangle. These large excess accumulations are "hallmarks" of Alzheimer's disease.

Then the researchers put what is called a *physiologic dose* (meaning the amount that is usually there by nature) of testosterone in the petri dishes with male neurons, and physiologic doses of estrogen in the petri dishes with female neurons. What they observed was amazing: The rate of accumulation of the intracellular garbage just mentioned went down by nearly 90 percent.

SS: What does that mean?

JW: It means that the sex-specific testosterone and estrogen were inducing the formation of a protein that we could think of as the head of the janitorial crew that cleans up the cell. All cells take in nutrients and make waste like whole bodies do. In these cells before adding the hormones, the waste—again, in Alzheimer's the waste is beta-amyloid, tau protein, and neurofibrillary tangle—wasn't being disposed of properly, but with the addition of testosterone for male neurons and estrogen for female neurons, the waste was suddenly being disposed of efficiently, not perfectly, but more efficiently.

SS: So if those neurons were actually "people," they most likely would have contracted Alzheimer's disease because the waste was accumulating like trash being stuffed into a garbage can, and damaging the brain? But I can hear my readers right now, "But what if I get cancer from those hormones?"

JW: Of course, a good question. There is evidence that bioidentical estrogen actually *lowers* the risk. As you have informed us so well in your prior books, Suzanne, bioidentical estrogen means that it is identical in every way: size, shape, molecular structure, quantity, in timing, in everything to what our bodies naturally produce. Bioidentical estrogen is associated with a lower risk of cancer than any of the phony estrogens, meaning synthetic hormones. On the male side, Professor Morgentaler from Harvard . . .

SS: Yes, he is a great guy, smart guy, and he is featured in this book, another Harvard guy like you. Sorry I interrupted . . .

JW: Yes, and he shows us evidence that the lower the testosterone, the higher the risk of prostate cancer for men. For years, dogma made it impossible to question the unproven theory that testosterone causes cancer. It took Professor Morgentaler to show through scientific dogma that this wasn't the case.

SS: And does this theory go for women also?

JW: If they have their balance of estrogens correct, and that is key. Balancing estrogen for females is even more important than balancing testosterone for men. For women, the balance needs to be firmly anti-carcinogenic, which happens when the woman's body makes sufficient estriol greater than the quantity of estrone and estradiol, the ratio of

2-hydroxyestrogen is higher than her 16-hydroxy estrogen, and her body is making sufficient amounts of 2-methoxyestradiol.

Estrogen is a blanket term for the dozens of estrogens our bodies make. The three most important are sometimes called *classical estrogens*. They are

Estrone, which is procarcinogenic
Estradiol, which can be procarcinogenic or anticarcinogenic
Estriol, which is anticarcinogenic, as is 2-hydroxyestrone and
   2-methoxyestradiol, which is profoundly anticarcinogenic

SS: You discovered that my body doesn't make estriol, an estrogen that protects against cancer. That protection along with the right ratios, stay with me, of 2-hydroxy and 16-hydroxy estrogen and enough 2-methoxyestradiol is why hormones won't give us cancer when these ratios are correct, but it takes a qualified doctor who specializes in bioidentical hormones to correctly interpret these ratios. The fact that my body for some strange reason wasn't making estriol is most likely why I got breast cancer, and I imagine twenty-two years of birth control pills couldn't have helped either, but that's another story. Your making this discovery about my body has most likely prevented a recurrence.

What about the other profoundly protective estrogen you were telling me about?

JW: Yes, that would be *2-methoxyestradiol*, which is a very, very potent *anti*carcinogenic estrogen. If the ladies out there would like to put into the search engines of their computers the number "2" sometimes they will find 2-methoxyestradiol. Every woman's body is supposed to make this estrogen, and nearly all women's bodies do. This natural metabolite of estrogen is such a potent anticarcinogen; for instance, if you were to have chemotherapy and took, in addition, 2-methoxyestradiol, you wouldn't need nearly as much chemotherapy. But even all by itself it works against breast and prostate cancers. It actually works against just about any cancer you can name: blood cancers, all kinds of cancers. When taken, the cancers either regress on their own, or get better in combination with a therapeutic agent. This has been studied at a number of universities now.

A woman's body makes 2-methoxyestradiol, and it is so potent that another researcher found it was able to inhibit fibroid tumor growth.

SS: Are fibroid tumors then a result of a deficiency of 2-methoxyestradiol?

JW: Yes, that would be one of the causes . . . adding it to an estrogen protocol has been very useful in shrinking fibroids.

SS: So instead of surgery to remove fibroids, all she would have to do is take 2-methoxyestradiol and the fibroids regress? How long does she take it? Is it known yet?

JW: There's no published research on that point yet, but it likely would take years if the fibroids have been there for years.

SS: Why do women get low in 2-methoxyestradiol?

JW: One major reason women deplete this valuable anticancer estrogen component is stress. When we are under stress, our bodies make more cortisol and also more adrenaline. Making more adrenaline-related molecules requires more methyl groups—from methylfolate, methylcobalamine, trimethylglycine, anything in our food and supplements that contains a methyl group—so the methyl groups are no longer as available to make 2-methoxy (there's that methyl group again) and more 2-methoxyestradiol. If stress is long and unremitting, it can open up the body to cancer because it depletes so many methyl groups to make methylated catecholamines (that's medicalspeak for methyl groups "stuck on" adrenaline-like molecules). So 2-methoxyestradiol is made in very low quantities—those adrenaline-like molecules have preference—and 2-methoxyestradiol goes way down.

SS: Okay, that's a lot to grasp, but it shows you again that we are in control of not getting cancer. Managing stress is as important as eating.

Luckily for me, you found that my body doesn't make the estrogen component called estriol, and lack of estriol is also a pathway to cancer, right?

JW: That is correct. It's all chemistry and getting the ratios correct.

SS: What about young women and cancer?

JW: The majority of young women metabolize their estrogen properly and have more anticarcinogens than procarcinogens; a minority don't have this ratio, and these are the women who are much more likely to get cancer.

SS: So all women should test for the right ratios, including estriol and 2-methoxyestradiol?

JW: Yes. If bioidentical hormones are done properly and balanced properly and followed carefully with very careful testing of all the things I mentioned, plus a bunch more, then it's a much safer path.

SS: I mentioned cancer, so let's talk about it. I hear over and over that women and men are afraid to take hormone replacement because of their fear of cancer.

JW: The risk of cancer is much less if hormones are balanced properly with bioidenticals. There is also less risk of osteoporosis and fractures because bioidentical hormones build bones, plus there is less risk of heart attack and stroke.

SS: Those are pretty huge benefits. Bioidenticals are so terribly misunderstood. I attribute my lack of a cancer recurrence (I had cancer before I was taking hormones but didn't realize it) and my superb health, bone strength, lack of plaque, vitality, and strong libido to replacing my missing hormones all these years. I have been cancer-free for twelve years at present.

JW: Of course, and surprisingly enough, researchers have found that the bone effect, heart attack, and stroke risk reduction are due to the same molecule in both men and women.

SS: When you say "molecule," you mean hormone, right?

JW: Yes, it's called estradiol. Estrogen protects women's arteries and bones and so does progesterone. Recently it's been discovered (in just the last few years) that for men when testosterone gets to the bone, it's transformed into estrogen that builds bone strength. Testosterone is also transformed right in the walls of the arteries into estrogen and that helps combat cardiovascular disease for men.

SS: So bioidentical hormone replacement protects against cancer, protects bones, reduces heart attack and stroke, stimulates the libido, and makes you look better . . . which all affects the aging process. Sounds pretty great to me.

JW: And you already know this yourself, but the women I work with who've been on bioidenticals for ten years simply look significantly younger than women their same birth year who aren't taking replacement. For women it really makes a significant difference in their appearance. It has effects all over the body; for instance, hormones stimulate collagen, which is what keeps the skin thick and prevents it from getting thin.

SS: Thin skin is very aging.

JW: Absolutely. It's also important for lung health, and it literally stimulates better oxygen–carbon dioxide exchange. At the Lung Biology Laboratory at Georgetown University, some doctors (Massaro and others) have done a series of experiments with animals, and now with people, and found that the enzyme that exchanges oxygen for carbon dioxide is stimulated to work more effectively by estrogen. Also, the gradual breakdown in the lungs that happens naturally with time and aging is slowed down by estrogen.

SS: How is that?

JW: You always hear when a woman is pregnant she's eating for two, but what you don't realize is she's breathing for two.

SS: And this is because of her high estrogen levels when she is pregnant?

JW: Right; she's got to get enough oxygen not only for her but also for the baby, especially when it gets into the second half of pregnancy.

SS: Very interesting. Is estrogen replacement for a menopausal woman essential if she wants to stay athletically active?

JW: Yes, if she wants to be as athletically active as she can. And here's another thing affected by estrogen or testosterone depletion: our voices. We all know our voices change through puberty because that's when the hormones rise dramatically. When a man or woman begins to decline in hormones, their voices change once again.

SS: Wow. That's true, as men age their voices get higher, and weaker, sounding old, and women's voices get deeper, like Lauren Bacall's.

JW: Right, but with hormone replacement that doesn't happen. For instance, your voice, Suzanne, sounds very, very young.

SS: Interesting. One of my dear friends said to me recently, "You should record before you lose your voice." I hadn't thought of that because I've noticed no change in my sound. But come to think of it, older singers' voices get deeper.

Here's the big debate with taking bioidentical hormones correctly . . . Women hate to get their period back. Can you explain the importance of this natural function?

JW: There is a five-year scientific study on this. Researchers at USC recruited women to take estrogen and progesterone together in a *cycling* fashion. The first group took estrogen and progesterone in amounts to make a period just like in nature. The other group took estrogen and progesterone in a *cycling* fashion but not enough to make a period. The first group were very brave women because they agreed to have endometrial biopsies (scraping the inside of the uterus) done at regular intervals to really examine what was going on. They also had regular breast exams.

SS: What happened at the end of the five-year point?

JW: To start with, no one had an abnormal biopsy, and, second, no one had more breast abnormalities than the other group; the researchers concluded that it didn't make any difference as long as they cycled the women, meaning giving them a three-day pause.

SS: Every time you say that it scares me.

JW: Why?

SS: You need to convince me, because I am so hormonal that if I even take my hormones late in the day, I can feel it. But what is significant is that you use the word *cycling* as opposed to *continuous combined*, which means taking estrogen and progesterone every day of the month. Cycling is taking estrogen every day and progesterone for two weeks of every month.

JW: Yes, even in animals that are given just a balanced combination of estrogen and estriol, and not given a break after a period of time (could be a year or more), the anticarcinogenic estriol starts to become a problem and can actually *induce* procarcinogenic changes.

SS: So by not giving yourself a three-day break from hormones each month, you can set yourself up for cancer? This is new information. This is not what I've been saying in my books. My readers are going to react.

JW: You raise your risk a little, yes. If it's too difficult to go "cold turkey" because of symptoms of low estrogen, then take the tiniest amount during those three days that you can to take away the symptoms and to feel good.

SS: Or send my husband away once a month!

JW: Today most people recognize that we need to go deeper into hormones than just estrogen, progesterone, testosterone, and DHEA in order to live longer and healthier and to combat the dangers present in our world today. For instance, let's talk about thyroid.

SS: Oh good. You see, I have this bad habit of analyzing people on television as to who has thyroid problems and who doesn't . . . I think I upset a news anchor on Fox News because I mentioned to him he should have his thyroid checked! He took it in good humor. But it's easiest to recognize with men because you can see their eyebrows, and they usually don't wear makeup so their entire face is exposed to show the symptoms.

JW: It's because the problem is so common that the abnormal looks normal. We're not supposed to be purple, have sagging skin, and all the other symptoms. Unfortunately, many people just don't realize the value of iodine replacement.

SS: Okay, now explain why iodine and thyroid have a relationship.

JW: We have an iodine shortage in our diets, and iodine is key to a balanced thyroid. In the United States, Mexico, and Canada, we have an iodine shortage in our food and what little iodine there is, is very minimal. The countries with the most iodine in their diets, namely Japan and Iceland, have the least breast cancer. And iodine—among very many other things—is responsible for combining with lipids in the breasts and killing breast cancer cells. Iodine also modifies estrogen metabolism so that we have more estriol, which is the anticarcinogenic component of estrogen.

SS: But aren't people getting sufficient iodine from iodized salt?

JW: Hardly . . . In the 1950s, "authorities" stuck a tiny bit of iodide (with no iodine) into the wrong kind of table salt, "plain" sodium chloride. I am not talking about sea salt, which is what everyone should be consuming if they use salt, because it has at least a little bit of many missing trace minerals.

SS: I agree. People buy table salt because it's cheaper and then spend money on mineral supplements where they could be getting some of their trace minerals from consuming sea salt, and it tastes so much better. But I digress . . .

JW: I agree with you . . . So with iodized salt everybody falsely felt they were protected. In the 1800s, if you lived in the Midwest, it was common to develop a goiter.

SS: Goiter sounds so "unsexy."

JW: True, but, as we said, a goiter is a swelling of the thyroid due to an iodine deficiency. In fact, that area of the country was so deficient they called it the "goiter belt." Also, unfortunately, city and state officials have allowed toxic chemicals like chlorine and fluoride in the water supply, and even though we have systems available to clean our water by ozonation and ultraviolet radiation, which eliminates toxins, those officials in charge have chosen not to use these methods.

Here's the problem . . . chlorine *displaces* the iodine in the thyroid gland. Fluoride is actually fluorosilicic acid, which originated in the waste dumps outside of the Alcoa Aluminum plants, and also comes from Florida phosphate fertilizer mills. We have been told this fluoride "prevents tooth decay," which is mostly a falsehood.

SS: I am aware of that myth. Fluoride does not prevent tooth decay; in fact, it encourages decay and bone mottling.

JW: Right, and fluoride is even worse at getting into the thyroid gland and messing up thyroid function.

SS: Pretty incredible because the thyroid is a major hormone. If it is too high or too low for too long a time, a person won't live very long. That's how important the thyroid is to human function, yet this lack of understanding, or may I say greed, accounts for our iodine deficiencies, then putting carcinogens like chlorine and fluoride in our water truly boggles the mind.

JW: Particularly when there are inexpensive, safe alternatives to prevent tooth decay such as the natural sugar-alcohol xylitol. There's really good research about that.

But back to fluoridation and chlorination: Research done in Germany shows that in chlorinated communities, on average the people's thyroid function isn't as good as in the unchlorinated communities. So once again, because everybody has these symptoms, and because it is so widespread, we don't see it. The other problem relative to thyroid is that doctors who test for thyroid problems with lab tests are not treating the individual. In medical school, we were taught not to treat the lab tests but to treat the individual. So you, Suzanne, are correct; you look at symptoms: color of skin, sagging skin, and missing eyebrows. There is a wonderful paper on this by Dr. Denis St. John O'Reilly.

SS: Okay, an Irish guy; one of mine!

JW: Yes, thanks to him, he carefully pointed out that the whole structure of checking thyroid is based on two flawed studies done at the Mayo Clinic. The Mayo Clinic is very prestigious so everyone believes everything that comes out in their name. But here's the flaw: Those studies did not include any details of the clinical examination of the patients, just a statistical analysis of the lab tests.

SS: Meaning, no one was looking at the patients, just their numbers?

JW: And, as you know, many doctors have had their licenses removed for doing just that, looking at the patients and diagnosing them without following conventional testing.

SS: Yes, look at what they did to Dr. James Forsythe, who prescribed HGH to his patient by carefully looking at and examining him. He was raided, taken to jail, and finally won in court because the lab test came back and indicated that, indeed, the doctor had been correct; the patient was HGH deficient.

JW: Yes, tragic what happened to him . . . and in medical school, we are trained to look at the outward physical signs, listen to the symptoms, and then diagnose. Lab tests can help, but the signs and symptoms should never be ignored.

SS: Dr. Ron Rothenberg told me in my book *Ageless* that in medical school they are taught to diagnose the patient while speaking with them in the exam room during the first five minutes, that humans show symptoms outwardly in many cases, and these are signs and indicators of problems and conditions.

JW: That is true.

SS: Would you tell my readers why antiaging medicine gives them an edge for living longer, healthier?

JW: Antiaging medicine could also be called *physiologic medicine*, meaning using natural substances and natural energies in both the prevention and treatment of disease. Physiologic means following the normal patterns that the body follows and using the same molecules and the same quantity of molecules, plus using the same timing. In other words, it's life-copying medicine. There have been marvelous advances in diagnostic technology; for example, MRI scans, being able to see a tiny tumor in the brain that has never existed before, and other things. There have also been some surgical advances that never could have been accomplished without these improvements. But where all progress has come to a halt has been with the use of patent pharmaceutical medicines, meaning molecules that have never been found in nature or on this planet. I call them "space alien molecules"! How do we expect our bodies—which for hundreds of thousands of years were made up only of nature's molecules—to function properly with molecules that have never been found naturally occurring on the planet, but are of strictly synthetic origin and are never, ever found in nature? It's like trying to fix your Ford with Toyota parts!

These patent medicine molecules don't belong in our bodies and they have side effects, which is another way of saying they do bad things to the body. But if we use molecules found in nature, and I don't mean overly large quantities of them—for instance, water is natural and a bath is healing, but if we submerge in too much water we will drown—they restore and balance. Hormones and natural medicines must be used in physiologic quantities, and when that happens, they provide restoration and quality of life and health, and we are least likely to do any harm this way.

Over a hundred thousand people a year die of patent medicines (also called prescription pharmaceuticals). But in the last two decades only fifteen or twenty deaths have occurred as a result of natural medicine, and even those numbers are disputable.

SS: Have we hit the wall with allopathics?

JW: I think so. At Tahoma Clinic, we've found that the large majority of illnesses can be treated and often eliminated with natural substances and natural energies—mostly based on scientific research—and almost no allopathic patent medicines. Certainly surgery can be lifesaving, and sometimes there's no alternative, but there's no need for at least 90 percent of all patent medicines, if not more.

SS: So you are saying, simply put in your body substances that the body itself makes or that come naturally from nature?

JW: Yes. For instance, if there is something wrong with your Chevrolet, you use Chevrolet parts to fix it. If there is something wrong with our bodies, let's use from nature, for instance, anything from "I need a kidney transplant" to "I need a molecule of estrogen." Everybody is going to die someday, but we can live a lot longer and healthier, and not end up in a nursing home or relying on our kids to take care of us, if we follow the plan of nature and use natural substances and natural energies to the best of our knowledge.

SS: Very well said. That in a nutshell is antiaging medicine.

How important is supplementation?

JW: Exceptionally important. Unfortunately, just eating a good diet is not enough. The soil and food supply are now depleted of minerals, particularly. Everyone needs minerals and vitamins, and at the top of my list is taking 3,000 milligrams of vitamin C daily. That is based on research. Also important is vitamin D_3, and most adult people need to start at 5,000 units daily. Some people I work with need 10,000 units or even a little more. Depends on the individual; we prescribe vitamin D followed by blood tests to be sure no one is taking too much.

Vitamin C is the major detoxifier for nearly every living thing. Vitamin C is made out of blood sugar, glucose, and a series of four enzymes (this information goes back to Linus Pauling and Irwin Stone). If there is stress or a carcinogen or a patent medicine or anything bad that happens to an animal, then some of that glucose is taken out of the bloodstream and out the other end comes vitamin C. The human body, given the same stress or carcinogen or patent medicine, tries to make more vitamin C just like animals by passing glucose through this four-enzyme assembly line, but the last enzyme is not there, so the detoxifying vitamin C can't be made. When an enzyme is missing, it means a piece of the DNA is missing. That's the definition of a genetic disease, but since this is one we all have, it seems normal. Technically, the genetic disease we all have is called *L-gulonolactone oxidase deficiency*, which would be lethal if there weren't a little bit of vitamin C in our diets. But that little bit doesn't fully correct the problem.

Dr. Pauling said that one should take vitamin C three times a day because it's a water-soluble vitamin, meaning it runs through the body rapidly. You know if you are taking too much if you get gas or loose bowels. If you don't experience this effect, you probably need more vitamin C. You find your own limit.

Researchers at UCLA did a longevity study with several thousand people over a period of seven years. They kept track of what they ate and the vitamins they took. They found that men who took 800–1,000 milligrams of vitamin C a day could expect to live six years longer. For women, it was only one year longer, but then women usually outlive men by five or six years on average, so vitamin C might be an "equal rights" vitamin for longevity, anyway.

SS: Well, that's worth it right there; and I am sure these people had fewer colds.

JW: Actually, that is true. Regarding vitamin D: We don't get close to tropical optimal levels. Clearly the amount of vitamin D people take in from the tropical sunshine is very high and no one drops dead from it. These people are just healthier. There are two studies, one in Germany and one in Austria, with fifteen thousand people enrolled. Researchers checked participants' blood levels for vitamin D for nearly ten years.

THE PEOPLE WHO HAD THE HIGHEST LEVELS OF
VITAMIN D WERE THE LEAST LIKELY TO DIE OF *ANYTHING*...
HEART ATTACK, STROKE, OR CANCER.

It didn't matter. So the higher your vitamin D, the less likely you are to die of anything except trauma. Another longevity vitamin!

There was another Scandinavian study printed in the *Lancet*, a major medical journal, and the author was Dr. Elina Hyppönen. Researchers asked mothers to give their newborn infants 2,000 units of vitamin D daily. Some did, and some didn't. They followed these kids for thirty-one years. After all that time, the incidence of type 1 diabetes was 80 percent less among the children of the mothers who gave their children vitamin D.

SS: Why haven't we heard about this study?

JW: Because you can't patent vitamin D! Nobody can make crazy money on it, so no one is out there pushing it to the doctors. Vitamin D is beneficial for so many things. For instance, let's expand on diabetes; type 1 diabetes is known to be an autoimmune disease. In the United Kingdom, scientists published an article saying they found the very part of the DNA that, when there isn't enough vitamin D, allows multiple sclerosis to happen . . . yet *all* autoimmune diseases are rare among people raised in the tropics: lupus, Graves' disease, Hashimoto's thyroiditis, vitiligo, pernicious anemia, Addison's disease—there are more . . . a very long list of these diseases that are just not present nearly as much in the tropics. So, clearly, vitamin D prevents autoimmune diseases to a large degree. Also Dr. Michael Holick and others have told us that sufficient vitamin D helps to prevent infection as well as any vaccination does.

When vitamin D is combined with vitamin A, it has been proven in clinical trials to prevent childhood mortality from infectious disease. If we all took enough vitamin D with vitamin A, we'd do better than getting flu shots and vaccinations of all sorts. Vitamin D also cuts the risk of prostate cancer, breast cancer, and colon cancer by a significant margin.

SS: What else do we need to take as protection from the diseases and conditions of today?

JW: For sure, minerals, fish oil, vitamin E, resveratrol, and coenzyme Q_{10} if we're over forty, and for sure if we're past fifty. Depending on the individual, there are always others.

SS: I grow my own organic food and it thrills me. I know it's not possible for everyone, but I try to urge my readers to use community farms, window boxes, planters to grow food, even if it's just in the warm months.

JW: There is no substitute for fresh organic food. If you pick a fresh leaf and eat it immediately, you get all the folate that is in that leaf. But if you take that same leaf, put it in your refrigerator and leave it for a day, 50 percent of the folate is gone. It breaks down with heat, with cold, with light, or just by sitting there. When shipping food around the country from one coast to another, the folate is simply gone, and this is why folate is at the top of the list of vitamins we need to supplement. As you know, Suzanne, that's just so, so important for women who want to help ensure that their babies don't have birth defects.

SS: What about soil demineralization?

JW: Believe it or not, the only soil tested in the United States west of the Mississippi River—by the USDA in the 1960s or 1970s—that had adequate zinc was in Nevada, but hardly any crops are raised in Nevada. So zinc is an important supplement. Nonorganic farming takes the minerals out of the soil and replaces these vital elements with nitrogen, potassium, and perhaps phosphorus, and if we're lucky a very little bit of trace elements. But still it's not going to get into the plants without some of the organic material. So with soil demineralization, we lose essential nutrients. I said "essential," and there are many: B vitamins and vitamin E are only two of over sixty essential-to-human-life nutrients.

SS: Then of course we need essential fatty acids or fish oil.

JW: Yes, but how many of us eat very much fish? And any fish larger than a salmon is likely to carry more mercury than we want. So supplementing with good-quality mercury-free fish oil once or twice daily is essential.

SS: How about farmed fish?

JW: Well, those are not so good for us at all due to antibiotics and feeding these fish corn, which has never, ever been part of a fish's natural diet and helps cause infections in the fish.

SS: In essence, our food has been hijacked?

JW: Sadly, yes. For as long as there have been cattle and sheep—hundreds of thousands of years—they ate grass, weeds, growing plants. But around 1870, people decided it would be much more efficient to raise these animals in stockyards and fatten them up on corn, which was never part of their natural diets. It also made the ratio of omega-6 to omega-3 fatty acids in the animals go way up. If we eat corn- and grain-fed animals, then we also eat way more omega-6 fatty acids. Too many omega-6s are not good for our health. Omega-6 fatty acids are proinflammatory, and the anti-inflammatory omega-3 fatty acids in corn- and grain-fed animals are much lower.

SS: Also, this corn is most likely genetically modified, which in my opinion is "valueless" food. How did this happen?

JW: We weren't paying attention, and labeling of foods as genetically modified is deliberately not required, so we can't know without a lot of research which foods being sold are genetically modified.

SS: Imagine . . . Are you upbeat for the possibilities of aging well?

JW: In spite of interference by the government, which is currently trying to introduce "approval" of all new natural substances put into supplements after 1994, and that includes a very large proportion of all supplements (which would be a disaster), there are enough people out there researching natural molecules and what we can do with them. When organic food gets into Walmart, which it has, that is a very good sign. It means a very large number of us are beginning to understand the value of nutrition and the concept of "you are what you eat." This to me is very hopeful. Antiaging medicine is finding its voice. Your books, Suzanne, help tremendously. And more and more people are finding that aging well can be a positive, if you adopt a few new changes.

SS: It's that concept of turning the ocean liner around . . . takes a long time, but it is doable. Thank you, Jonathan. So much valuable information, and only so many pages.

For those who are interested in voicing concern about government interference in supplements, go to www.anh-usa.org, the Alliance for Natural Health.

CHAPTER 10

BOMBSHELL #6:
A SUPPLEMENT MAY HOLD THE SECRET
TO EXTREME LONGEVITY

> A bulldozer of change is charging over the planet, and if you're
> not part of the bulldozer, you'll become part of the road.
>
> —Frank Ogden, futurist

Telomeres and *telomerase*—these are two words that will change
the way you age!

So it's only fitting that they are the next Bombshell I'll introduce
you to. There is a new supplement that may turn the medical world
on its ear. It works by lengthening your telomeres, which appear to
be the key to the fountain of youth. And best of all, the supplement
that does this work is all natural.

> Telomere therapy won't change the speed of cellular aging: it will
> just change the number of years it takes for your body to grow old.
>
> —Michael Fossel, Greta Blackburn, and Dave Woynarowski, *The Immortality Edge*

Throughout history, man has been searching for the secret to immortality and now, spectacularly, scientists have unraveled the mystery specifically pinpointing the premier *cause* of aging! This is
science at its best and it earned researchers Elizabeth Blackburn,
Carol Greider, and Harvard geneticist Jack Szostak the Nobel Prize
for developing an enzyme that can actually *reverse* aging. They called
the enzyme "the little engine that could." That enzyme, called *telo-*

merase, determines a cell's ability to regrow or lengthen *telomeres*, which are the essence of life. Simply put, aging happens and accelerates with the loss of telomeres.

What exactly is a telomere? Here's the textbook definition:

> Telomeres are a short repetitive segment of nongenetic material that functions as a biological clock to determine the life span of a cell (meaning how many times the cell can reproduce before it dies). The telomere is also intimately involved with stabilizing the genetic material and is thus directly involved in the health of the cell and the entire organism.

Huh?

In layspeak, telomeres are the tails on the ends of our chromosomes. Each cell in our body has approximately fifty replications. Every time a cell replicates itself, the "tail" (telomere) gets shorter. By the time the cell has replicated fifty or so times, the tail is nonexistent and then the cell dies. We have over fifty trillion cells, and the process of dying cells is called *senescence*. Senescent cells promote the progression of age-related diseases, including cancers. Senescent cells in our skin make us look withered. In our immune system, they make us susceptible to the diseases of aging such as heart disease, heart failure, diabetes, and overall fragility; and even if we are lucky enough to avoid these conditions, eventually so many of our cells will be in a state of senescence the body as a whole will no longer be able to sustain itself. When that happens, we die of "old age."

The good news is that science, thanks to the Nobel Prize winners mentioned above, has found a way to reverse senescence. Around the mid-1970s, scientists were in general agreement that both ends of every chromosome contain relatively long strands of "junk" DNA called telomeres, and the primary function of these telomeres appeared to be to protect the DNA. So when chromosomes divide and multiply, instead of losing the DNA that matters, they lose only some of the telomere's DNA. With every replication of our DNA, part of the telomere sequence is chopped off. This is how nature protects the DNA in a chromosome. When cells divide and multiply, it is very important that the DNA in the chromosomes remains intact; otherwise, genetic defects can occur, some not so serious and others very serious (like causing cells to become cancerous).

To understand the importance of telomeres, let's look at those with the disease called *progeria*. You may be aware of children who are born "old." Those with this disease have short telomeres. They age prematurely and, sadly and shockingly, wither and die in a very short time. Shorter telomeres correlate with age and the state of your health. In a study of 780 patients with stable heart disease, people with the shortest telomeres in their immune cells had twice the risk of death and heart failure after 4.4 years compared to the patients with the longest telomeres.

As telomeres shorten they are like ticking genetic clocks in your cells. As you age and telomeres shorten, they cause certain of the body's systems to shut down. The systems that repair damage and keep your metabolism regulated have a drastic effect on aging once removed from action. Some of the key systems affected by diminishing telomeres are your endocrine system (in charge of releasing hormones, crucial to youth) and your all-important immune system. In addition, once some things are damaged, they can't be repaired very well, such as certain organs and joints and, of course, damaged cells.

Telomere length has been implicated in almost all aspects of normal aging. High levels of stress hormones, inflammation, insulin issues and high blood sugar, as well as habits and conditions such as smoking, poor diets, obesity, and sedentary living are all linked to shorter telomeres and lower telomerase levels. Cancer, atherosclerosis, Alzheimer's, osteoarthritis, osteoporosis, macular degeneration, cirrhosis of the liver, and AIDS are all related to having shorter telomeres.

Sperm cells divide millions of times and their telomeres never get short, because when you add the enzyme telomerase, it adds telomere DNA back to the cell's telomeres and keeps those telomeres as long as they have always been. That's why an old man can still father children. Again, nature is perfection and always has the perfect plan.

Aging well requires planning, and now you can add another tool to your kit; it is a new, sophisticated nondrug way of lengthening your life that allows you to remain healthy and vital while also maintaining your "edge." This new discovery just might make aging the enjoyable experience it should be. This advancement may extend life, and those presently using it enthusiastically report that they feel and look better. Results differ, but some say they notice those things that bug most aging people, like bad eyesight, hearing loss, stringy hair, brittle nails, sagging skin (have you noticed that suddenly your skin doesn't "fit" anymore?), all improve with it. If you have a magnifying mirror, you know there are days when you want to jump back in horror. Yipes! Who is that, you ask? Unfortunately, these changes in your appearances are manifestations of internal deterioration. To date, there has been little you can do about it.

Disease, unfortunately, is also part of the present template of aging. We "expect" we will be brought down by one of the big three—Alzheimer's, heart disease, cancer—and now add to them environmental diseases, which are so rampant.

But science has a plan . . .

THE DISCOVERY OF TELOMERASE IS THE MOST EXCITING
NEW ANTIAGING DEVELOPMENT OF THIS DECADE,
AND IT IS AVAILABLE RIGHT NOW!

Because of the amazing work of the Nobel Prize winners Carol Greider, Elizabeth Blackburn, and Jack Szostak, it is now possible to extend your life expectancy beyond 100 years to 120 years or more, while leading an active, robust, independent lifestyle, maintaining all the strength and vitality you had when you were much younger, and again, without the use of drugs.

Imagine being a centenarian looking half your age, playing outdoors with your great-great-grandchildren, dancing with much younger partners, enjoying new hobbies and pursuits, and, yes, still having a great sex life. All without having to worry about life-threatening conditions like cancer, heart disease, diabetes, chronic infections, dementia, poor eyesight, hearing loss, low energy, and other miserable conditions that plague too many older people. Imagine!

The paradigm of aging is changing. Rapidly.

The scientists who discovered telomerase realized that this enzyme provided a germ cell with an unending ability to reproduce itself. They found that telomerase keeps DNA tightly wound so the cell is not subject to the normal wear and tear that other cells in the body are subjected to; consequently, they proved that reproductive cells don't lose telomere length as we age. Why? For the same reason babies are born with telomeres that are long rather than short like those of their parents. Clearly human biology is about perpetuation of the species.

Long telomeres, long life!

So obviously, you want to figure out how to keep your telomeres longer.

> This new advancement comes with a hefty price tag, so if it's not affordable to you, there is evidence that fish oil, vitamin D and multivitamins, and healthy lifestyle choices may slow the rate of telomere shortening as well. This helps explain why people who take care of themselves and use the proper supplements enjoy such profound health benefits.

> The key to extreme longevity is turning the telomerase gene from "off" to "on"!
> –Michael Fossel, Greta Blackburn, and Dave Woynarowski, *The Immortality Edge*

TA-65: THE ENZYME THAT PROVIDES A FAR BETTER WAY TO AGE

T.A. Sciences, in New York City, has created a supplement in pill form that the company claims has been lab tested and shown to *turn on telomerase and lengthen the shortest telomeres!* This is critically important because it takes only one short telomere to send a cell into crisis.

The makers of this supplement can't stop talking about it. They report "new skin," a clear and visible smoothing and "reverse aging" of the skin. Others report improved vision and hearing, shinier hair, and stronger nails.

The product is called TA-65. It contains a single molecule from the astragalus plant, which has been used in Chinese medicine for thousands of years, often in combination with other herbs to strengthen the body's immune system. TA-65 is the *only* telomerase activator that is available right now. T.A. Sciences purifies the rare and expensive substance through an extensive process that also factors into its high price, which begins at around $2,000 a year. Hopefully, as people start using it the price will come down . . . Read Noel Patton's section that follows on this exciting supplement, then review Dr. Andy Jurow's interview, as he is a prescribing doctor for it. Both Mr. Patton and Dr. Jurow are beyond excited, and I have to say those I've spoken with who are using it are ecstatic. The theory behind TA-65 is beyond making you look good; it's about the possibility of reversing aging by releasing the enzyme telomerase. This is a major Bombshell to hit the antiaging world, and Noel Patton has brought this supplement to the market. Read what he has to say.

NOEL THOMAS PATTON
OF T.A. SCIENCES

Noel Thomas Patton *is a businessman, a visionary, and an entrepreneur. He is the founder of T.A. Sciences and responsible for bringing TA-65 to the public. A graduate of Indiana University (1969) with an honors degree in philosophy, Noel furthered his studies on the East Coast and is an alumnus of the Harvard Business School. His interest in telomere biology began in 1999, when he heard a lecture that explained how an enzyme called telomerase had the potential to rejuvenate human cells and keep them from dying of old age.*

The importance of telomerase for changing the way we age was emphasized in 2009 when its discoverers won the Nobel Prize for medicine.

SS: Thank you for your time, Mr. Patton. You own the company that makes the incredible new supplement TA-65. Can you give me your explanation of how it works and why this is so revolutionary?

NTP: Thank you, Suzanne. What we are talking about today is telomere biology and how our product TA-65 can lengthen telomeres, and what that means in our quest for life extension. Telomeres are the ends of the chromosomes. We have 23 pairs of chromosomes in every cell in our bodies; 23 from your mother, and 23 from your father and all the genetic material is on those 23 pairs of chromosomes in every cell.

SS: In other words, it's who we are?

NTP: Correct. It's critically important that the genes on those chromosomes are kept intact and in good health. At both ends of every chromosome are sequences of DNA that are not like other genetic material and these are the telomeres.

SS: These are the little tails on the ends of the chromosomes?

NTP: Correct. They act as protective tips at the ends of the chromosome to protect the integrity of the genome, like the plastic tips at the ends of shoelaces. One of the most important scientific discoveries of the last twenty years was learning that these "ends" act as the aging clock for nearly every cell in our bodies, because every time a cell divides, the ends (telomeres) get shorter. When they get to certain critical shortness, cells can no longer divide and they become senescent (nonfunctioning/sick) and then die. For the cell, this is a crisis, like falling off a cliff. But there is a long downward spiral before this crisis happens. This telomere shortening is what is driving the aging process. Changes in telomere length signal certain genes to either turn on or turn off. This is called *changing gene expression*. Which genes are turned on and which ones are turned off is what dictates the functionality of the cell; this is the fundamental aging process.

SS: Like a shutdown. Little by little the functions give out on us.

NTP: Right, so even before your telomeres get so short that the cell no longer functions or dies, along the way, telomere attrition is causing aging of the cells. This is consistent with recent studies by Dr. Ronald DePinho when at Harvard that showed telomere shortening to be one of the root causes of aging.

In November of 2010, Dr. DePinho published an important paper in the scientific journal *Nature* where he showed for the first time in history that the aging of a mammal was reversed. Notice that we are not talking here about life extension; we are seeing actual *age reversal*. He started out by engineering mice that had no telomerase to be the equivalent of eighty-year-old humans, and then he activated telomerase in those mice.

SS: Again, you are speaking of the enzyme that is responsible for *lengthening* telomeres.

NTP: Correct. So when Dr. DePinho *added back* the telomerase to these eighty-year-old mice, they essentially became young adults again.

SS: As you say this, I'm thinking that throughout history humans have been searching for the elusive fountain of youth . . . is this it?

NTP: We are not there yet, but we are on the right road. Telomere biologists have a lot more work to do, but we are having very significant results. I got interested in telomeres more than ten years ago because I was an aging human being and I didn't like it. And now ten years later, we are seeing real results in human beings like me. I don't have all the answers on this very complex subject of aging, but aging clearly correlates to a shortening of telomeres, and it's becoming more and more apparent that this telomere shortening is one of the fundamental causes. So, personally, I agree with Dr. DePinho that a lack of telomerase, which causes the shortening of telomeres, is the root cause of aging.

We can take a human cell in a petri dish and by activating the enzyme telomerase, we can make that cell immortal.

SS: What do you mean by "immortal"?

NTP: By immortal, I don't mean in the religious sense, but that the cell won't die of old age as long as you keep feeding it and keep the telomerase gene activated so that the cell can continue to keep making its own telomerase.

SS: So is this telomerase something you can inject or put in a pill?

NTP: No, it's made inside the cell, and TA-65 turns on the gene that makes it, which normally is turned "off" in almost all cells of an aging person. Going back to your "fountain of youth" question; the idea is not entirely science fiction. If you activate telomerase within each cell and keep it activated, then, yes, we may be able to make those cells immortal.

SS: That takes my breath away.

NTP: There's a lot more we have to do and know about. Also, as far as expecting a miracle, you have to remember that it took us a long time to get to the age we are now, so you are not going to regress overnight.

SS: Okay, I'm breathing again. [Laughs.]

I interviewed Dr. Andy Jurow for this book. He is an antiaging doctor in Burlingame, Northern California, and is certified to prescribe your supplement. He and his wife have been taking your supplement TA-65, and they are talking about amazing skin changes—smooth, young skin . . . noticeably so. My sister ran into them in downtown Burlingame and was blown away by how different they both looked. He also reported that his eyesight was better, and both say their hair is looking better. I feel that skin and hair are good indicators of interior health.

NTP: The results vary with different people. My eyesight has gotten better since taking TA-65, but my hair has not gotten darker, although it looks healthier and plentiful.

SS: How long have you been taking it?

NTP: I've been taking it for four and a half years. When I turned fifty (I'm sixty-five now), I started to notice the effects of aging and, like I said, I didn't like it: stiff joints, low energy, and so on. So I started looking into antiaging medicine strictly to help myself. In that process, I heard a speech by Dr. Jerry Shay, a professor at the University of Texas Southwest, who talked about telomeres and telomerase and how it was possible to immortalize human cells.

After his talk, I asked the professor where I could get some of this immortalization stuff. He laughed and said his university had licensed all their patents to a company called Geron in Menlo Park, California, and that they were developing this technology for telomerase activation. The very next day I called the CEO of Geron, flew out to meet with him, and ended up investing in the company through a private stock placement. That investment helped to finance the development of what we now call TA-65, and later I licensed all Geron's telomerase activation technology for nutraceutical and cosmetic applications.

SS: Why wouldn't Geron have kept this license for themselves? I mean, they are a giant pharmaceutical company.

NTP: They ran into some financial constraints at that time. They had a lot of good science, but not enough money to properly develop all of it and had to decide what to emphasize and which to cut back on . . . they decided to eliminate telomerase activation and instead went forward on cancer drugs. Today, I think Geron is surprised and probably regrets having given me the license for TA-65 and all their telomerase activation technology.

SS: Does TA-65 cure disease?

NTP: Even if we did studies proving TA-65 cured or prevented diseases, we would not be able to make those claims because we are selling a nutraceutical and not a drug. To make any disease claims, you have to go through the full FDA drug approval process, which can take up to ten years and cost hundreds of millions of dollars. I don't have that kind of money and even if I did, I would not want people to have to wait years to be able to take TA-65. We are helping a lot of people right now and very glad to be able to do so.

Geron on its own has been pursuing research for drugs that are telomerase activators. There is definite reason to believe that telomerase activation can be beneficial in a number of disease states, and Geron, which is a drug company, has kept those rights for itself. A few years ago the company announced it was developing a drug for HIV AIDS, which is actually a telomere-shortening disease that wears out your immune system. What happens is that the immune system senses that the HIV virus has gotten into CD4 immune cells, and certain other "killer" immune cells then attack those infected cells. The immune system keeps fighting this virus until the immune system becomes "worn out." When that happens, immunologists believe that a person goes from being HIV positive into having full-blown AIDS. As you know, AIDS stands for acquired immune deficiency syndrome. The reason the immune system wears out is because the killer cells keep dividing to fight the virus, and every time any cell divides, its telomeres get shorter. When the telomeres get too short, the immune cells can't divide anymore and you end up running out of immune cells.

SS: Well, I imagine the only reason a drug company would pursue a product with the hopes of curing a disease is to get FDA approval and sell it as a drug. They are not normally into supplements, which I imagine is why they gave you the license. Lucky you.

NTP: Yes, they are going for the drug or drugs that cure or assist in disease management. They can then apply for a patent and own the discovery.

I am involved because I got interested in the antiaging effect of TA-65, the thinking being that if you don't age, you won't get the diseases of aging.

SS: It's a theory that makes sense. It certainly has me intrigued. My inclination would always be to go for the nondrug first.

NTP: Yes, but you are not the average person. You are much more informed and knowledgeable about medical advances. The average person who gets sick goes to his doctor and the doctor tells him what to do and he does it.

SS: Just like they are children! And why not; we've been trained to think of doctors as gods. I remember my mother would never dare question a doctor. But that thinking has got to change because no one is going to care as much about your health as you, and with toxicity and environmental diseases at epidemic proportions, you have to be the one who is in charge of your own body. In that sense I definitely am different. I have my own ideas of what old age will look like, and it's a very nice picture. I think my doctors like that I am informed. That's why I write my books—so people have the information, so they can start connecting their own dots to their health. I believe doctors should actually be thought of more like mechanics you hire to fix your body. That attitude would get you better service. When you take your car in to the mechanic, you are not afraid to ask a lot of questions; you want to know what they are fixing and why and how. Right? I mean, after all, it's your car. And in this instance, it's your life!

NTP: Absolutely.

SS: How do you take TA-65?

NTP: I take a full dose of four capsules a day, two in the morning and two in the evening. One of our doctors, Dr. Ed Park, recommends that people take all four at the same time and in the evening. We offer three daily dose levels varying from one to four capsules; low, medium, and full.

SS: I met with Dr. Park and was amazed by his transformation since taking TA-65. He showed me a picture of himself ten years ago, overweight and looking much older than the way he looks today. He makes the same claims: more hair, tremendous weight loss, energy, vitality, and better lung capacity. It was quite remarkable.

Do you take different amounts of TA-65 depending on your age?

NTP: Generally, yes. If you are under fifty, take one pill a day; if you are from fifty to sixty-five, then take two; and if you are seventy or older, we recommend the full dose of four a day. But if you know the length of your telomeres, these age guidelines are not applicable. One person we tested was twenty-five years old, but her lab results showed that her telomeres were that of a fifty-year-old. Because of this we have given her two daily tablets, and she seems to be benefiting from it.

SS: What caused her to age so rapidly?

NTP: She had a tremendous amount of stress in her life, both emotional and physical; she had various disease problems along with severe emotional distress.

SS: So in her case it is not only life extending, it appears to be lifesaving.

NTP: Hard to tell at this point if it is life extending. Even with the telomeres of a fifty-year-old, at twenty-five she could still easily live for another forty years. Forty years from now would mean she might end up dying at sixty-five instead of living on into her nineties. At present, it is impossible to get statistical information on actual human life extension.

We recommend that everyone have their telomeres measured, but it's not always necessary. If you are seventy years old, all I have to do is look at you and I know you are not forty anymore. Forty is the age when everyone should start to do something about their telomeres.

SS: We measure our telomeres by taking a test. What are these tests? Is it the telomerase chain reaction test? The PCR test?

NTP: There are now three different commercially available tests that measure the length of telomeres; this way we get a baseline. SpectraCell is a U.S. lab doing it, and there is a company in Canada called Repeat Diagnostics; both of these companies measure the mean (or average) telomere length.

There is also a third company, called Life Length, formed by María Blasco, head of the Spanish National Cancer Research Institute in Madrid, Spain. Life Length has a more expensive test, but it can measure the shortest telomeres. This test has recently become available in both the United States and Europe.

Ideally, people taking TA-65 should do a test that measures the shortest telomeres. It only takes one cell with short telomeres out of the ninety-two telomeres in every cell to send it into crisis (apoptosis), which is programmed cell death.

There's another company called Telome Health in Menlo Park, California, formed by Professor Elizabeth Blackburn, the Nobel Prize winner who discovered telomerase, and Dr. Calvin Harley, who was the chief scientific officer at Geron. They are currently only doing work for academic institutions, but by the time this book is published, they expect to be doing testing for the general public. It will be interesting to see exactly what tests and pricing they will offer.

TESTING FOR TELOMERES

The standard test to measure your telomeres is called a *polymerase chain reaction test* (PCR test). It is a blood test done by SpectraCell labs in Houston and costs around $350. This test can determine the median length of your telomeres in relation to your age. The supplement must be prescribed by a qualified certified doctor, and the supplement itself can be obtained from MedQuest in Salt Lake City.

There is a gene called the *hTERT gene* (the "h" stands for human). This gene gets gradually turned off in normal aging. By the time we are adults, the hTERT gene has been turned off in almost all the normal cells in our bodies. We at T.A. Sciences want to turn it back on. TA-65 is able to turn on hTERT genes in healthy cells.

Cancer is caused by a series of mutations that cause the cells to lose growth control. These bad cells would soon die from telomere shortening, but they stay alive because the hTERT gene gets turned on full blast and they are able to continue to divide indefinitely because they are telomerase positive. But TA-65 does not turn on the gene in cancer cells; it is already turned on by a mutation—a mutation that may in fact be caused by telomeres getting critically short.

To illustrate that telomerase itself does not cause cancer, let's look at some healthy cells that also have telomerase turned on full blast: our germ line cells. These are our reproductive cells, eggs and sperm. Telomeres do not get short in reproductive cells because babies have to be born with baby-length telomeres, not the shorter telomeres of their aging parents. So the fact that you have that gene turned on all the time in healthy cells like eggs or sperm is a good thing. Telomerase simply allows cells to stay young and live longer; it doesn't make them cancerous. While people get testicular and ovarian cancer, no one ever gets egg or sperm cancer.

As I have said, turning on telomerase makes cells younger and extends their lives, and we want to do just that for the fifty trillion aging cells in our body.

Another point: TA-65 rejuvenates the immune system, and a strong immune system fights cancer. We have thousands of people taking our supplement and we have not heard of even one person coming down with cancer after starting to take TA-65.

SS: So TA-65 can rejuvenate and strengthen an aging immune system. Seems it's worth it if only for that.

NTP: To back up this theoretical argument, we and others have done in vivo studies and found that TA-65 did not accelerate cancerous growth or cause increased initiation of cancers.

SS: Going back to the importance of strengthening the immune system, has there been any clinical testing?

NTP: Luckily for us, strengthening the immune system is not considered a disease treatment by the FDA, so we can honestly tell people that taking TA-65 rejuvenates the immune system. We are also proud to report that there are several scientific studies on TA-65 that have established both efficacy and safety. One of them was published in 2011 in the English journal *Rejuvenation Research*. That trial showed that the shortest telomeres got longer in people taking TA-65 and their immune systems were rejuvenated. There were other good health benefits associated with TA-65 that are currently under study as we speak. We will have to talk again to update your book once those results are published.

If we do not get hit by a bus, all of us will get some form or fashion of a disease. It is just a part of getting older. However, supporting cellular health and the immune system should go a long way in contributing to our overall health and longevity.

SS: Well, I see this supplement as a step toward health and away from the present dismal aging paradigm.

NTP: That's the whole point of our business. The TA-65 molecule is found in the astragalus plant. It's a very rare molecule. We spent five years testing for safety and developing the technology for extracting and purifying it before we introduced it to the market for human consumption. Even though it's an extract from a plant, what we end up with is a single molecule. It's not a normal extract. There are more than 2,000 molecules in the astragalus plant and we take out the other 1,999 so there's only one left.

SS: Does one take TA-65 for life?

NTP: I will. But it's not like the hormones that you write about so eloquently. As you know, with hormones, once you start taking them you have to take them for life or you go right back to where you started. That's not the case with lengthening your telomeres. Here is a hypothetical example: If I take TA-65 for a year, and I lengthen my telomeres the equivalent of ten years and then I stop, my telomeres won't immediately go back to where they were when I started. They will start to age again, but it should take ten years to get as short as they were when I started.

SS: I see; it's like rolling the clock back.

NTP: Exactly. If you take TA-65 for one year or even six months, you'll get a benefit and that benefit will last.

SS: Will I notice a difference right away?

NTP: Not necessarily. Some people do and some don't. A major effect of TA-65 is rejuvenation of the immune system. But how do you know if your immune system is stronger? You don't necessarily feel any different at all; you would need a series of blood tests to track changes.

Similarly, how do you feel if your telomeres are longer? You don't feel that, either. It's a long-term lengthening of the telomeres that's going to have the effect. But a lot of people do notice things like sleeping better, having more energy, better sexual performance, and so on.

SS: Who is taking it?

NTP: I'm not at liberty to name names without specific authorization, but I can say this; we have Nobel laureates, famous actors and actresses, professional athletes who are trying to prolong their careers, and a lot of people who are simply not willing to be packed off to the nursing home.

SS: So you are making cells young again. It's actually a fantastic dream. Can any doctor prescribe it?

NTP: No, we only sell through doctors and health professionals who we have licensed. There are more than 250 in the United States and more are being added each week. To be licensed by us, health professionals have to pay a licensing fee, sign a legal document, study our fifty-page manual on telomerase activation, and, finally, pass a written test. Only then will we certify them. TA-65 is not just another supplement; it addresses the fundamental root cause of cellular aging. We don't want it sold by anyone who doesn't understand at least the basics of telomere biology.

SS: Is there a resource list so people from all over the country can access one of these doctors?

NTP: Yes, all our licensees are listed on our online website: www .TASciences.com.

SS: And how much will this cost?

NTP: For older people or those with short telomeres who take the full dose of four pills a day, it costs about $4,000 for a six-month supply. If you are younger and need a lower dose, it will be less. The low dose of one pill a day costs $200 a month. That's not too bad; many women spend more than that for cosmetics.

SS: Not everyone will see the same results. What complaints have you gotten?

NTP: Well, the worst case that I can think of was not actually so bad. We had an eighty-year-old client who took TA-65 for two years and then we noticed he had stopped reordering. So I called and asked him why. He said, "Well, I've been taking it for two years and I don't think it's doing me any good. I feel exactly the same as I did before I started taking it." I then said to him, "John, you've gone from eighty to almost eighty-three with no deterioration, feeling exactly as you did before; don't you think that may be a benefit in itself?" He said he hadn't thought of that, and then he said, "Actually, come to think of it, I haven't been feeling as good as I was when I was taking TA-65 every day." So I said to him, let's retest you and objectively see what has happened. Luckily, he had done blood work to establish a baseline before he started taking our product so we could make a comparison. He took a follow-up blood test and we found that his immune system had quite significantly improved so he went back on the supplement.

SS: How does TA-65 affect stem cells?

NTP: Stem cells are like every other human cell in that every time one divides, the telomeres get shorter. But they are different from most cells because they have some telomerase, which is why they can make enough new cells to keep us alive. Unfortunately, when stem cells get old, they can't produce enough telomerase anymore, and their capacity to make new cells decreases. The result is obvious; we lose regenerative capacity and eventually succumb to old age. But TA-65 activates telomerase in all types of cells we have studied, and we expect it is active in stem cells as well, keeping them functioning longer.

We are talking to stem cell people who multiply stem cells in their labs with the idea of using TA-65 so that all that cell division does not end up severely shortening telomeres. Clearly it is not a good idea to put back stem cells that are older than they started with, and that's what happens when cells divide if they don't have telomerase activated at the same time. I would like to see stem cell therapy one day using adult cells that in addition to having been multiplied have been made younger.

Let me say a few words about telomere lengths over the course of a lifetime. Did you know your telomeres are the longest at conception, not at birth? Remember that every time a cell divides, your telomeres get shorter. When we start out as an embryo, we consist of only one cell. Then that single-cell embryo starts to divide. By the time a baby is born, the cell numbers have increased billions of times to get all those cells to make a fully formed baby. Telomeres in an embryo start out being about 15,000 base pairs of DNA long, and by the time the baby is born, telomere length is down to about 10,000 base pairs. We all lose about one-third of our telomere length by the time we are born. Over the next eighty or so years, we lose another 5,000 to 7,000 base pairs. Then when a telomere gets down to about 3,000 (it doesn't have to get to zero), it's too short to do its job of protecting the chromosome. You get double strand breaks and fusions of different chromosomes that cause various mutations. At this point, telomeres are so short that the cell can no longer divide; it becomes senescent and goes on to die.

Short telomeres are literally the "kiss of death."

SS: Thanks, Noel. This is intriguing and fascinating. It feels as if we are at the brink of what Ray Kurzweil refers to as "a fantastic voyage." No one wants to age unless we can do so in perfect health and remain vital and energetic. The benefit of aging and why we want to age is that with age comes wisdom, and the planet is in dire need of wisdom. So I see this as a possibility for longer life and more wisdom.

NTP: Thank you, Suzanne. It's been my pleasure to have this opportunity to talk about telomeres and TA-65.

ANDY JUROW, M.D.

Dr. Andy Jurow *is a strapping, good-looking gynecologist and obstetrician as well as an antiaging doctor who moonlights at night as a SWAT team cop. I attribute his fantastic health and energy (he's a bit of an overachiever) to following the regimen he recommends to his patients in order to live life in optimal health. He was educated at Michigan State University Medical Center and did his residency at the University of Southern California Medical Center. He has obtained fellowships with the American Academy of Anti-Aging Medicine and is presently enrolled at the University of South Florida College of Medicine studying metabolic and nutritional medicine. He is excited about the possibilities of living longer and makes sure he keeps up with all the most up-to-date information and studies. He is smart and compassionate, as well as passionate about reversing aging and longevity. He is located in Burlingame, California.*

SS: Good morning, Dr. Jurow. You are one of those "combination doctors," a gynecologist with an antiaging medicine practice who specializes in bioidentical hormone replacement, and now you have been certified as a specialist in testing and prescribing TA-65, the telomere-lengthening supplement. Do your patients understand the advantage they are getting from you relative to aging well?

AJ: Thank you, Suzanne. My patients understand and that's why they come to me, but I do experience resistance and criticism from my peers. Some doctors in this area have not branched out and do not agree with antiaging medicine, and my approach may threaten them.

SS: Crazy, isn't it? I would think they would seek you out for instruction on the new ways to help people make their way through the toxic soup we live in and the longer lives we've obtained through technology.

AJ: Yes, but most of the information they get is from big pharma, and that general literature and information turns them against these new ideas. It's frustrating. Even though we do have the data on bio-identicals, they still fight it. They take their patients off the hormones I have prescribed to them. Even though those patients are feeling great, they take them off and then they become miserable again.

SS: Are the women just afraid to go against their GP?

AJ: Most of the women stay with me because their quality of life is so improved on bioidentical hormone replacement (BHRT). But I'm constantly fighting misinformation. Women will come to me and say, my doctor told me to stop taking estrogen because it will cause breast cancer. In my opinion, there is no data to support that BHRT properly administered will cause breast cancer. I know these doctors are not trying to harm their patients, but they respond to the misinformation of the media who interpret things negatively and incorrectly. There are studies that support what I am saying. For instance, the famous Fournier study; Agnes Fournier is a wonderful French investigator, and she reviewed data on some eighty thousand patients over an eight-year period. It showed there was no increased risk in breast cancer for women on bioidentical estrogen. There are many other studies that back up the positive nature of hormone replacement.

Also, as part of my regenerative protocol, I stress to my patients the other important components of aging well; they of course are nutrition, lifestyle, exercise and sleep, managing stress, and avoiding toxins. We also go after cleaning out the body to detoxify from all the pollutants that contaminate all of us; we give them appropriate nutrients and supplements, and then we balance their hormones.

Women and men educate themselves, mainly by reading your books. I often encourage my new patients to read your book *Breakthrough* to educate themselves. It makes my job easier, and when they are armed with current information, they are more responsive to complying with my protocol. It doesn't take long before they start feeling fantastic. For me, after all these years as a general gynecologist and an OB and not having been able to do anything for the debilitating symptoms of menopause, hormonal loss, and aging, to now actually be able to naturally improve the quality of life for my patients is very rewarding work. Bioidentical hormone replacement is life changing for these patients. Hormones enhance their immune system; estrogens improve neurotransmitters, allowing the brain to remain healthy to maintain their thinking and memory. Hormones also certainly help with vaginal health and, no small thing, by taking BHRT these people become sexually functioning again.

SS: Sounds like a no-brainer to me. And we know a healthy person is a sexual person; an unhealthy person has no interest in sex. My sister is one of your happy patients by the way, and I appreciate that you take such good care of her. Do you consider yourself a gynecologist first and an antiaging doctor second?

AJ: Good question. I started out as a gynecologist. Now I have an additional office for my regenerative patients. My passion is this new regenerative medicine. If you feel better emotionally, physically, and mentally, you are going to get more enjoyment out of life. For me, this new specialty is a matter of paying attention to what's available and being on top of the research. It's changing and updating all the time. I review the literature on a weekly basis if not more often, to see what's out there that's new. For example, a federal task force came out with a thousand-page study not favorable to vitamin D. Even though there are numerous studies showing the tremendous benefits of vitamin D, this report focused on a negative study from thirty years ago. It was a very small group and the participants were smokers. Yet there are many other studies showing the benefits of vitamin D, which has been proven to improve the immune system, improve diabetes, and reduce cancer risk. So if you are not out there keeping up with all the recent studies, you could be doing your patients a disservice. I had a patient who lost her hair; literally all of it. She went from doctor to doctor, and finally the third doctor she went to tested her vitamin D level and found it was one of the lowest the doctor had ever seen. The patient was put on a vitamin D regimen and her hair returned. So keeping updated is essential; it's a matter of being aware, and watching what's out there.

SS: Yes, you are right. Doctors must keep up with the changing medicine or they will find themselves left in the dust. As people catch on that there is now another way, that it's not all about pills and that their end point does not and should not be the nursing home, then regenerative medicine, or as I call it advanced medicine, will become the way it's done.

AJ: This is the new education. Regenerative medicine is difficult for some physicians to pick up on because it is a different concept of complete care. In medical school, we are not taught a true model for health. We are not taught about nutrition and prescribing hormones. We are taught to treat diseases.

Regenerative physicians do an extensive panel of blood tests, a complete analysis from head to toe, from the thyroid to the gonads, bowel function, gut function . . . it's all essential. We test for malabsorption, dysbiosis, and yeast overgrowth because all these things affect the bowel, and the bowel is one of the entranceways and the primary resource we have to maintain our immune system and get nutrients into our bodies. Regenerative medicine is a complete approach to true health, and it also requires that you listen to the patient.

The void in traditional medicine is that doctors don't have time to spend with their patients. Ten to fifteen minutes per patient is simply not enough. My first interview with a new patient lasts at least an hour to listen to them and see their symptoms; this directs me as to whether the patient's problem is thyroid, hormonal, or a combination of many different things, including food allergies or toxicity. I do the easiest, simplest, most cost-effective protocol possible for each patient. I do not want to overwhelm them.

SS: Are your patients receptive to supplementation regimens?

AJ: I explain to them, when you are twenty years old, you haven't spent much time in our toxic environment so you don't need supplementation as much, plus the younger body is better able to absorb things than when the body is older. Some of my patients require only, maybe, ten pills a day, others need forty a day, which is a lot, but it's always determined by blood tests showing the patient's unique deficiencies. They all need vitamin D, and I cannot emphasize fish oil enough; it's good for cholesterol levels and aches and pains, and it helps with neurotransmission and depression. With a few simple changes in the way my patients live their lives and by taking hormones and supplements, I can get them smiling and happy. The rest is fine-tuning.

SS: The goal being optimal health?

AJ: Yes, that's the goal; but it has to be done in baby steps. Otherwise, it overwhelms the patient. In the beginning I'd send new patients home with forty or fifty supplements, they'd take them, they'd throw up—and they wouldn't be very happy with me. Now, I start slowly. I work together with my patients. If a patient comes in who is heavy and asks, "Can you help me?" I say, "Yes, I can help but if you don't change your diet and lifestyle I can't do much." I stress eating organic food if they can afford it. I teach the value of nutrition: that you don't diet to get skinny, that you change your diet to promote optimal health, and that prime health and thinness go together. In today's world, we know that toxins are hurting us. Pesticides allow for bigger, more beautiful-looking fruits and vegetables, and pesticides allow for more yield per acre, but at what cost to us?

SS: When we were kids, there was no organic food because it never entered our minds to spray poison on our *food*!

AJ: Yes, the food didn't look as good back then when we went to the market; the apples and oranges looked a little grungier, but they were natural. Now when you go to the nonorganic section of the supermarket, everything is so pretty. And the meat is so red with all its dyes and preservatives, but again, at what cost to us?

SS: Let's talk about TA-65. For anyone interested in antiaging, this could be the biggest breakthrough of all time.

AJ: Yes, this is a tremendous advancement in medicine. TA-65 was based on the Nobel Prize winners' discovery of the enzyme telomerase that actually lengthens telomeres. The length of the telomere on each and every cell in our trillions of cells determines our health and aging. With each replication of each cell the telomere gets shorter. Once it reaches critical mass and the telomere no longer works, then that cell dies. Along the way with shortened telomeres, the body gets older and less healthy. This new supplement actually lengthens short telomeres through the use of telomerase, and the effect is to enhance wellness.

SS: Is the advantage of the TA-65 supplement that it is the only telomere-stimulating substance on the market? And is this going to allow us to live till we are two hundred? [Laughs.]

AJ: Well, it's a start. We are seeing very few side effects with it, and there are so many advantages. Although more research is needed, telomerase certainly has the potential to extend life and in many ways reverse aging. If we increase the life span and if, in fact, telomere length determines the state of your health, people will no longer retire at sixty or sixty-five. They will be healthy people, and healthy people are productive people.

SS: So that answers the question of what will they do with themselves? You think as a result, we will have all these healthy productive people running around with good brains and the wisdom that only comes with age? Currently, our planet is sadly devoid of wisdom, so this would be a good thing.

AJ: It would be a good thing . . . I'm not going to retire at sixty-five. I'm not going to retire; I don't want to. I want to be healthy and contribute. TA-65 is multifactorial, a combination of advantages. Your mental clarity is sharper, your skin changes are slowed down, and you don't have the same degeneration of your joints and muscles, so you can be ambulatory. You can be cognitive, you can be intelligent, and you can be sharp. Also, we like the way we look with this supplement plus a complete individualized supplementation program. With TA-65 you can glance in the mirror and see that you are looking better and your muscle mass is more cut and defined. It could be the end to walkers, and drooling, and the present template of what we think of as aging.

SS: Yes, and the present paradigm of aging is something so unappealing. Is TA-65 something you can take if you have active cancer?

AJ: So far there has been no downside to TA-65, but we do not have any information on its effect on active cancer. But if you think through what telomerase does, I can see where it could actually prevent cancer by lengthening the telomeres. When you think about it, cancer already has telomerase. That's why cancer cells are immortal. So there is no way to make these cells any worse. TA-65 lengthens telomeres and that boosts the immune system so you have positive factors at work. The best way to prevent cancer is to have a strong immune system. Any organism with an optimal, balanced immune system tends to be stronger. We produce cancer cells in our bodies almost from the time we're born, yet we don't get that many cancers because our system destroys the cells. So an immunologically enhanced individual is just not going to have as high a cancer risk.

SS: The concept makes sense to me . . . We need something new, and to now have a supplement to possibly boost the immune system, we may be at the dawning of a new day. What are the advantages and the disadvantages?

AJ: The advantages: a small study showed that it significantly boosted the immune system, lengthened short telomeres, showed an increase in sexual function, skin got better, eyesight improved, and hair growth was significant. These are some very, very substantial advantages. The disadvantage: It's expensive, starts at about $2,000 a year depending on your age.

SS: Frankly, for all it does, considering what women in particular spend on beauty products and treatments—expensive visits for Botox and other injections, plastic surgery going into the thousands, facials, peels, liposuction—it all adds up. The beauty business is red-hot even in this bad economy. A supplement touted to make you healthier, possibly protect you from cancer and build up your immune system is pretty spectacular, but then add in the other benefits of fewer wrinkles, shinier hair, better eyesight, better sexual function, better working brain and it becomes a very appealing supplement to take. The supplement, however, is expensive to make as Noel Patton explained in his interview. Obtaining the ingredients is difficult and the process of making TA-65 is complex, so for now, it keeps the price high.

Some people are just not going to be able to afford it, but if it is the miracle it seems to be, wouldn't it make sense that our health care system would provide this to prevent all the expense down the road for diseases from our toxic environment and debilitated immune systems?

AJ: I couldn't agree more. Perhaps when Geron pharmaceuticalizes it, then there's a possibility that insurance would pay for it. But then it will be a drug. To obtain a patent they would have to alter the molecular structure. What I like about TA-65 is that it is a pure nutraceutical that isn't chemicalized in any way. TA-65 does not put environmental or toxic stress on the body as do some drugs.

SS: I hear that you and your wife, who is also a doctor, are taking the supplement. My sister Maureen said she saw the two of you on Burlingame Avenue and she couldn't believe the difference she saw in both of you. In fact, she thought you both had face-lifts, but then she said that the skin on your hands and arms was also young and different. Younger! She said you both look phenomenal. How long have you been taking it?

AJ: We've been using it for about six months and have noticed a significant improvement, and that's saying a lot because my wife and I are very balanced. We walk our talk and use what we encourage our patients to take. My wife says that her skin feels like it has been plumped. In fact, she was scheduled to have a face-lift in September and she canceled that because the effects of this supplement have been so dramatic.

By the way, your sister Maureen looks great.

SS: I know, because she is doing all of this. She's in her early seventies and looks, and better yet feels, fifty!

AJ: She is a great patient. In my experience, people who are on antiaging regimens are just brighter and sharper, and they feel better.

SS: Well, your results with this supplement are very exciting. A natural way to boost health and beauty potentially.

AJ: Well, who doesn't want to look and feel better? With telomerase, instead of cells dying, we can maintain them. I tell my patients, you can start a healthy program including TA-65 now and jump-start your regenerative health, but it's expensive. Or you can wait ten or more years for the pharmaceutical version so that insurance might pay for it.

SS: I guess you have to look at this as a luxury. Maybe instead of a trip you wanted to take or remodeling your kitchen or whatever, you decide between that or what you would get the most enjoyment out of. Not being sick, run-down, looking better, having better hair and eyesight, plus being sexually functional . . . all pretty exciting.

AJ: I tell my patients that I can get them back to balance, and if they stay with me, they can expect improved overall health and mental health. I can restore their quality of life without growth hormones or TA-65. But if someone can afford those things, then I certainly recommend it if indicated. Not everybody needs growth hormone and not everyone needs TA-65, but you are right—if you can afford it, it's a true luxury and benefit.

SS: What about the argument that you are messing with nature—that a sixty-five-year-old is supposed to feel like a sixty-five-year-old—and you should stop interfering with the natural course of life?

AJ: If that were the case, then we should stop all technology. We should stop MRIs and sophisticated blood testing and get rid of all the modern technology that has allowed us to live longer than ever before. Does it make sense that we are supposed to live longer but in total deterioration? One of the articles I read concerning TA-65 is a philosophical discussion of what we will do if this really works.

SS: What *will* we do?

AJ: Society will adjust. We'll work longer, harder, we won't use Social Security, and the economic system will adjust to it. But certainly ethically, morally, and even religiously, no one has ever said that we shouldn't make optimal use of our life span.

SS: What about the environment? The chemicals, the pesticides, the fluoride, the assault that every living human on the planet cannot help but be exposed to? Is TA-65 a protector, because it strengthens the immune system to put up a resistance to the invisible and in many cases visible enemy?

AJ: It helps with strengthening the immune system, and a strong immune system is the best line of defense. We have to keep educating. People have to get involved and realize that the body was never meant to handle so many toxins and that the liver is not able to clear the body of them when under such a bombardment. Every time I educate somebody, they go out and tell their family members who then tell their friends. Hopefully that groundswell will help us.

SS: And that's our journey . . . how well can we be in a sick world? As a healthy sixty-five-year-old I realize I am valuable to society. Older people who have taken care of themselves provide value and do not drain society by their sicknesses and ill health.

AJ: You may not remember, but I've also been in law enforcement for years, and I recently left my department to apply for another one. When I fill out my form, it's going to ask my age and I will say sixty-two and they are going to say, wait, a cop? SWAT? Sixty-two years old? But I know that I compete in all the physical agility tests with all the twenty-five- and thirty-year-olds and I not only keep up, but I'm often ahead of them.

SS: Do you think it's the payoff because you practice antiaging medicine?

AJ: Yes. It has paid off. I don't feel any older than I was when I was considered young. I think this direction of medicine has given me a new sense of enjoyment about my craft. I was getting to the point where traditional medicine wasn't satisfying to me anymore. I was putting Band-Aids on patients; I'd be able to help them a little bit, but no one got really well. No one was able to slow the course of nature. This new arena is so much fun. The reward I get is listening to my patients talk about how great they feel. My lot in life is to make my patients feel the best that they can. It's not a big moneymaker. Fifty percent of antiaging doctors go out of business in the first year. You do it because it's rewarding and fulfilling.

SS: Yes, but all people have to do is look at you and your wife and they will want what you have. You both look like movie stars! Actually that's the basis of the Al-Anon program, that by attraction, others will want what you have. So just by being so healthy and well and beautiful, you inspire others to want the same.

AJ: Thank you, Suzanne.

BOMBSHELL #7:
THE CHEMICALS KILLING OUR BRAINS—
AND WHAT WE CAN DO ABOUT THEM

If you want to know what's wrong, look down at the table. It's staring back at you.

—Andrew Saul, *Food Matters*

We are surrounded every day by an invisible sea of synthetic chemicals, and our bodies absorb them like sponges until we are toxic. We consume foods that have been depleted of essential natural healing nutrients. These nutrients have been replaced by synthetic chemical additives.

These additives in our processed foods interact synergistically in our bodies with synthetic chemicals absorbed from our water, our air, and our consumer products, weakening our immune systems. Once weakened, we become susceptible to illnesses and diseases that medical practitioners treat with synthetic chemical drug compounds that often prove even more toxic to us. And this cycle in our culture and in our lives repeats itself over and over.

—Randall Fitzgerald, *The Hundred-Year Lie*

There is no greater assault to our health than environmental toxicity. Chemicals are everywhere—in our food, water, the air we breathe, our household cleaning products, from the formaldehyde outgassing from our carpets, electromagnetic rads, and more—and we are getting sick as a result. The overabundance of chemicals thrust on the human body are life shorteners. Our livers are groaning trying to process substances they were never designed to filter. We are not supposed to ingest chemicals.

Dr. Russell Blaylock is a renowned neuroscientist I have featured in several of my other books. He has devoted his life to understanding the effects of toxicity on health and the human brain. He allowed me to interview him yet again and what he has to say is truly a Bombshell.

RUSSELL BLAYLOCK, M.D.

Dr. Russell Blaylock *and I have become very good friends over the years I have been interviewing him. The first book of his that I read was* Natural Strategies for Cancer Patients *and I thought,* This is interesting, an oncologist, a brain surgeon, and a neuroscientist writing a book about natural strategies? *Clearly this is one special man.* His accomplishments are too many to list; they would go on for pages. To name just a few, though, he is a board-certified neurosurgeon, an author, and a lecturer. He attended the LSU School of Medicine in New Orleans and completed his general surgical internship and neurosurgical residency at the Medical University of South Carolina in Charleston. During his residency, he ran the neurology program for one year and did a fellowship in neurosurgery after his residency. For the past twenty-five years, he has practiced neurosurgery in addition to having a nutritional practice. He recently retired from both practices to devote himself full-time to nutritional studies and research.

Dr. Blaylock was one of the first neurosurgeons to utilize high-intensity nutritional supplementation in trauma patients, which met with great success. He has written and illustrated three books: Excitotoxins: The Taste That Kills, Health and Nutrition Secrets That Can Save Your Life, *and, as I said above,* Natural Strategies for Cancer Patients. *He has written over thirty scientific papers published in peer-reviewed journals on a number of subjects.*

He lectures widely to both lay and professional medical audiences on a variety of nutritional subjects. He also has a monthly nutrition newsletter, published by NewsMax.com, The Blaylock Wellness Newsletter, *and he is a member of the Association of American Physicians and*

Surgeons, the American Nutraceutical Association, the International and American Associations of Clinical Nutritionists, the American College of Nutrition, the American Association for Health Freedom, the National Health Federation, the American Academy of Anti-Aging Medicine, and the Price-Pottenger Nutrition Foundation. He was recently appointed as a member of the scientific advisory board of the Life Extension Foundation.

How he has time to do it all boggles the mind . . . He is indeed a national treasure, a font of accurate information, and a source I go to regularly to back up my facts. I am proud once again to feature him in another of my books.

SS: Hello, Dr. Blaylock, so good to have this opportunity to speak with you again. You always inspire, not only me, but also my readers, with your knowledgeable information about the dangers of toxins. Yesterday I was reading about a forty-year-old woman who says she is a healthy eater and who exercises, yet has a very bad brain tumor. How can that be? Doesn't a good diet provide protection?

RB: There is a very definite link to women (and men) developing brain tumors who are using aspartame in increasing amounts. They think they are healthy, and they do in fact eat a healthy diet, but they are drinking diet sodas and sweetening with aspartame, which is strongly linked to brain cancer in experimental studies and is also very strongly suggested in our observations.

I'VE HEARD FROM A NUMBER OF WOMEN FROM ALL OVER THE UNITED STATES WHO HAVE DEVELOPED BRAIN CANCERS, AND THE COMMON DENOMINATOR IS THAT THEY ARE ALL HEAVY USERS OF ASPARTAME.

Secondly, there is a strong connection with the huge exposure to pesticides, herbicides, and fungicides. Unfortunately, all these products have a tremendous financial bottom line that the manufacturers don't want the public to know about for fear they will be frightened off from using them. For instance, take formaldehyde, which outgases into your house from a number of construction products and releases this known carcinogen into the air.

SS: Where else do we get this chemical, from carpeting?

RB: Correct. Plus the fillers they use in different cements and building materials. In addition, aspartame in your food breaks down into formaldehyde.

WE ARE NOW BEGINNING TO APPRECIATE THAT WE ARE BEING EXPOSED TO A NUMBER OF VARIABLY TOXIC COMPOUNDS THAT, WHEN COMBINED IN OUR BODIES, CAN TRIGGER A NUMBER OF DISEASES, WHICH INCLUDE CANCER AND DEGENERATION OF THE NERVOUS SYSTEM.

SS: Yikes. When you say fillers, do you mean you can buy a brand-new house and not realize you are buying into a toxic environment?

RB: Yes. For example, I had a patient who built a brand-new beautiful home but had severe chemical reactions to the released toxic components in the house. It was so bad that he was unable to move into it.

SS: Are you talking about drywall?

RB: That and most all the new manufactured products, many of which have components that some people are extremely sensitive to, like vinyls, composite woods, certain glues, and other man-made products that are used. In addition, carpet adhesives, solvent, and caulking glues all contain a number of compounds known to produce neurological damage; in particular, formaldehyde is pervasive and powerfully connected to brain tumors. So what probably happened to the woman you mentioned was exposure to a number of toxic chemicals over a period of time. She could also be getting exposure from food. Even though she's eating vegetables, if they are not thoroughly washed, you can get exposed to a fair amount of pesticides and herbicides.

SS: This information makes eating organic foods even more important.

RB: Even organic foods can get contamination from herbicides and pesticides in the atmosphere, or, in some cases, the organic growers think they are using natural pesticides but it might be a fluoride compound and that is toxic as well. If you are eating organic food but the plant itself isn't healthy (if it has spots and damaged areas on it), then the plant will secrete carcinogenic substances trying to kill the fungi or viruses that are attacking the plant, so even if you eat organic foods, you have to be sure they are healthy organic foods.

SS: A person reading this could get pretty discouraged; I mean, if even the organic food isn't completely healthy, what are we supposed to do?

RB: I'm just trying to make people aware of the need for vigilance. It's important to wash your fruits and vegetables and choose healthy-looking organic foods. Another thing related to brain cancer is the dental amalgam. Mercury is a potent inducer of brain cancer and brain tumors. So if this unfortunate woman had dental amalgam fillings, which contain almost 50 percent mercury, or if she's been vaccinated with mercury-containing (thimerosal) vaccines or lives in a part of the country where there is high atmospheric mercury, like west Texas, she could have trouble. *Eating certain fish could also add to your mercury burden, and these things increase your risk of developing a brain tumor.*

Sadly, there are many, many different environmental toxins that can lead to a tumor. We are under such a terrible inundation by chemicals in the atmosphere and in our food that we really need a higher level of protection than just eating a good diet, which of course is crucial and the foundation of good health.

SS: So what can we do?

RB: What you can do to help is:

- Eat at least five servings of fruits and vegetables a day to derive any benefit. It takes ten to fifteen servings to get maximum benefits. That is a lot of fruits and vegetables. The reason it takes so many is that only about 30 percent of vegetable nutrients are absorbed with eating. This is because the nutrients in vegetables are locked within the cells of the plant and we do not have enzymes to dissolve the cell walls of vegetables. This means that you either have to chew the vegetables extremely well or grind them up in a blender—which I do. Running vegetables through a blender releases 80 percent of their nutrients for absorption.
- Because of the high level of toxic chemicals, we need additional antioxidants, such as flavonoids (mostly brightly colored fruits and vegetables, but also in some colorless vegetables) and the

basic vitamins and minerals that maximize your ability to neutralize these toxins. For instance, green tea has been found to
be a very potent neutralizer of benzene, which is a major carcinogen.

SS: Where are we getting benzene?

RB: Unfortunately, benzene is rather ubiquitous; you get it from
oil products. For instance, in the Gulf right now it was recently found
there were high levels of benzene in the seafood. Also, an orange
drink that was popular was found to have significant benzene levels.
Plus they found high levels of benzene in a carrot juice used for infants. It is the young people who are at the greatest risk.

SS: How could this be?

RB: When you ultrapasteurize fruit juices, it converts things like
beta-carotene, phenylalanine, and terpene into benzene. Also when
you cook with foods that have aspartame in them, you produce high
levels of benzene, which is linked to lymphoma.

SS: Then we need to connect the dots . . . chemicals and their
association to cancer.

RB: Absolutely; for instance, there is more benzene in foods than
anyone realizes because of the heating process and widespread use
of aspartame. By people using and cooking with aspartame, they are
producing not only the formaldehyde carcinogen but also benzene.
Lymphoma has the fastest-growing incidence of any type of cancer in
people under age thirty.

No one is paying attention to the literature showing this powerful connection and also the possible connection to the weed killer
Roundup. These products, combined with many others used around
most homes, produce a tremendous increase in hematologic malig-
nancies like multiple myeloma and non-Hodgkin's lymphoma and
leukemia.

SS: And these weed killers have now created a new generation of
superweeds and superbugs that have developed that are immune to
this herbicide. Yet from lack of knowledge, people are deliberately
consuming these foods and naively spraying these poisons around
their homes. Tragically, the children play in these same yards, as well
as their pets, and then bring that poison into their homes.

RB: Yes, and as a result their bodies now contain high levels of carcinogenic chemicals that can persist for a lifetime. Pregnant women
are walking in their neighborhoods where Roundup is routinely used,

as well as other pesticides, and they are breathing it in and absorbing it through their skin.

SS: What will happen to their babies?

RB: Clearly they are now exposed.

OF GREATEST CONCERN ARE NEWBORNS AND SMALL CHILDREN, NOT ONLY BECAUSE OF THE CANCER RISK BUT ALSO BECAUSE MANY OF THE COMMONLY USED CHEMICALS HAVE AN ADVERSE EFFECT ON BRAIN DEVELOPMENT AND FUNCTION. REMEMBER, THE HUMAN BRAIN UNDERGOES A CONSIDERABLE AMOUNT OF DEVELOPMENT AFTER BIRTH UNTIL AGE TWO YEARS, AND SOME PARTS OF THE BRAIN (CONTROLLING HIGHER BRAIN FUNCTIONS) CONTINUE THEIR DEVELOPMENT UNTIL AGE TWENTY-SEVEN YEARS. THESE CHEMICALS CAN CAUSE ABNORMAL WIRING OF THE BRAIN AND TRIGGER CHRONIC BRAIN INFLAMMATION.

SS: What is the effect of genetically modified (GM) foods on the human body?

RB: There is an interesting Russian study in which researchers found after the third generation of consuming these GMOs [genetically modified organisms], test animals developed kidney problems, liver problems, adrenal problems, and heart failure from eating GM corn and soybeans. With the widespread use of Roundup, you are not only getting the effects of the GM soybeans, but you are also getting a lot more exposure to the Roundup itself. As weeds become resistant to this pesticide, farmers are forced to use even more of it. So it's a triple threat. The plants have higher levels of pesticide contamination, as does the atmosphere from the vaporization of these massive amounts, in addition to the harmful effects of the GM plants themselves.

In my studies from looking at what we know about Roundup, it's a potentially powerful inducer of lymphomas and leukemias. This is being ignored because of the massive money made by Monsanto, the maker and leader in the industry of GM foods. European countries won't use any GM foods or seeds. Africa tried to resist it, but the United Nations and the International Monetary Fund used their power of the purse to force them to accept it.

SS: And we do know the United States is saturated with Roundup. I read that 90 percent of all corn is genetically modified, and 80 to 90 percent of soy is genetically modified.

RB: Plus a lot of the rice; it's quite tragic. More and more of our crops are ending up genetically modified, and of course legislators get legislation passed that doesn't require labeling of GM foods, so no one knows when they are eating it. In addition, once the foods are contaminated, there is no way to restore what has been lost—that is, natural foods.

SS: Unless you are buying organic.

RB: Correct, but so much of what people are consuming today are processed foods, and most all processed foods have soy flour in them so it's almost impossible to avoid GM soy if you are going to eat processed foods.

SS: And please tell my readers about the realities of soy, which has been sold as a healthy food to consumers.

RB: Soy, even in a natural state, is not a good thing to eat. It's very high in fluoride, manganese, and glutamate. It's always been considered something that is not good for human consumption—until a massive propaganda campaign by the industry. They have figured out how to use it with clever processing methods, for example, soy milk; and then to add insult to injury, they've sold soy as a breast cancer preventative and a generally healthy food choice.

SS: And women think, If a little soy is good, then a lot is better?

RB: Yes, so they are buying soy in all different forms. Over half the children born in this country are drinking a formula rather than breast milk and most of it is soy formula and these babies are getting, in my view and others, brain toxic levels of manganese. This has been published in major pediatric journals.

SS: I'm a little confused; manganese is a mineral that is good for us, right?

RB: Only in trace amounts. It's extremely brain toxic in higher amounts as in the amounts found in soy, so if you are drinking soy milk and particularly if you are giving it to babies, it has high enough levels to produce brain damage. Then if you are combining it with fluoride (through drinking water and the soy itself) and glutamate (a powerful brain toxic chemical), which is also found in the soy and many processed foods, you are greatly compounding the toxicity to many organs, especially the brain.

SS: Our poor babies. At present they are already born with 287 different toxins, 180 common to all of them.

RB: It's pervasive. Even people in the North Pole have been found to have large numbers of these pesticides and herbicides in their bodies, plus industrial solvent residues in their tissues. Babies get it passed through the mothers' placenta. When researchers biopsy the fat from the breast tissue or abdominal fat of women, they find hundreds of these compounds, known carcinogens and known neurotoxins. They damage the brain and particularly the developing brain.

SS: But no one is telling the mothers. It's the biggest-held secret in the United States. And when it comes to people's homes, no one wants a single insect, so they have the exterminator come in and regularly service their houses. Factor in having a child born into this environment that's virtually saturated with these carcinogenic chemicals, and the result is an explosion of damaged livers and immune systems.

RB: Yes, and many of these pesticides are known to also produce autoimmune diseases. In addition, many produce abnormal development of the brain. We are saturating ourselves to the point where it's seriously impacting health. We are seeing a rise in all kinds of cancers and neurological degenerative diseases. Studies show that vaccines do not cause brain damage or autism and that the autism groups made a mistake saying it was because of the mercury, which is a neurotoxin, but even if you remove the mercury from a vaccine, you will still get the same effect. There are also other toxins that are a bigger problem in vaccines than mercury, like aluminum. But the fact is that all these toxins are stimulating immunity excessively. Our children are being given six or seven vaccines during a single office visit, and this is very damaging to a developing brain.

If you gave the same thing proportionately to an adult, which would be around thirty-six to fifty vaccines, no adult could tolerate it. You'd be so sick, you'd think you were dying, plus you would risk developing all sorts of things like MS and other serious autoimmune disorders. You wouldn't be able to think, your joints would ache, and your body would break down. So no adult would ever accept getting that many vaccines in one office visit, yet that's what we do to children every day in this country. Several studies have shown that the vaccination process soon after birth can dramatically increase the sensitivity to exposure to a pesticide later in life. We call this *microglial priming*. This could increase the child's risk of developing a disease, such as Parkinson's disease, at an earlier age. It can also increase the child's sensitivity to the toxic effects of exposure later in life to illicit drugs, such as cocaine and methamphetamine.

SS: And the children are already toxic from all the other chemicals plus fluoride and soy formula, then add in dioxins and phthalates from plastic baby bottles and it's a recipe for disaster.

RB: Exactly, plastics are leaking out BPA and other toxins, and these are endocrine disrupters. We are seeing an explosion of thyroid dysfunction in this country from plastics, pesticides, and fluoride—all known thyroid disrupters. In our research, we know that if you have reduced thyroid function, it is the leading cause of elevated cholesterol. Textbooks will tell you that.

SS: But people can take a statin. All the doctors know that! [Laughs.]

RB: Well, that's the craziness of all this kind of modern, so-called evidence-based medicine. They sell the patients a drug, a statin, when all you have to do is get them off the endocrine disrupters and get the thyroid functioning again. In addition, there are many ways to naturally reduce your risk of a heart attack or stroke that far exceed the efficacy and safety of statin drugs.

SS: Interesting. I was on a major news show last year and the newscaster and I were discussing vitamins and supplements (he thinks they should be government controlled), and he lashed out at me over red yeast rice, saying that it raised his liver enzymes so he went back on Lipitor. I looked at him and all his apparent low-thyroid symptoms—missing the outer third of his eyebrows, sagging skin on his face, poor coloring, thick through his abdominal region—and I realized just how "off" today's medicine can be even for people like this successful man who thinks he is paying for the best advice. I'm sure no one connected the dots to realize that most likely he didn't need cholesterol-lowering drugs but that his thyroid needed attention.

RB: He would be better off checking his T3 and T4, putting reverse osmosis filters on all his water faucets, getting off Lipitor, finding out why his enzymes were elevated, and eliminating chemicals from his life.

A researcher named Dr. Beatrice Golomb did a comprehensive review of the side effects of statins, and it is very extensive. Everything from memory loss, brain dysfunction, increased cancer rates, peripheral neuropathy, and increased risk of ALS (a highly fatal disease) are all conditions caused by taking a statin and the effects are devastating. It gets crazier; now many doctors are urging nearly all forty-year-old men to take a statin. The fact that a person with normal cholesterol would get on statins is insane. Manufacturers of statin drugs even suggest putting statins in the drinking water, which is frightening because statins are also a powerful immune suppressor. If you have over two hundred million people in this country regularly taking statins, including children, for a lifetime, that means they are immune suppressed for a lifetime. They are going to catch every cold, virus, and bacteria; and they will have difficulty overcoming these infections plus have a high rate of cancer. Early observations with statins are that they increased the cancer rate because they suppress immunity. Yet, I suppose the manufacturers feel this will justify even more vaccine recommendations.

SS: Plus, statins suppress testosterone.

RB: And deplete coQ_{10}. Did you know that every cell in your body is absolutely dependent on coQ_{10}? So when a statin suppresses coQ_{10}, a person can go into heart failure. It has been proposed in research that the widespread use of statins is responsible for the dramatic increase in heart failure cases over the past twenty years. The brain, one of the most metabolically active tissues, is also highly dependent on coQ_{10}, and this explains why we are seeing more cases of an amnesia-like syndrome in people on these drugs.

SS: All for taking a drug that is supposed to prevent heart failure???

RB: Crazy, isn't it? One of the big problems with taking a statin is that patients complain of having no energy. Some can't even get out of bed. And then there is the potentially fatal disease rhabdomyolysis, which has been linked to statin use. Studies have shown that even short of this syndrome, statins are associated with pathological damage to muscle fibers.

SS: Rhabdomyolysis?

RB: Yes. It's a disease of the destruction of the muscle and it's fatal. Many patients who were on statins and did not take coQ_{10} died.

SS: What do statins do to the brain? I have friends on statins who can't remember the conversation we had the night before.

RB: If you look at the research on physiology on the effect of lowering brain cholesterol, it shows that you lose memory. Some people are proud of having excessively low cholesterol, as in 150 or lower. The brain can't function at that low level. Even in studies that physicians quote to support statin use, evidence shows that at that extremely low cholesterol level you increase death rates from brain hemorrhages. The cholesterol theory is badly flawed and this explains why over 50 percent of the heart attack deaths occur in people with perfectly normal cholesterol levels, and this includes diabetics.

SS: Well, that's a difficult sell because many doctors have convinced their patients, especially men, that they cannot live without statins.

THE TRUTH ABOUT CHOLESTEROL ACCORDING TO RUSSELL BLAYLOCK

The truth about cholesterol is that this brainwashing has been around so long it's now dogma, and it's wrong. Cholesterol is not what causes heart attacks. If you study the research (I went back to the 1930s and 1940s) in which they came up with this idea of cholesterol, it's not what the research showed; they made a mistake.

The research actually showed that the number one cause of atherosclerosis was consuming too much sugar and eating too many processed carbohydrates. At the time they were feeding the research rabbits cholesterol, but rabbits don't eat meat, and when they do, they develop atherosclerosis. The research showed if you fed the rabbits only cholesterol, they did not develop atherosclerosis even if you injected it. But the researchers ignored this valuable and important bit of information that the cholesterol was not the problem, but the problem was oxidation of all the fats in the blood vessels. They focused on cholesterol because it was the one you could measure. It is interesting to note that in these early studies, they mixed the cholesterol with corn oil. When the corn oil was removed, the animals developed very little atherosclerosis. Newer studies have now shown that the very type of oils recommended by medical authorities and the government, the heart-healthy polyunsaturated vegetable oils, increases atherosclerosis as well as inflammation throughout the body.

Atherosclerosis is an inflammatory disorder of the blood vessel lining, not a disorder of cholesterol, and this is the inflammation that is produced by all the polyunsaturated vegetable lipids: the omega-6 fats and oxidized cholesterol. Fats oxidize, and oxidized fats are very, very irritating. They produce high levels of free radicals in the walls of the vessel, and the body recognizes this and starts sending white blood cells in to gobble up the toxic oxidized fat. Then the white blood cells get filled with fat (these are your so-called foam cells), they subsequently break and release fat into the wall of the vessel, and you get plaque. At this point the body tries to protect itself against the inflammation (plaque) and that's when you get calcium deposits.

SS: So wait a minute . . . sugars and processed foods are the problem?

RB: Processed foods and sugary foods are made with omega-6 oils, like corn oil and safflower oil. If you feed animals omega-6 oils—corn oil, safflower oil, sunflower oil—they develop rampant atherosclerosis. The only way researchers were able to produce atherosclerosis in rabbits was to mix cholesterol with corn oil. If you didn't mix it with corn oil, they didn't develop the disease. So it's the corn oil causing the problem.

SS: But corn oil has been recommended as a "heart-healthy oil" for the last fifty years!

RB: Yes, and it's wrong. Corn oil is polyunsaturated oil. You never should cook in polyunsaturated oil because it oxidizes the oil; but people are cooking fries, chicken, and other things in these oils, and the food is oxidizing. Fast foods are notorious for cooking in cheap omega-6 oils and people are eating massive amounts of it. In most fast-food restaurants, the oil is used over and over, and this results in a highly oxidized oil ending up in your food.

SS: So Americans are consuming massive amounts of already oxidized oil and they are developing atherosclerosis?

RB: Yes, but it's not cholesterol doing this to them. I don't care if you have a level of 280. If it isn't oxidized, then it's not going to produce a problem.

SS: Is there a test to show if it's oxidized or not?

RB: Not clinically, but you can do it experimentally. Doctors never look at experimental studies; they only look at clinical studies, but a great number of the clinical studies are doctored to sell statin drugs. If you look at all the major studies that have been done on the benefit of statin drugs, you will see that very commonly the authors of the papers will have to disclose that they are getting paid by the statin makers. Actually, in several instances it has been proven that the studies were written by the pharmaceutical companies and the doctors just put their names on them, having never seen the paper prior to attaching their names. So it's tainted research. If you look at the actual research on atherosclerosis, it's saying just the opposite of what all the clinical studies are interpreted as saying.

Atherosclerosis is an inflammatory disease; if you want to stop it, stop inflammation. Here's the secret of statins I wrote about years ago . . . the only reason a statin reduces heart attacks at all is because it's an anti-inflammatory. It's an immune suppressant. It has nothing to do with lowering cholesterol. We know this because other drugs that do not lower cholesterol, but reduce inflammation, reduce heart attack risk even more than statins.

If you want to prevent and reverse atherosclerosis, there are a lot of natural anti-inflammatories that are far better than statins and far safer: curcumin and quercetin, pomegranate extract, garlic extract, omega-3 oils, extra-virgin olive oil, vitamin E with high gamma E tocopherol, tocotrienol, and vitamin C. The preceding are powerful antioxidants that prevent excessive blood coagulation, reduce inflammation, block excitotoxicity, detox toxins, and, as a result, are inhibitors of atherosclerosis. Ellagic acid, as found in pomegranate extract, is one of the powerful flavonoids known to not only prevent atherosclerosis but also reverse it.

Ellagic acid as a natural product is not harmful, but of course the pharmaceutical industry would rather sell you a toxic drug that is also a powerful immune suppressant, one that increases cancer and leads to brain degeneration.

SS: We've talked about this before and I know from experience, even in the light of reading this, most people have such fear of going against Western medicine that they probably will take Lipitor or one of the other similar statins anyway.

RB: People have been taking them for the last twenty years and yet the incidence of heart attacks and stroke has not decreased until recently when the doctors started recommending coQ_{10}, but the entire time they were just on statins there was no decrease in the death rate from heart attacks and strokes.

SS: If a person is taking a statin and coQ_{10}, then is that person protected from inflammation?

RB: Yes, but at the risk of chronic immune suppression, which increases their risk of infections of all types and cancer.

Look at Bill Clinton: He had a heart attack and his doctor put him on a statin; he had another heart attack and he was put on more statins. The doctors raised his statin level and he still has heart disease. And now he's not taking supplements because he's been advised they are no good. He thinks being on a vegan diet is going to save him. But now there's the danger of being B_{12} deficient and deficient in amino acids without sufficient protein, which will cause a whole host of other problems.

SS: What happens when a person is B_{12} and amino deficient?

RB: These deficient amino acids are called *essential* amino acids, because the body cannot manufacture them from other metabolic products (such as sugars). These make the building blocks of cells and tissues as well as enzymes. The B_{12} deficiency is associated with a high incidence of heart disease, and this is because it leads to high levels of homocysteine. Homocysteine is an excitotoxin and breaks down further into even more excitotoxins. Excitotoxins can cause atherosclerosis (blood vessels have a number of glutamate receptors). B_{12} deficiency also leads to extreme fatigue and weakness.

SS: So the answer to plaque in the arteries is to take curcumin (turmeric), quercetin, ellagic acid, and omega-3 fish oil, plus eat a good diet?

RB: And avoid chemicals, processed foods, and cut out the sugar.

SS: Okay, next I want to talk to you about something you said about the dumbing down of Americans. What did you mean? Is there a sinister plot?

RB: There is a book called *The Molecular Vision of Life* written by a scientist, Lily E. Kay; it chronicles the history of molecular biology in the United States. It all started with the fundamental idea that elites felt they needed to socially engineer society, the theory being that most people are too stupid to take care of themselves and that they (the elites) needed to be the ones who design society. They were the money and the force behind the eugenics movement back in the '20s and '30s. Rockefeller was one of the leaders of this movement who believed they needed to control society because they knew best. This author had access to the Rockefeller family's archives and found that these elites had purchased pharmaceutical companies and then changed the curriculum in medical schools so as to emphasize pharmaceutical treatments of disease. They did this by funding what is known as the Flexner Report.

SS: This is where they sent Abraham Flexner to offer financial incentives in perpetuity to medical schools and universities to teach only allopathic.

RB: Correct. That is when they were able to get rid of all instruction concerning nutrition and only teach about pharmaceutical medicines. Cold Spring Harbor Laboratory was one of the major ones, but also Caltech was another big center, and then the University of Chicago joined in along with Johns Hopkins and others. Rockefeller made sure all professors appointed as heads of departments and presidents of universities were in agreement with their philosophy. They were all eugenicists; they all thought that science should be redesigning humanity so only perfect people could exist. Everybody else would be weeded out.

SS: Sounds very Hitler-ish.

RB: Actually, Hitler heard about this and sent his people over to be trained in the theories. Also, emissaries were sent to Hitler's Germany to learn his techniques. This is all documented.

It used to be that John D. Rockefeller was anathema. Nobody ever wanted to admit they knew him because he was so unscrupulous. He had a friend who advised him that to remove the black mark against his name he should start being philanthropic: build museums and give money to educational institutions. Rockefeller did this and it worked. He became respected.

SS: I guess you could say this is a brilliant business template . . . if you own pharmaceutical companies, and create what is now our sole approach to medicine, then you are going to sell a lot of drugs.

RB: Right, then eugenics started to backfire. Because of Hitler's actions, the world suddenly realized that people like Hitler were sick monsters. So Rockefeller told his people never to use the word "eugenics" again. Instead he called it "social engineering" or the "new man," and that was when he hit on the idea of molecular science or molecular biology based on new studies coming out of science laboratories. Then Rockefeller poured huge amounts of money into major medical universities to set up departments of molecular biology, which would use eugenics to accomplish the same thing; that is, create genetically perfect people and weed out those who were not perfect.

SS: What was the big idea behind all this and how are we affected today?

RB: By dulling down people, we won't be paying attention to what the elites are doing. Look at how people are ignoring fluoride, formaldehyde, and pesticides, herbicides, and GM food. People have their heads in the sand about toxins in general, and look what is happening. Sickness is everywhere. Cancer is soon to be the biggest killer in the world; the number of autoimmune diseases are climbing drastically; and debilitating conditions not only abound but are occurring at an earlier age. When traditional medicine practitioners are asked why? they just shrug their shoulders.

SS: I say this over and over . . . connect the dots. But you think this is a sinister plot?

RB: I think the original idea has gotten out of control and now we are all at risk. It's really all a matter of worldview. Historian Eric Voegelin has shown that the idea that has captured the world is one that sees a handful of elites as the ones who should design society and move people about as if they were chess pieces. This worldview began as gnosticism. The great mass murders of the twentieth century were engineered by men who held this worldview—Lenin, Marx, Hitler, Mussolini, and Mao. Others were less bold and carried this idea out much more subtly and with a scientific flair. Most people I speak with don't want to know the realities of what is really going on. They just want to play tennis, watch sports events, and play with their electronic devices.

SS: Okay. So what should we do?

RB: Here's the reality: Supplementation alone is not the basis of good health; it is diet and exercise that matter most. Supplementation can improve the odds if there exists a severe deficiency, or if one's underlying problem is inflammation. You have to build your health on a good foundation. Your foundation is a good clean life:

- Make good friends.
- Concentrate on your spiritual life.
- Engage in regular exercise.
- Do mental exercises.
- Try to eat organic foods.
- Avoid the major toxins.
- Cut down omega-6 fats dramatically.
- Increase your omega-3 fats substantially.
- Consume meats from animals that are fed grasses and have no antibiotics or growth hormones.

If you do all this, you will return to times when people lived a very long life.

SS: Can we live a long time and still have a brain that is working well? After all, you are a brain scientist. You would know.

RB: There are actual studies that show once you reach age ninety-two, your body doesn't age anymore. The brain will last if you follow the basics: don't drink to excess, don't smoke, try to keep your spirits up, and keep a strong family and good friendships. Most elderly today look terrible; they are incredibly frail, they have thin, transparent skin, broken and bruised, with red watery eyes. So even though we have medicines and technology that can force them to live longer, they become very frail quite early in life and as a result, they are chronically ill. The human brain has the potential to work efficiently well past the age of one hundred.

SS: And of course supplementation is important?

RB: Yes, as part of the program, to handle the toxic burden and aging in general, your body needs more than it can get from diet only. You want to take higher doses of vitamin C. I generally recommend 1,000 mg three times a day taken between meals, so as to prevent excessive iron absorption.

SS: That's a lot.

RB: Vitamin C is a potent stimulant for absorption of iron. As you age your body accumulates iron, which is a powerful generator of free radicals. Iron also plays a major role in cancer development and degeneration of tissues. You don't want to increase your iron absorption, which is why it is important to take the vitamin C between meals. This is well researched.

I also recommend two kinds of vitamin E as a mixed tocopherol with a high gamma E component. Tocopherol is what vitamin E is made of and it has four components: alpha, beta, gamma, and delta. Tocopherol is a chemical name. Gamma is the only one that's been shown to have anti-inflammatory properties. Tocotrienol is also part of vitamin E and it has four different parts: alpha, beta, gamma, and delta. Tocotrienol is a very potent cancer inhibitor and protector of the brain. So if you take both, it's important to take them at different times of the day. The usual dose of mixed tocopherols is 400 IU twice a day and 50 mg to 100 mg of the mixed tocotrienols.

Also, coQ_{10}, nanosized coQ_{10}, 100 mg daily, because nanosizing breaks the molecules down into a much smaller size so that you absorb a lot higher levels. A lot of the studies originally were done on coQ_{10} and found that 600 mg is the most effective dose for protection of the brain, heart, and other organs. It is also a potent cancer inhibitor, and research on lab rats implanted with human tumors as well as humans with widespread cancer metastases demonstrated that if you supplemented them with coQ_{10} they lived a lot longer.

Vitamin D_3, 10,000 IU daily, has also shown to be life extending for some cancer patients. When researchers looked at cancer patients, many of them had very low vitamin D_3 levels, and in particular patients with the worst kind of brain cancer, glioblastoma, yet a number of the people in this study lived three to five years after their diagnosis, which is significant. Then there's curcumin, 500 mg to 1,000 mg three times a day. This is an extract of turmeric and has a profound effect on inhibiting cancer. It is a powerful antioxidant, and the actual level needed to protect the brain is very small, which includes protection from Alzheimer's and Parkinson's. One of the major problems is the poor absorption of curcumin from the gut. Dissolving curcumin in olive oil increases the absorption capabilities, and several brands of high absorption are available—such as the Super Bio-Curcumin from the Life Extension Foundation.

SS: I take turmeric, mixed with olive oil, and rub it all over chicken and then roast or bake it and it makes the most delicious-tasting chicken.

RB: If you prefer to take it as a liquid or to mix it with your food, mix one tablespoon of extra-virgin olive oil with 500 mg to 1,000 mg

of curcumin. Take it three times a day. Curcumin stimulates emptying of the gallbladder and is a very powerful protector of the liver. It
also stimulates detoxification enzymes in the liver. It is being extensively tested against a number of cancers, including pancreatic cancer, and the results are dramatic.

SS: Cancer doctor Nick Gonzalez is a big proponent of olive oil
to stimulate emptying of the gallbladder and protecting the liver.
Can you substitute turmeric in olive oil and get the same results?

RB: Curcumin is the active component in turmeric. The spice
turmeric itself contains only about 6 percent to 8 percent curcumin.
It's a remarkable supplement. People are living longer and Alzheimer's is a big concern. Curcumin supplements are protective, but they
also interact with other important supplements to enhance their effectiveness; for example, as with resveratrol, quercetin, ellagic acid.
Together, they are quite potent.

SS: Curcumin is also an inhibitor for something called mTOR.
What is mTOR?

RB: This is what we call a *cell-signaling molecule,* whose job it is to
transfer information inside cells—like a messenger service. This molecule, mTOR, which stands for "mammalian target of rapamycin,"
regulates protein synthesis.

If mTOR is overactive, you won't live very long. If you inhibit it,
you not only inhibit cancer but will live much longer. So this simple
supplement protects against cancer and lengthens life span. Curcumin
targets cancer cells, and like a magic bullet it causes cancer cells to die
but protects against cell damage caused by chemotherapy.

SS: That is an incredible statement. What drug can do that?

RB: None that I am aware of. If a patient is taking chemotherapy,
it dramatically improves the effectiveness of the chemotherapy while
at the same time protecting normal cells and tissues from chemo
damage. It also protects the brain from chemotherapy damage.

I have a doctor friend whose wife had stage IV breast cancer. It
had spread to her bones, liver, and elsewhere. Her oncologist said
she wouldn't live but a few months at best. Her husband, a cancer
researcher, put her on curcumin, high concentrations, and it's been
fifteen years, she's alive and doing well. She stopped the chemotherapy also.

SS: Well, you suggested curcumin to my girlfriend, Susie, who
has lung cancer and I notice she has no brain loss at all; sharp as a tack.
We both agree the curcumin was vital.

RB: Anyone having radiation would also be well protected from damage by taking curcumin. This is especially important if you insist on getting yearly mammograms or you require diagnostic x-rays or a CT scan.

SS: A lot of my friends are being diagnosed with breast cancer, mostly DCIS. What do you think is causing it?

RB: Most likely pesticides and industrial chemicals; it could also be from their makeup, which has parabens, benzene, toluene, and other carcinogens. A lot of those chemicals get concentrated in the breast ductal tissues because special enzymes concentrate these toxins to dangerous levels locally. Also, women need to understand that cancer loves sugar.

SS: That's a problem for menopausal women because low estrogen makes you crave sugar.

RB: Yes, and it's difficult to make people understand that cancer will starve to death if you have no sugar of any kind in your diet.

I recently found a case report in a medical journal of a man with an advanced pancreatic cancer. After a short time on curcumin, one of the man's tumors shrunk 75 percent. As long as the patient stayed on curcumin, the tumor did not grow. What is interesting about this is that he was receiving a small dose because they didn't use olive oil to enhance absorption. So if it was that powerful against pancreatic cancer in a small dose, imagine if it was used with olive oil to enhance absorption. Researchers found that curcumin protects against every kind of cancer they've tested: the leukemias, lymphomas, multiple myelomas, and pancreatic, breast, and brain cancers.

The third important thing to know is that once you develop cancer, you must avoid all glutamate, which includes MSG. Most processed foods contain some form of hidden glutamate, such as caseinate, natural flavoring, hydrolyzed protein, soy protein isolate, autolyzed yeast, et cetera. Tumors have extensive glutamate receptors on their membranes, and studies have shown that glutamate stimulates the growth, and even more important, the invasion of the cancer. If you deny the tumor glutamate, its growth is significantly slowed.

SS: What foods have glutamates?

RB: Red meats. It doesn't matter if it is grass fed or not, plus the iron in red meat is a potent stimulus for cancer growth. Some designers of cancer treatments have used iron chelators with great effectiveness against cancer. It binds the iron so the cancer can't use it.

Curcumin also binds iron in tissues so cancers can't use it to grow, but allows you to have normal functional use of your iron.

SS: What other foods?

RB: You'll be surprised to know, tomatoes. If you pureed a tomato, it releases a fair amount of glutamate; also soybeans and mushrooms—portobello and mushrooms in general have a lot of glutamate. That's why they taste so good, so you have to avoid them if you don't want to stimulate your cancer's growth and invasion. Cheeses also have a lot of glutamate, especially Parmesan cheese. Soy, as stated earlier, also has relatively high glutamate content.

SS: But again, women feel soy is cancer protective.

RB: Studies have found that soy makes breast cancer grow faster because it is a powerful stimulant for aromatase, an enzyme that stimulates cancer growth. Also, the glutamate and the fluoride in the soy stimulate cancer growth.

SS: Does that include soy sauce?

RB: Yes. Soy sauce is also extremely high in glutamate.

SS: It's a bummer about tomatoes.

RB: A whole tomato is fine, because if you eat a whole tomato, it releases the glutamate very slowly and most of it is used up by your muscles.

Again, curcumin is the best protection of all for cancer as it inhibits cancer at every stage; it's a powerful preventive. If you take curcumin, quercetin, ellagic acid, and resveratrol and avoid sugar, your chance of developing cancer falls dramatically. And if you do develop cancer, it's going to be a lot more benign than if you eat a typical Western diet. What people don't realize is that they can change the aggressiveness of cancer through these powerful supplements.

If a patient continues to have a bad diet and consume a lot of omega-6 fats, he or she will stimulate a very aggressive cancer.

Diet does make a difference, but you never hear oncologists talk about nutrition. When I was in medical school and residency training, nutrition was never part of any protocol.

SS: Up until I began with alternative Western doctors, I never once in all my life had a doctor advise me about nutrition. Okay, let's talk about the obesity epidemic and health.

RB: I am absolutely convinced that obesity is due to the high level of excitotoxin additives in foods, particularly when fed to small children. These chemicals produce lesions in the brain that in lab animals produce gross obesity and metabolic syndrome. Until adults stop feeding children soy products and the high level of glutamates found in other foods, we will be plagued by this obesity problem. I strongly suggest getting rid of high fructose corn syrup as well. I would also reduce the massive sugar intake seen today among our youth, which greatly compounds the obesity caused by glutamate. Feeding animals glutamate makes them prefer high-carbohydrate diets and sugar. I would encourage children to eat healthier food. The problem is that these poorly nutritious foods are full of glutamates (which taste scrumptious) and sugar and that's all kids want once they taste it.

I tell my patients, don't eat corn oil and safflower oil and it's not just when you are cooking at home; it's in all the commercial baked goods. Chips like Doritos are cooked in it. Most people are consuming massive amounts of these harmful oils, which are known to accelerate degeneration of the brain, possibly contributing to the degeneration seen with Alzheimer's and Parkinson's disease. They're known to worsen heart failure and damage the liver and kidneys. They produce atherosclerosis and lead to cancer by triggering inflammation throughout the body. If you have cancer, these oils will make it grow much faster and become more invasive—that is, more likely to spread (metastasize). Canola oil is no better; it's a mixture of omega-6 and omega-3 oils and it's polyunsaturated. Like omega-6 oils, canola oil is easily oxidized and has been shown to promote cancer growth. One should never cook in canola oil.

SS: There's a lot of talk about the benefits of coconut oil.

RB: Yes, it's fine because it's saturated, so you can cook with it. You can also put turmeric in with the coconut oil and it protects both the coconut and olive oil from oxidizing. It is best to use extra-virgin coconut oil and extra-virgin olive oil. The unprocessed olive oil is best. It should be made from fresh olives and made by a cold press process. Heat destroys some of its protective compounds.

SS: Do you feel hopeful about the future?

RB: I fear that people are distracted, and they have been dumbed down from all the chemicals they are exposed to, as well as the ever-growing number of vaccines and poor dietary choices. But there is hope because here, and in many foreign countries, people are starting to figure out the flaws in the traditional medical system. They are getting fed up and frustrated with an increasingly cold and uncaring system, which treats them as ignorant children. I hear a lot of complaints about doctors becoming more arrogant. People are not getting well, and the medications they take often do not work and make them sicker. What those of us who study natural healing methods are trying to do to improve health is backed up by hard science.

For many years, alternative medicine was associated with health food stores and girls wearing prairie dresses. Now we're as legitimate as so-called traditional medicine and I believe more so because our science often is much better. In the past, traditional medicine relied heavily on natural treatments.

What people don't yet understand is that we have the capacity to cure most of the really bad diseases in our society, such as type 2 diabetes, which could disappear tomorrow with dietary changes and the use of a few supplements. Cancer rates would drop 70 to 80 percent if we utilized what we have learned from our research. Degenerative disorders would be reduced if people would just do the simple things we've talked about in this interview. Many don't understand the enormous impact of these dietary changes and supplements. By making the changes we've spoken about here, we can far exceed what present orthodox medicine can offer, especially for chronic degenerative diseases. Heart disease would be drastically reduced. Science is now finding that almost all diseases go back to chronic inflammation, everything: heart disease, cancer, degenerative brain disorders, kidney failure, diabetes. All these conditions and diseases have as a central mechanism inflammation, and guess who has the best weapons against chronic inflammation? Alternative medicine!

While traditional medicine is excellent in treating acute disorders, it has a dismal record in treating chronic disorders. Very few of their drugs address inflammation in a safe way at all. We have the most powerful weapons against chronic inflammation. We are now learning that even diseases related to genes can be altered, that our diets can turn off harmful genes and turn on beneficial genes. It goes back to genes being turned on that produce chronic inflammation. It's changed the entire spectrum of what we used to think. It's not about genetic predispositions; it's about turning on other genes that nullify that negative effect.

SS: What about our thoughts? Can we heal ourselves by thinking good thoughts?

RB: Absolutely. Your attitude can change genetic switches as well. With prayer, diet, and exercise, we can see dramatic effects on our health.

SS: So there is hope for humanity as far as health is concerned?

RB: Yes, by educating the public. We are fighting the forces of these enormous pharmaceutical companies and their influence with the media and medical universities. Every year I lecture to doctors, many of whom are specialists, and they tell me that much of the information I share with them from research studies is material they have never heard of before. For many, it has opened up their eyes to new ways of looking at human health. So that's hopeful; if we can educate the doctors, it will go a long way in turning around the toxic problem.

SS: Thank you for enlightening all of us.

RB: My pleasure, Suzanne. I appreciate all you do, and you do a tremendous amount. You are a leading voice out there.

SS: Well, I couldn't do it without you.

CHAPTER 12

BOMBSHELL #8:
THE NATURAL, EFFECTIVE
ALTERNATIVE TO BYPASS SURGERY

Chemicals have replaced bacteria and viruses as the main threat
to human health ... The diseases we are beginning to see as the
major causes of death in the latter part of this century and into
the twenty-first century are diseases of chemical origin.

—Rick Irvin, Texas A&M University

If you have any expectations of living longer and healthier, then waking up to and accepting the horrifying effects of toxic contamination
is a must. Dr. Blaylock just laid out the effects of the toxic assault,
and it is clear that the answer for adverse effects of pesticides and
chemicals is not more toxic drugs. In this chapter, Dr. Garry Gordon
will explain ways of detoxing so that we can win the fight against
this environmental assault. Recently a report came out that making
even a small effort to reduce home and garden use of pesticides provides potential benefits, including lowering the incidence of cancers
(including leukemia), as well as lessening cognitive disturbances and
disturbed behavior.

Dr. Gordon explains the benefits of preventing toxicity by utilizing oral and IV chelators such as high-dose vitamin C, fiber, zeolite,
and daily greens throughout life. Sadly, toxicity is not going away.
You have to wage your own war, and as the toxins come in, you must
know how to get them out.

Organic food will provide substantial benefits. It is tragic that one out of four children is on drug treatment for some illness—including autism, ADHD, OCD, cancer, hypertension, obesity, and diabetes—by the time they start school. When did we become so complacent? Why aren't we terrified that our children are so affected by toxins that these stats exist? As adults we are climbing uphill relative to our own personal toxic burdens. We are accepting cancer, autoimmune diseases, brain fog, bone deterioration, and general lack of energy as part of aging. Sadly, you are being done in by the chemicals, drugs, pesticides, and poor-quality contaminated food. The body requires fuel to operate, and it requires top-octane fuel at that.

As you have just read in Dr. Blaylock's interview, and now as you will hear from Dr. Gordon, you can fight this assault. It is definitely not hopeless. In fact, you can create perfect, optimum health in spite of the damaged planet if you involve yourself and your family in the changes and protocols advised in this book. Remember, no one is ever going to care as much about your body as you, and no one will be sorrier than you if in the end the chemicals win.

To live a long healthy life with quality, it's past time we look toxicity in the eye. The chemicals are not going to go away, at least not in our lifetimes. But we can win the fight against toxins and secure the health of our bodies with commitment and determination. If you are one of the ones who gets sick in the end, you will wish you'd taken this seriously.

Dr. Gordon is loaded with enthusiasm. He is for hire as a consultant if you so wish, but just reading his interview here will inspire and teach you to find his methods on your own. His supreme protocol is chelation, a method not understood and widely dismissed by establishment medicine. Chelation cleans the blood of heavy metals and toxins. Why is that controversial? It requires no drugs. It can be done by IV at your antiaging doctor's office or by oral supplements. But read on, he will explain it much better.

GARRY GORDON, M.D., D.O.

Dr. Garry Gordon *is an internationally recognized expert on chelation therapy and antiaging medicine. He is also a consultant for various supplement companies and the coauthor of* The Chelation Answer, *and he lectures extensively on the topic "The End of Bypass Surgery Is in Sight." He is on the board of the Homeopathic Medical Examiners for Arizona, is cofounder of ACAM (the American College for Advancement in Medicine), and a board member of the International Oxidative Medicine Association. He received his Doctor of Osteopathy in 1958 from the Chicago College of Osteopathy in Illinois and completed his radiology residency at Mt. Zion in San Francisco in 1964. He was the medical director of Mineral Lab in Hayward, California, a leading laboratory for trace mineral analysis worldwide. He does telephone consultations for patients from around the world, offering second opinions on any type of health issue, from his offices in Arizona. Dr. Garry Gordon is dedicated and passionate about educating doctors and patients about the harmful and devastating effects of environmental pollution, and he provides documented alternatives for any health condition. He wants everyone to feel as good as he does at age seventy-six, having restored himself to optimal health in spite of suffering from serious illnesses for most of the first thirty years of his life, including genetic heart disease.*

SS: Thanks for your time, Dr. Gordon. What troubles you about people's health today?

GG: I am troubled that none of us are reaching our full potential. I am troubled that we are passing down to our children diseases and conditions that will keep them from realizing a full, happy, and healthy life. I am troubled how we as a people are losing our personal freedoms, and rights to our health, and how we are becoming enslaved by our governments and global corporations out of greed. There are so many breakthrough therapies and treatments for illnesses and disease that do not involve taking harmful drugs, yet we don't hear much about those things because finding a natural cure or an actual effective treatment doesn't make money.

My life's work is about giving everybody the opportunity to achieve health and realize their full life's potential. The more people we get feeling as good as I feel, the more people will understand that it's simpler than what orthodox medicine has made it out to be. With my detox program, I have witnessed people who were always very negative about change becoming much more positive. My program is an approach to life that is healthy, teaching people to take personal responsibility for their own health, appreciating it, respecting their bodies, and understanding the need for seriously taking proper care of it.

We have the knowledge today to live a far healthier life for many more years than most of us dream possible. I get true joy from helping people heal and seeing them get their energy and vibrancy back. It's all possible—that's the great part. I did it for myself and was able to change the course and quality of my life. It is possible to live a long healthy life in spite of the toxicity, but you have to know how to do it. That's what I like to do for my patients.

SS: Well, that's what I want you to tell us. How are we going to survive? You emphasize chelation, and I suspect it plays a huge part in the detoxification of the body. In fact, you are known as the "father of chelation." It is a treatment that is really not well understood. Can you explain its importance relative to detoxification and why it is so healing and useful for a healthy and a long life?

GG: My pleasure, Suzanne. Chelation is a natural process without which life would not go on. In other words, if our bodies didn't chelate the iron in our red blood cells, we would die rapidly.

Unfortunately, today we have so many toxins built up in our bodies that we are unable to detox naturally, as we've said. Chronic preventable diseases are now the world's leading cause of mortality. In today's toxic world, where no one is safe from toxins and environmental pollutants, the ability of the body to detoxify is extremely essential to one's health. Toxins damage the immune system and inhibit our natural ability to heal. Toxins are the single most common underlying factor contributing to *all* diseases.

Chelation therapy is a detoxifying process used to rid the body of poisonous toxins and heavy metals like arsenic, lead, and mercury or organic pollutants like BPA, PBDEs, Teflon, dioxins, and pesticides. We use a chelating agent, EDTA, a synthetic amino acid that binds to and traps the toxin, causing it to become inert while it is safely excreted from the body.

SS: Sounds like something everyone needs to do, knowing we are under such a tremendous toxic assault. Tell me how you came to learn about chelation.

GG: I became interested in chelation therapy because I was very ill for the first thirty years of my life. As a young man, I had not been able to be athletic in any way. In fact, I was never allowed to participate in physical education or sports because I had a significant heart issue—I was born with a congenital heart condition called an AV conduction block. I also suffered from total achlorhydria with associated malabsorption, leading to dangerous mineral deficiencies, including magnesium deficiency, and was toxic with mercury poisoning from dental fillings. With all these issues, I suffered from chronic disabling fatigue and could not even swim one lap in a standard swimming pool. At age twenty-nine, I was so ill I had to stop practicing medicine. Then I discovered chelation therapy and it dramatically improved my health after I received only the first eight IV chelation treatments. Because of that experience, I decided to make detoxification and chelation my life's focus. Suzanne, my health improved so much I was literally able to run up the side of a mountain, gaining two thousand feet of elevation over a distance of two miles, without collapsing! But I did wear out my two-year-old Irish setter who was with me. Chelation helped turn me into Superman.

My vision was that if I could learn how this therapy worked, I could help teach it to other doctors, who would then offer it to their patients, and then everyone could enjoy the amazing benefits I have experienced. Beginning with this first personal breakthrough, I have gone on to discover and review over seven thousand published articles on EDTA, have cofounded ACAM, and have literally helped thousands of patients worldwide to avoid bypass surgery and heal from a myriad of chronic illnesses through detoxification—and that's how I became known as the father of chelation. We even have a $29 million NIH-funded five-year study, known as the TACT study, Trial to Assess Chelation Therapy, going on now to assess my treatment. It's not only detoxification that is necessary in today's world;

we also have to replace the lost minerals, so our bodies have the components necessary to rebuild and maintain health.

When I was a young doctor, I went to a bariatric conference to hear a lecture on trace minerals by John Miller, Ph.D., a former chief of research for Roerig and Pfizer pharmaceuticals. At that time he was the editor in chief of *Chemical Abstracts*, which is one of the most prestigious chemical journals in the world. He had developed the first mineral/vitamin combination, which probably doesn't seem extraordinary, but until he did this it was thought that minerals could not be packaged along with vitamins because they might cause interactions and lead to exploding jars in the pharmacies.

Dr. Miller demonstrated how a garden could have mineral deficiencies, leading to unhealthy produce, which is more subject to crop diseases. After determining the soil mineral deficiencies, and replenishing the soil with the needed minerals, extremely disease-resistant crops could be raised. However, the minerals needed to be chelated first, possibly with some amino acids, to alter their charge. That avoids toxicity to the plant. He demonstrated that as a result you could have large, healthy, award-winning flowers, and he demonstrated huge roses that were opening on a snowy day in Chicago.

SS: So from an understanding about gardening and mineral deficiencies, and your personal experience with chelation, you put two and two together?

GG: Yes. Dr. Miller's lecture started me thinking. I decided to work with Dr. Miller and use his concept of testing soil for deficiencies and adding the needed chelated minerals. My brother and I had a 440-acre "ranch" in Northern California. We wanted to raise livestock, but had been told by the Department of Agriculture that the land would not support even one goat per acre or support any meaningful crops. The only thing that was growing there was manzanita on the old gold mining property, and a resinous creeping ground cover called "bear clover," or mountain misery, neither of which was considered very commercially useful.

But by applying Dr. Miller's approach of improving soil by determining mineral deficiencies, my brother and I turned our land into a veritable park! We were able to grow alfalfa deep enough to support a large herd of Black Angus cattle. So I decided to utilize these same principles in treating my patients. I started doing mineral analysis of hair, blood, and urine. These tests established not only the mineral deficiencies, but I also discovered that excessive amounts of toxins such as lead and mercury were found in almost all my patients. So, although adding things like zinc and magnesium is often a vital step toward optimizing health for anyone, I soon realized that adding good minerals to the body would only have a limited benefit.

SS: What do you mean?

GG: I mean, if the body continues to be poisoned by lead, mercury, aluminum, cadmium, and other toxins, it limits the success of any nutritional support program. Finding toxic levels of heavy metals in most of my patients led me to understand that it was *essential*, for maximum benefit, not only to put minerals *in* the body but also to offer chelation therapy to remove the toxins *from* the body. Harvard does testing for lead levels in the bone, and through this we know that everyone born today has approximately a thousand times more lead in their bones than we had a few hundred years ago, before the industrial age poisoned our planet.

SS: The toxic assault is overwhelming . . . I truly fear for humanity. How do you remove these toxins? In other words, how does chelation work? I understand that there is oral chelation and IV chelation?

GG: Right, chelation can be done orally, which will do the job for almost everyone if the correct chelators are used for a long enough period of time. However, to deal with more acute poisoning, or for deeper initial cleansing, IV chelation is used. IV chelation is what helped me so much at age thirty. I was so sick I wound up ultimately taking nearly two hundred of these intravenous treatments. My continued research led me to conclude that we all can live far longer, and can eliminate most fatal heart attacks, by simply ingesting an oral EDTA-based nutritional program I call BC-I, which I'll explain in a bit. This is because we are being bombarded by toxins every day.

THERE IS NO SAFE LEVEL OF LEAD OR
MERCURY FOR THE HUMAN BODY.

SS: Is detoxification something we are all going to have to commit to do for the rest of our lives in order to combat the toxic burden we carry around?

GG: Yes, I believe it's necessary for everyone to commit to a life-time detoxification program. Bones take an average of fifteen years to remodel, and IV chelation will not pull the lead out of bones. Therefore, we must take protective steps *every day* to prevent the lead and other heavy metals stored in our bones and tissues from leaching into other tissues like our heart, brain, and eyes.

I worked with Dr. Lester Morrison, then director of the Institute for Arteriosclerosis Research in Loma Linda, California, on an answer to preventing heart attacks that would be all natural without using drugs such as Coumadin, Plavix, or aspirin. My oral chelation program is based on natural, safe blood thinning and continuously helps get lead out. We are constantly bombarded, because our environment is polluted through coal-burning emissions, waste incineration, mining operations, volcanic eruptions, and soil erosion, and then we take in toxins daily from our water, food, and air. Oral chelation helps to rid our bodies of toxic lead, while preventing more lead from getting in. At the same time it works synergistically along with the Morrison Institute Formula to eliminate fatal heart attacks and strokes. That is why I developed my chelating vitamin/mineral formula that is based upon Dr. Morrison's Institute Formula, but with EDTA added. It is called Beyond Chelation Improved, or BC-I, which is a regimen of nine capsules that includes three very powerful mineral/vitamin tablets and three Essential Daily Defense capsules—they are a combination of EDTA, garlic, and sulfated mucopolysaccharides from carrageenan—one omega-3 capsule, one 1,300 mg capsule of primrose oil, and one capsule containing ginkgo biloba and phosphatidylserine.

THIS FORMULA PROTECTS AGAINST DYING FROM HEART ATTACKS AND STROKES!

As a by-product, this same formula also helps maintain vision and memory, which is a nice side effect. If you do this program, you can expect to live long and healthy into old age.

SS: What about bones? . . . You mentioned that chelation therapy doesn't remove lead from bone. Can you explain a bit more?

GG: Chelation takes the lead out of your heart, kidneys, and soft tissues so you feel fantastically improved, but it doesn't remove lead from the bones. Even IV chelation with EDTA does not pull the lead from the bones, and as we are all excessively lead burdened from the day we are born, our bones can poison us just like welding or working with lead can. When bones start to thin, as they do when we are injured and unable to move about, or when menopause starts, lead is leached from our bones into our bodies, along with the calcium losses. That is why women at menopause often see blood pressure going up, as a direct result of lead being released from their bones.

SS: That's serious. If we can't get lead out of our bones, what can we do?

GG: It's a problem; getting the lead out of bones is a lifetime endeavor since everywhere on earth our water, food, and air give us more lead. That is why I never go a day without some kind of heavy metal chelator like the EDTA that I have in my BC-I to clean the blood. Vitamin C is a chelator, and also an active fiber, just as stabilized rice bran is a chelator. Other products are zeolite, garlic, DL methionine, organic vegetables, and sea greens. There are many natural substances found in our diet that can help; daily exercise is also vital, as without exercise bones thin and any bone loss is a real danger—not just fracture risk, but because lead is stored in bones, and if it gets released, it poisons our tissues and other organs.

SS: So keeping the blood clean keeps the lead in the bones and not released?

GG: Yes. Lead is known to be dangerous for everyone, and there are no safe levels. All causes of illness and death can be associated with levels of lead in the body, as reported in an article called "Low-Level Environmental Exposure to Lead Unmasked as Silent Killer," which was published in the American Heart Association journal *Circulation*.

It's a proven fact that the lead levels in our bodies are toxic and dangerous, yet there is little interest by mainstream medicine in lowering lead; instead traditional doctors have their patients brainwashed into covering up their symptoms by taking statins and other harmful drugs to lower their cholesterol. I do not use statins with any of my patients; instead I offer natural anti-inflammatories like curcumin. We know cholesterol is not the problem, so why risk the proven side effects, including increased incidence of diabetes that is reported as a result of statin therapy?

SS: I would imagine the statin/diabetes connection is due to the testosterone depletion from statin use. Low testosterone, according to Dr. Abraham Morgentaler, can cause diabetes.

GG: Yes, and we all know that the real problem with arteriosclerosis is inflammation and toxicity. I have not had a single patient die of arteriosclerosis in over ten years while taking my oral chelation formula twice a day. I have little interest in lowering my patients' cholesterol, since cholesterol is *essential* for all our cell membranes and maintaining healthy hormone function. Elevated cholesterol levels indicate an underlying problem, where the body is producing more of it as a protective measure. Lowering it or stopping the body's production is actually causing further harm.

SS: I hear this from doctor after doctor; that statins mask the problem until so much damage is done that the patient eventually experiences the catastrophic event.

GG: Correct. I recommend canceling stenting and bypass surgery on almost all my patients, as my background in radiology taught me that what looks like a serious obstruction in a blood vessel on the angiogram often has already made collateral vessels not visible on angiograms, so it's missed. Most cases do just as well with medications. I tell my patients that I feel they should cancel their heart surgery for blocked blood vessels and get on my program. My program has not harmed anyone, and it carries low to nil risk. We have documented improved blood flow in at least 85 percent of patients with IV chelation, and once patients are out of the woods and back to an active life without symptoms, they can go on my oral program. They have no need for any prescription blood thinners, even if they have skipped beats, arrhythmias, or even atrial fibrillation, and now with a new hydrogen supplement, many find their heart rhythms become rock solid over time.

SS: That is spectacular information, an all-natural way to clear out obstructions in the blood vessels! So many people my age are on blood thinners like Coumadin. What do you think of these drugs?

GG: Patients with arrhythmias are usually told that they must take anticlotting drugs like Coumadin. Anyone on Coumadin needs to know that it is rat poison.

SS: Really?

GG: Yes, really. They need to learn the published side effects, like bleeding into the brain and calcification of blood vessels. The number of people admitted to the hospital with bleeding and other complications from using Coumadin makes it one of the most dangerous drugs prescribed by doctors. It is never needed by any of my patients who are on BC-I.

When I have someone on Coumadin, I always recommend that they switch to far safer and even more effective enzymes such as Boluoke (lumbrokinase), which helps the body break down and digest blood clots safely. This is an all-natural enzyme extracted from a Chinese earthworm and it specifically targets fibrins in the blood. Another similar and beneficial enzyme called nattokinase, is derived from fermented soy that the Japanese call Natto. Nattokinase is a slightly weaker alternative to Boluoke, but it is effective and more affordable. I put all my patients on EDTA and my BC-I regimen so they are getting the anticlotting effects. It was proven in research that came out in the 1960s that the ingredients in my BC-I were more than adequate to stop most fatal heart attacks.

Today we live in an even more polluted world due to hundreds of new power plants in China, plus toxic dusts from the wars overseas, and these toxins and pollutants are still blowing all around the atmosphere. With the added pollution from this and other sources, the nutritionally depleted, pesticide-ridden foods we consume today, and the increased stressors we all deal with, I feel that if patients can afford to add either nattokinase or Boluoke to my basic BC-I program, then they have moved from 90 percent protection against fatal heart attacks or strokes to more than 98 percent protection.

Dr. Roger Bick, a pathologist at the University of Texas and author of the definitive medical textbooks on blood clotting, has lectured at my conferences, stating conclusively that statins were useless because people die of blood clots at least in 85 percent of all vascular deaths, so lowering cholesterol is not as important as they pretend, unless it is oxidized cholesterol, where the antioxidants we put in BC-I are helping.

SS: What about the benefits of turmeric (curcumin) as an antioxidant and anti-inflammatory?

GG: Turmeric is a powerful anti-inflammatory, and it is also included in my BC-I formula along with vitamin K_2, which helps lower the levels of calcium in the arteries. Vitamin K_2 is so valuable that when patients take 90 mcg of it daily, I no longer need to keep them on my standard three-hour IV chelation protocol that I developed thirty-five years ago when I cofounded ACAM, although that chelation protocol has had an amazing track record and has safely helped many, many patients avoid heart surgery, strokes, even amputations.

But now that we have vitamin K_2 to help us have strong bones and soft arteries, even when patients are old, they can change from the three-hour recommended treatment time for IV chelation to a five-minute treatment time by using *calcium* EDTA instead of sodium EDTA. This approach is even better for lowering lead levels in the body, and it has the advantage that it is painless.

SS: Well, and frankly, most people don't have three hours to spend in a doctor's office having regular IVs.

GG: Right, and we no longer need to do that. IV chelation treatments do help give a deeper cleansing. The IV treatment is all absorbed, while oral is only 5 to 15 percent absorbed, but since we can take it twice a day for life, this is a great preventive approach and enough to save lives. Also, the oral approach helps millions who cannot locate a chelation doctor in their area. The older three-hour chelation treatment has helped thousands of patients, and it is still the preferred method if you have seriously calcified tissues.

However, I believe everyone today needs vitamin K_2, at least 90 mcg a day, if you hope to avoid the hardened, calcified arteries that we see in nearly everyone by age eighty. By this time in our lives, our aorta, which is the main blood vessel coming out of the heart, has turned to stone! We have, on average, 140 times more calcium in the aorta than was present at age ten, while at the same time our bones are getting weaker and losing calcium. Vitamin K_2 is one of the keys.

SS: What else can we do?

GG: Since my patients are not dying of heart attacks or strokes, they are going to be alive well into their eighties, when Alzheimer's can affect 50 percent of those over eighty-five. So I also include phosphatidylserine in the nine-pill BC-I packets, telling my patients that with phosphatidylserine, they will still be able to find my phone number when they are eighty-five. This provides an essential component of cell membranes, helping prevent age-related decline in mental function, and it even improves athletic performance.

Also I recommend my patients implement a one-to-one ratio of calcium to magnesium, not two-to-one as everyone else is using, which is too much calcium without enough magnesium. When you don't have enough magnesium, you will end up with more rapid pathologic accumulations of calcium in tissues, and hardened arteries lead to hypertension. Americans are taking far too much calcium, I advise at most 500 to 700 mg of calcium daily, but always with the same amount of magnesium to control the calcium.

SS: That's very interesting, because in my earlier years when I was taking calcium alone, I felt sick all the time. Then I added magnesium, and I felt great.

GG: Magnesium is essential to balance the calcium. Also, if you really study the American diet, people are getting more phosphorous than calcium. Now if you were to do that to horses or humans for very long, they will develop secondary hyperparathyroidism and that leads to abnormal calcification of the tissues. As an antiaging doctor, I know that by age eighty the average human aorta has a 140 times increase in calcium. It can be plainly seen on x-rays. As we age, our tissues are calcifying while we are losing the calcium from our bones. That is why I feel so strongly about preventing bone loss with the natural support of some form of bioidentical hormone therapy, which you have done such a good job of educating the public about, Suzanne.

SS: Thank you.

GG: I have found a plant in northern Thailand called *Pueraria mirifica*, or Thai kudzu, and it is from this plant that we make HRT. Plus, HRT stands for Herbal Remedy from Thailand, and *Pueraria mirifica* is the reason that northern Thailand has the lowest level of breast cancer in the world. It seems that this plant stops the proliferation of breast cancer cells because it acts as a SERM beta, or selective estrogen receptor modulator of the beta receptor, which stops bone loss and helps prevent heart disease and breast cancer at the same time. *Pueraria mirifica* is far more specific than soy or red clover for the estrogen receptor—and it is the *beta* receptor that we want to modulate to stop vaginal dryness, depression, insomnia, and bone loss, and it's even beneficial in maintaining a healthy prostate in men. It really is a miraculous healing herb. These natural products are key to my osteoporosis program, where I safely reverse osteoporosis with no drugs.

SS: Interesting; my oncologist, Julie Taguchi, wrote me about *Pueraria mirifica* recently as being important with my supplemental program, since I once had cancer. Now you are saying you are reversing osteoporosis. Is this because your supplementation program stimulates osteoblasts, which are what produces bone building and formation?

GG: Yes, along with other nutrients, such as aggressive doses of vitamins D and K$_2$, all work particularly well if used concurrently with my BC-I oral chelation formula. By constantly assisting the lead-removal processes of the body, we help bones and arteries restore their capacity to repair themselves. Today we have the ability to stop bone loss and prevent osteoporosis and the associated pathologic fractures in everyone, again without the need for prescription drugs.

SS: What else do you give your patients?

GG: I give garlic, which is vital for heart health. One form I recommend is Kyolic liquid garlic from Japan. They have done studies at UCLA proving it reverses arterial blockages in coronary vessels. A high-quality garlic is a major component for detoxing and heart protection, and garlic is one of the components included in my Essential Daily Defense (EDD) formula in my BC-I.

Also, I mentioned a sulfated mucopolysaccharide from carrageenan, which comes from a particular type of seaweed, and it looks to the body like heparin. It is a natural extract I incorporated to help prevent blood clotting, although it barely works alone, and for effectiveness, it must be used in concert with EDTA, which is also in my EDD formula. EDTA is so important to stop blood clotting. For example, in order to draw blood for a complete blood count, clotting must be prevented, so the tube used to draw the blood in every lab around the world contains a tiny amount of liquid EDTA in the bottom of the tube. It's in there for a reason . . . so the blood won't clot.

EDTA GETS THE LEAD OUT SO YOU CAN LIVE LONGER!

This BC-I formula is what I use to thin the blood instead of drugs like Coumadin, Plavix, or even aspirin, which kills over three thousand people a year due to internal bleeding. Those drugs are very weak at preventing fatal heart attacks, and they have so many negative side effects.

SS: Yet millions of people are taking these dangerous and harmful drugs blindly because their doctor says so. This is why I keep stressing with my readers . . . get informed! Take charge of your health. Learn how your body works! It's your body and it's your life! For instance, you mentioned aspirin, and I know many people think that taking some aspirin every day helps prevent heart attacks. Why do you believe otherwise?

GG: I believe aspirin gives people a false sense of security. Thirty percent of people do not get any antiplatelet effect from aspirin. It never was an anticoagulant, and the facts prove that it kills over three thousand people a year, so I don't like to use it. Experts agree not everyone should take aspirin, depending upon their current state of health, and to prove it, just listen to the rapid commercial disclaimers on TV; the dangers still exceed any tiny benefit.

SS: Methylation is a word that comes up again and again in my interviews. Why is it so key as one of the reasons that we age?

GG: Methylation is a key to detoxification, and to making new cells that are identical to the ones they are replacing. You want to live a long time, then you want to constantly detoxify your body; the high levels of toxins found in everyone today, such as bisphenol A, or BPA, have been shown by Randy Jirtle at Duke University to convert healthy lean brown mice, called *agouti mice*, into pale yellow, obese, and diabetic mice all within a single generation. Clearly, all these toxins are devastating to our health. This change is called an *epigenetic* change, meaning the genetics are changing in one generation, instead of the genetic changes that previously occurred over the course of many generations. Toxin-induced epigenetic changes disable certain genes, affect hormonal functions, and decrease the body's ability to deal with stress. Methyl-based nutrients, such as MSM (methylsulfanomethane) and TMG (trimethylglycine), help us overcome the impaired methylation processes we are seeing happen in so many today—all which lead to changes in our DNA and prevent the brain from properly handling stress. Methylation deficiencies are linked to heart disease, hypertension, obesity, depression, et cetera.

I find that when a child is not developing properly, or is suffering from seizures, he or she may need to be treated with a methyl form of folic acid. This particular form of folic acid is expensive, so it is not widely available and found in fewer than 1 percent of multiple vitamins. But recently the *New England Journal of Medicine* (*NEJM*) wrote about cerebral folate deficiency syndrome and that because of this deficiency children were experiencing serious neurological issues, including seizures. I've been saying this could happen for years.

SS: Must be frustrating to have to wait so long for mainstream medicine to catch up or catch on.

GG: It is frustrating, and the sad thing is that the usual blood tests doctors do for folic acid come out normal, so doctors fail to diagnosis and treat it properly.

SS: Why? Because they don't know what to look for?

GG: Yes, exactly. I recommend supplementing folic acid in a separate tablet called Beyond B_{12}. It's formulated with methyl B_{12}, and I have my patients take this in a sublingual tablet form with excellent results.

Now we have this *NEJM* study saying low levels of folic acid are only detectible in the cerebral spinal fluid. Well, who wants to remove spinal fluid from a child? We have determined that there is actually a problem with the folate receptors, which is why conditions like autism will finally become recognized as yet another toxicity-related, autoimmune disease. It's terrible . . . we have over a hundred of these conditions today; autoimmunity is epidemic, and I am referring not just to MS, lupus, or type 1 diabetes, but to hundreds of autoimmune-related conditions that specialists struggle to treat with dangerous expensive drugs that do little if anything to help.

SS: It's overwhelming, Garry . . . this book is to give my readers information on how to live longer with great health and to instill the seriousness of the damage being done to us by toxins of all sources. Toxins are the real enemy today, and if we want to live longer and healthier, we have to do whatever it takes to *detoxify*! Wars are going on around the world, yet here at home not many are noticing the real enemy and that we are being done in by this insidious killer. Like a night prowler, it gets in our food, our water, all the places you mention. People have to comprehend that we can no longer escape, that Western medicine is at a loss and doctors don't know what to do, and that detoxification is the only way we can save our lives.

GG: I agree. I developed my "F.I.G.H.T. for Your Health" program, as described in detail on my website, www.gordonresearch.com, to help deal with these conditions naturally, without all the dangerous drugs being used today that only ignore the causes and mask the symptoms.

We now have published research proving that the conditions created by toxicity are not being adequately treated with pharmaceutical drugs. Most people often only need competently prescribed nutritional therapy. The folate deficiency mentioned is just one of myriad conditions where methylation issues are involved, and in these types of conditions, drug therapy is generally useless. My F.I.G.H.T. program helps put MS, lupus, Parkinson's, autism, and other chronic conditions into remission almost all the time.

SS: What you say makes sense: clean out, detoxify, build up nutritionally, and change diet and lifestyle. But you see the answer seems too simple for most people to take seriously and certainly for the orthodox medical community. I believe at some point we have to realize that what we've been doing is just not working and that it's time to look in another direction.

You know that definition of insanity: If you keep banging your head against the wall and are getting no results, at some point you have to stop doing it or it's insane. That's what has been happening. We keep banging our heads over and over and over to the point of insanity. It has to stop. These diseases and conditions are impairing and paralyzing people's health and, sadly, in many cases killing them.

GG: Yes, it is insane. It goes on; there are many gene-related issues today that are being ignored, like the new gene test panel from Australia, called *smart DNA* (smartdna.net.au). For $425 you can be tested and have seventy-two genes interpreted. This test enables me to offer tomorrow's medicine today, and it helps me pinpoint issues such as this epidemic of methylation-related problems that are currently being observed in over 30 percent of all chronically ill patients.

We have the tools; these patients need a targeted supplement program, and the smart DNA gene test helps me to further personalize my F.I.G.H.T. program for my individual clients' health needs. I am able to provide proper treatment that helps them overcome these methylation issues. Without correct gene-based treatment, they will have a far lower level of health throughout their lives and possibly even impaired health for their children.

Unlike other mammals, humans do not make their own vitamin C. We need to get it from our food. Massive doses of 10 grams or more of oral vitamin C are needed daily to help overcome life-threatening conditions, and when treating very advanced or serious illnesses, in high enough doses, oral and or IV can be lifesaving.

SS: Vitamin C . . . another one of the pieces of advice that keeps popping up in my interviews. All of you are concerned about the inadequate levels of vitamin C.

GG: Yes, it's because we are living on a polluted, toxic planet. We have to help humans who wish to achieve their maximum life span and enjoy optimal health by offering meaningful information about toxins—where they come from, how to avoid them, and then how to lower the body burden of these substances that we all carry from birth. We must deal with the hundreds if not thousands of different toxins that affect us on hundreds of different levels. It's not just mercury and lead; toxins include other metals such as cadmium, arsenic, and uranium; fluorine; and *organic* substances including dioxins, PCBs, and many, many more toxins that are released into the environment and have subsequently been found in the human body.

Clearly we have poisoned our nest, and there is nowhere left to run. It was the Environmental Working Group that conducted a test called "Ten Americans" that showed no one is toxin-free no matter how well you try to live—even babies are acquiring toxins in their mothers' wombs. Because of the prohibitive cost of this test, many doctors ignore it and just prescribe drugs to control symptoms, which just makes you even more toxic and does nothing to deal with causes.

It's criminal; doctors prescribe drugs that the American Medical Association itself has admitted are now the fourth-leading cause of death in America. *Drugs are killing us and causing new diseases and conditions!*

SS: Imagine!

GG: It is sad that one out of four school-age children is taking a prescribed drug for some health conditions, even cancer.

I am extremely upset about this, because if we could just treat the underlying causes, we would have much less disease and suffering and death. We must always lower toxins, identify food sensitivities, find the hidden infections, treat with recommended protocols, and when needed, add some oxidative therapies like ozone, HBO, or UVB.

If we did this, all the dangerous drugs we are force-fed today would not be needed. Very often, once started on drugs like proton pump inhibitors or antidepressants, or painkillers and NSAIDs, there is almost *no way* to get off them. Patients become dependent on them, often for life.

SS: So what do people do?

GG: Use natural alternatives to drugs plus detoxification therapy.

SS: You often mention zeolite. What is it?

GG: Zeolite is a natural volcanic rock, and there are different grades or types used in a myriad of different ways—from water treatment to medicinal uses. I have located a highly micronized form with a quality so high it can be used for space travel, as the ultimate filter, to permit astronauts to recycle all fluids on a spaceship, including urine. Zeolite is a safe natural alternative to the chemical process of chelation that can even help handle toxins that chelation does not touch. Zeolite under magnification looks like a sponge or a honeycomb. The tiny holes, or cages, have a negative charge, and since toxins and harmful metals are positively charged molecules, the zeolite attracts them like a magnet. The toxins become caged within zeolite's honeycombed structure and are safely excreted from the body. People often see improvements in their health and the way they feel just after a few weeks. Often the dose of any drugs they are on can soon be lowered, and over time, many of the drugs would no longer be needed when the total body burden of all toxins is substantially lowered. With toxins being lowered, the body can start to heal itself and the conditions that required drugs are no longer needed.

SS: What about cancer and chelation? Is it effective?

GG: Chelation is essential for treating cancer. The American Medical Association's own literature states that all causes of morbidity and mortality are tied to low lead levels that are kept throughout life, and *JAMA* published the Harvard research showing the level of lead in bones determines how soon you go blind and also how soon you get heart attacks. Detoxing the body is essential for cancer patients, as are increasing gentle daily exercises, infrared sauna therapy, lowering stress, getting more sleep and simplifying your diet, and using natural herbal immune support products. I find using cancer screening tests helps patients stay on their F.I.G.H.T. program because it motivates them to never run out of their recommended supplements, as this is a lifetime struggle. Testing also motivates patients to take care of themselves every single day, and avoid overindulging. The answer is proven; by lowering stress, simplifying the diet, and detoxifying, cancer can be managed—and even cured. We have detectable signs of cancer cells in our system for an average of about seven years before it expresses itself as a lump or a bump.

SS: I feel that prostate cancer is an overdiagnosed condition, that men are rushed into removing their prostates in the same way women are rushed into hysterectomies.

GG: Today, we have a federal panel that has determined that PSA testing is a waste of time and money because the treatments recommended do more harm than good. I recommend taking the test to motivate patients to start to take better care of themselves. The truth is by age fifty, 50 percent of all men have prostate cancer, yet it doesn't have to be the cause of death if the patient takes special efforts to enhance his body's overall level of function. Mainstream medicine uses elevated PSA tests to keep men living in fear and wastes tons of money on ineffective therapies for a disease that most likely will not kill them.

SS: What's the good news about cancer?

GG: The good news is you can reverse the outcomes of the cancer screening tests when they are done before you have developed the lump or bump stage of clinical cancer by lifestyle changes and detoxification. Now that we have affordable gene tests to help us further personalize the F.I.G.H.T. program, more and more patients can get on top of their genetic issues. The BRCA 1 and 2 genes, which normally indicate a predisposition to breast cancer, do not need to express. Patients can improve their environment so cancer does not develop. No one needs their breasts removed prophylactically. Everyone has some cancer in their bodies, but it is our toxic and malnourished environment that causes those genes to turn "on." If patients are willing to modify their lifestyles and live a healthy life with proper supplements, diet, and exercise along with a lifetime detoxification program, they need never suffer from or die from cancer. Some people will do it, some people won't. But cancer screening tests give people the chance to know that they are at risk, so some will make changes in time.

SS: It's interesting you say "manage" cancer. In my book *Knockout*, as well as in my most recent interview with Dr. Nick Gonzalez, he also used the word "manage." Cancer as manageable is an interesting concept. What about meditation and prayer? Thoughts are so powerful.

GG: Yes, I absolutely agree with that. There is a book by Bruce Lipton called *Spontaneous Evolution*, which is a follow-up to his *Biology of Belief*, and he describes how our thoughts and internal energies affect us on a cellular level and have a direct impact upon the quality of our lives and health. *Biology of Belief* makes it appear that thoughts are possibly the most important part of the equation. Thoughts are energy, and the form they take—negative or positive—does affect our health, as well as influence other energies and people around us.

Thoughts and emotions are extremely important to our health— and the health of our planet.

SS: What is the single most important factor necessary to survive in today's world?

GG: I urge everyone to detoxify daily for life, and then in addition take a week out of your life and go through an intensive detoxification program *every year*!

SS: So how does my reader access you? What does it cost and how do they find you?

GG: I schedule one- or two-hour phone consultations with each patient. My consultation fees are typically $300 per hour. During this time, I go over any old records patients were able to obtain and any new lab results they agreed to have done. Then I make recommendations for their health and healing regimen. Everyone needs supplements and a personalized care program to survive today's toxic world. Ideally, I like to have them do the gene test panel to help me maximize the effects from supplements they need. Then, I find a safe substitute for most of the drugs patients are taking, as we don't need 90 percent of the drugs prescribed today. They can detoxify using these new incredible protocols that you and I have been discussing in this interview. People can contact me through the Gordon Research Institute, by going to www.gordonresearch.com, or by calling 800-580-7587 and requesting a consultation.

SS: Thank you, Garry. After speaking with you, I am convinced detoxification, and in particular, chelation, is the premier way to remove toxins. In today's world there is a need for environmental medicine, to live longer and redefine aging as a pleasurable experience. I love your passion and a lot of people are going to find answers to their health problems through your work.

CHAPTER 13

BOMBSHELL #9:
STEM CELL TREATMENT MAY SOON
ERADICATE CANCER

A new scientific truth does not triumph by convincing its oppo-
nents and making them see the light, but rather because its op-
ponents eventually die, and a new generation grows up that is
familiar with it.

—Max Planck, Nobel Prize winner for his work in physics

Imagine...the answer to cancer, one of our two biggest age stop-
pers. Today, through stem cell protocols, stem cell treatments to end
cancer are in *human* clinical trials right here in the United States, and
soon this treatment will be a reality for all of us. Imagine eradicating
cancer and the present torturous treatment as we know it. Dr. Dipnarine Maharaj is a stem cell specialist and the work he and his team
have been doing is going to rock the medical world. His work with
Parkinson's at present is being lauded as spectacular in the conventional medical world, and his understanding of cancer stem cells and
eradicating them by building the immune system through stem cell
protocols is nothing short of miraculous. The information we learn
in Dr. Maharaj's interview brings hope and light to the nastiest of
all diseases. But his caution, as with all the doctors presented in this
book, is that the state of health of the patient determines whether
there will be a successful outcome. A frail unhealthy body will most

likely not be able to access these great breakthroughs. This is yet another reason to take your health seriously and do anything and everything to keep your body, your own personal Maserati, in great health. The body needs to be strong to combat the present-day assault of stress, toxicity, and rampant disease. Cancer is not a mystery: how we get it, how we manage it, and now how to eradicate it is what Dr. Maharaj is about to tell us.

DIPNARINE MAHARAJ, M.D.

I was originally *introduced to Dr. Dipnarine Maharaj through Ray Kurzweil, who said to me that if I was writing a book about living longer, then I needed to talk to Dr. Maharaj.*

Dr. Maharaj is the founder and medical director of the South Florida Bone Marrow/Stem Cell Transplant Institute, one of the few completely outpatient bone marrow/stem cell transplant facilities in the United States. He also helped in the establishment of bone marrow/stem cell transplant programs at the University of Miami and for other communities in Florida. He has been involved with clinical research studies using stem cells in the areas of cardiac regeneration, neurodegenerative diseases, and cancer treatments. Most recently, he has obtained investigator-initiated permission from the FDA to study a novel treatment of solid tumors, using only healthy white blood cells. Dr. Maharaj earned both his medical degree and research doctorate at the University of Glasgow Medical School. He is also certified in internal medicine by the Royal College of Physicians of the United Kingdom, and he has accreditations in hematology, specializing in oncology and bone marrow transplantation. He has been a lecturer on internal medicine, hematology, and bone marrow transplantation at medical schools and universities in the United States and Europe. He is a bit of an overachiever, lucky for us. What he has to say in this interview will not only blow your mind but give you even more incentive for healthy living today.

SS: Thank you for your time, Dr. Maharaj. Ray Kurzweil, for whom I have the utmost respect, told me about the work you are doing with stem cells, which is certainly the direction of the future. You are in a new and rare specialty as a stem cell transplant physician. What excites you most that is accessible to my readers right now?

DM: Thank you, Suzanne. I am so pleased to be included in this book. We all know that the earlier the disease of cancer is caught, the better the outcome. So often a patient comes to me and the thought goes through my head that I wish we had seen him or her sooner, and then we really could have made a difference.

SS: Early detection is certainly an advantage, but is the real answer to cancer in finding the cancer stem cell?

DM: Yes. The best model for that would be leukemia, which is caused by a *cancer stem cell*. Chronic myeloid leukemia is where the leukemic stem cell has the abnormality. When a cancer stem cell divides, it produces two exact replicas, and one of them goes into what we call a quiescent (dormant) state. The other divides and produces the cancer. Chemotherapy will kill these cells, but the one that is not dividing is not touched by the chemotherapy.

SS: And this is where the patient goes into remission and everyone gets excited. But it's really not over, is it?

DM: Correct. The only way the cancer cell that's dormant is kept from recurring as cancer is if the cancer protective genetic switch is turned back on, and that happens if the immune system is intact so that the *cancer stem cell* can be destroyed.

SS: Is this possible?

DM: It relates back to getting the patient earlier. If a patient gets chemotherapy, then goes into remission, and the disease recurs, then subsequent chemotherapy further degrades the immune system and eventually renders it useless. When patients come to us in this state, it's like trying to close the door after the horses have bolted.

I am a stem cell transplant physician and the work I have been doing is to restore the immune system of patients with blood cancers, with either their own stem cells or a healthy donor's stem cells. Clearly cancer is a result of a broken-down immune system. The environment, diet, and lifestyle all determine your health. Take it seriously.

Here is what I am advocating: If you want to be prepared for the future when your immune cells diminish, then right now, while you are healthy, collect and store your stem cells!

SS: I agree. For that very reason, in 2009 I banked my stem cells with NeoStem. I call it bioinsurance. I know that in the future they are there and available to use for a catastrophic event, or merely for beauty.

DM: Again, you are well educated in your thinking of being proactive. I've seen the improvements that patients can get from using their own healthy stem cells.

This is the hope for the future. This is what excites me. If people store their stem cells when they are healthy, as you have, they are actually storing a healthier immune system than they could possibly have if they did develop cancer. So when we give them a stem cell transplant, it's best if done with banked stem cells that are in good health. It's a huge advantage.

SS: What else can be done with banked stem cells?

DM: We can repair and regenerate tissues instead of having to be dependent on a reactive process of using drugs and medications to treat chronic diseases.

SS: Does this mean I can eat junk food and chemicals and crap and not exercise, because I've got my stem cells banked so, yippee, it's a free ride?

DM: [Laughs.] NO!

SS: Can't blame a girl for trying.

DM: Seriously, the idea is that we want to improve our immune systems so we live longer with quality of life. In order to do that, you have to make the necessary lifestyle changes. Now, if as a result of your genetic inheritance and/or environmental effects, you do get some chronic disease in later life, then you've got your banked stem cells to counteract the disease processes that can be treated or prevented.

SS: So you are saying, the healthier we are entering the future, the better the shot we have at a longer, healthier life with quality.

DM: Correct. That is my belief.

SS: What is legally allowed at present in the United States regarding the use of stem cells, banked or otherwise?

DM: Approved treatments using stem cells from the patients themselves or from a donor can be used for treating blood cancers and disorders of the immune systems. That is the standard of care. I am able to do this on a day-to-day basis. We can repair a person's tissues utilizing a patient's own stem cells, and it is safe (these are adult stem cells).

My area has been focused on how we can optimize an individual's own stem cells so we can repair tissues. We've found that there are certain patients who we've been able to treat with very good results for blood disorders. In our research for treating patients with other diseases such as neurologic disorders, including Parkinson's disease, we have been working to develop a new noninvasive treatment allowing the stem cells from patients' own bone marrow to be released into their bloodstream. Those stem cells can go to the brain and repair it, and the patients show improvements in neurologic function. We are also doing the same type of research work in the area of diabetes by noninvasively using the individual's own stem cells.

SS: Can you explain the difference between embryonic stem cells and induced pluripotent stem cells?

DM: Induced pluripotent stem cells are formed when four genes called the *Yamanaka factors* are inserted into a mature cell, such as a skin cell, to convert it into an embryonic-like stem cell. Scientists are getting very encouraging results in the lab. But of course this is five to ten years off before we may see the benefit of this type of research. Embryonic stem cells are obtained from a five-day-old embryo. The embryo has to be destroyed to get these cells. This is where the ethical and moral issues come into play.

SS: But what about the problems that patients are having today?

DM: To use stem cell treatment today we have got to focus on safe treatments, and that would be using a patient's own stem cells.

SS: We have within our adult bone marrow, embryonic-like stem cells, right?

DM: Yes. These cells have some of the same capabilities of being pluripotent, just like embryonic stem cells that would come from embryos, with none of the controversy.

SS: And are these safe to use?

DM: Absolutely; the adult embryonic-like stem cells are safe because they are the patient's own.

SS: You mention Parkinson's, which is a devastating disease. Michael J. Fox comes to mind and through his courage, we've all seen the toll it takes on people of all ages. What kind of success have you had with Parkinson's?

DM: Parkinson's is a chronic neurodegenerative disorder caused by inflammatory processes in the brain. Any toxin or virus, or any process that induces inflammation, can cause chronic damage. It is similar for Alzheimer's disease or other neurodegenerative disorders. I believe these conditions are toxin related. The toxin can be viruses, or increased blood sugar, or pesticides, or environmental exposure, but there is a small percentage of people who unfortunately carry genes that predispose them to get these diseases. Our objective is to develop treatments to reduce the inflammatory processes and regenerate the tissues damaged by the inflammation.

SS: What about the gut? The second brain? Is there any connection from the gut to these diseases?

DM: I think so. If you look at chronic inflammatory disorders like diabetes, or if you look at the predictors of stroke or heart attacks, you will see that increased abdominal girth is a predictor. We think the reason is that toxins are being absorbed from the gut, causing inflammation; this results in increased abdominal fat, which predicts for these chronic diseases.

SS: People are getting weird bacterias, like *H. pylori*, from different sources, one being nonorganic chicken.

Is there an end point to having multiple bacteria in the gut? These things cause inflammation to one degree or another and they can lead to serious disorders, yes?

DM: Of course, anything that causes inflammation is not good.

SS: This is another reason to make good food choices. I grow my own organic food and only buy organic, but I'm on the road . . . a lot. Sometimes you just can't get good-quality food. I believe strongly in detoxification. I have an infrared sauna, and I also take detoxification measures through IV treatments with my antiaging doctor. Talk to me about detoxification.

DM: When I was in Scotland working on my doctorate, we discovered that the patients whom we were treating with the apheresis procedure for stem cell harvesting or plasmapheresis were receiving an albumin solution that was highly contaminated with heavy metals and toxins such as aluminum as a side effect of the manufacturing process. Because of these heavy metals, the patients' disease state was actually being made worse by these toxins. Part of my thesis was figuring out a way to remove those heavy metals from the solutions we were using. We were able to treat the patients who had developed heavy metal toxicity using chelating agents.

SS: I'm glad to hear you mention chelation because you are an orthodox doctor and so often chelation gets dismissed as antiaging quackery. But from where I see it, what else can we do when we are exposed daily to mercury, cadmium, aluminum, arsenic, dioxins, and PCBs? Does chelation, which cleans the blood of these contaminants, help control the inflammatory process these toxins create?

DM: Yes, you are correct. Certain heavy metals can circulate in the blood and then get deposited in the tissues, and this has been associated with Parkinson's. Chelation is effective in accomplishing the removal of heavy metals deposited in the tissues. The body responds to heavy metals by producing an inflammatory response, causing damage to the tissues, and that is when you can get disease. The problem with Parkinson's disease, or many other diseases, is often financial and related to approval of the treatments. For example, a patient goes to the doctor and is given an approved drug that insurance will cover, and most often that is the only option a patient has regardless of the effectiveness of that drug. Another example is with cancers, for instance, pancreatic cancer, where the drugs clearly are not producing cures but are covered by insurance and it is therefore what the patient is going to get. If you look at the survival rates of this disease and the effectiveness of these drugs, it's measured in months. There are many other ways these patients could be treated, but they are not given options because the reimbursement system through the insurance companies does not allow the physician to prescribe other treatments that could be effective.

SS: Yes, I know that the survival rate for stage IV pancreatic patients is 2.4 percent if they take conventional chemotherapy—2.4 percent! That is a total failure of a protocol. Give me hope . . . You think the answer is in stem cells?

DM: Well . . . yes. [Laughs.] As a stem cell transplant physician . . .

SS: [Laughs.] Sorry, of course . . . you *are*, after all, a stem cell transplant physician!

DM: I have discovered that patients who had neurological disorders, such as Parkinson's and stroke, may be able to recover with their own stem cells. The procedure we are researching is noninvasive, and the exciting part is that these patients can release their own stem cells from the bone marrow into their blood circulation, which then goes to the different areas of damage. In a small number of patients, improvements of about 55 to 60 percent have occurred and as an added plus, their medications are being reduced. Unfortunately, these patients are often on three or four different medications, and it's often the side effects of their medications that can delay the improvements in their condition.

SS: What about diabetes, that other big killer disease?

DM: Yes, we are doing similar research with diabetes as well as with people with liver failure.

SS: This is very exciting. It's not just about overcoming the disease; it's a return to quality of life. After all, what is a long life without quality?

DM: Right, and what excites me is finding a solution to these devastating problems. If we can regenerate the tissues, then we can repair the damaged tissues and we can continue improving a patient's condition. We can also reduce inflammation, which prevents further destruction; and by doing this we improve the lifestyle of the patient. And you are correct; it truly is all about quality of life. I'm seeing it on a day-to-day basis.

SS: Unfortunately, there are limitations in the United States. In what is currently allowable, how far away do you think we are (in terms of years) from being able to fully utilize the full potential of stem cell therapy?

DM: If we focus on patients' own stem cells (which is a safe way) and from current research, I think it will be allowable in the next few years. As far as the embryonic stem cells and induced pluripotent stem cells, I think that will take longer, maybe five to ten years.

SS: When you talk embryonic, do you mean actual fetuses or adult fetal stem cells taken from the adult bone marrow?

DM: We use adult fetal stem cells taken from their own body. By embryonic, I'm referring to cells grown in culture from the cell lines of embryos.

As I mentioned, we obtain pluripotent stem cells that are produced when cells taken from the skin have four genes inserted to produce a cell like an embryonic stem cell, called an *induced pluripotent stem cell*. I refer to adult stem cells as the stem cells taken from adult bone marrow.

I differentiate embryonic and adult stem cells so individuals who are not advocates of fetal stem cells do not become confused. I am familiar with very small embryonic-like (VSEL) stem cells. One of my collaborators, Dr. Mariusz Ratajczak from the University of Louisville, was one of the first to describe VSEL cells. You are correct. We can find these cells, which have characteristics of embryonic stem cells and also pluripotent capability, within our own bone marrow.

If we continue to develop the treatments for patients using their own stem cells, we will be able to bring this therapy to the general population at a faster rate with less controversy and few, if any, side effects. When we use our own stem cells, we do not have to worry about rejection. We don't have to worry about using immunosuppressive drugs that carry with them other diseases and problems from complications from the drugs themselves.

The public has to become educated as to the potential of stem cells, and to be as proactive as possible. It's important to bank your stem cells for future use when you are healthy. Frozen stem cells do not age, so when we do thaw them and use them for a procedure, we are actually putting back cells at the age at which they were when they were collected. Your body will continue to age but your frozen stem cells will not, which will be a huge advantage when they are put to use.

There is research coming out of Stanford and Harvard that involves taking old mice and young mice and connecting their circulatory systems; the young stem cells from the young mice will go into the old mice and repair the tissues. These are genetically identical mice. Using the same idea, if we have our own stem cells collected when we are young, then when they are put back at a later date, the younger cells will have the potential to repair the older tissues.

SS: So it's putting a younger *you* back into *you*! This is a true turning back of the clock and redefining what we think of as aging, the possibilities being that we can eradicate these particular diseases you have mentioned that are killing us now, using stem cells from our own bodies. Could this eventually be the protocol for any human ailment, for instance, heart disease?

DM: Yes, let's take the common heart diseases such as heart failure following heart attacks, chronic heart failure due to damage to the heart from other causes, hypertension, or cardiomyopathies where the heart is damaged.

STUDIES ARE NOW SHOWING THAT BY USING AN INDIVIDUAL'S OWN STEM CELLS AND PUTTING THEM BACK INTO THE PATIENT, THE HEART CAN RECOVER.

It is possible that all the chronic diseases can be eradicated, that tissues can be repaired, and in the future, stem cells will be able to regenerate organs. There will be no worry about rejections, or having to be on antirejection drugs or using somebody else's tissue. The catch is the healthier you keep yourself, the better your outcomes overall. We need to deal with chronic diseases proactively, to prevent and slow down the aging process so when we need stem cells, we use them only for the dramatic cases, where it requires an immediate fix of the tissue that's damaged.

SS: So the hope with stem cells is that we can tweak and fix all the parts of us that are worn out and repair them and also, in time, tackle all the major diseases?

But what about cancer? It is known that chemotherapy kills cancer cells in some cases but it can never kill the *cancer stem cell*, which is why most of the time the cancer comes back. Is anyone close to unlocking the key to killing the cancer stem cell?

DM: If you have a normal cell, a mutation occurs in the DNA that causes that cell to become a cancer cell. That mutation can be a single mutation, like say, chronic myeloid leukemia, or you can have ten thousand mutations, as in the case of a very aggressive cancer like a pancreatic cancer. If you introduce a drug that blocks a mutation and the effects of that mutation, you can treat the disease effectively. A good example of that is a drug called Gleevec, which has been very effective in treating chronic myeloid leukemia. It has improved survival and works well, until the patients become resistant to that drug. But recent research shows that Gleevec does not kill the cancer stem cell. So this drug can control the disease, but not kill it.

WHAT REALLY KILLS CANCER IS STEM CELL
TRANSPLANTATION, WHICH REPAIRS THE
IMMUNE SYSTEM, THEREFORE BLOCKING THE CANCER
STEM CELL FROM PROLIFERATING.

SS: And stem cell transplantation would allow the patient, say, with leukemia, to stay on that drug indefinitely?

DM: Without stem cell transplantation the disease can be controlled by the drug, but research shows that, ultimately, if the immune system is compromised and no longer effective, the cancer stem cell eventually will switch on and will no longer be controlled by the Gleevec.

SS: And then the person's disease recurs or relapses?

DM: Yes. The only treatment we have at that point is a stem cell transplant to repair the weakened immune system that allowed the cancer stem cells to grow in the first place.

SS: But why do some cancer patients who take chemotherapy survive? Are they simply time bombs?

DM: I have patients who have been cured of cancer. The answer that keeps coming to me is that their immune system was repaired. I have collaborated with Dr. Zheng Cui, a cancer biologist at Wake Forest University. Dr. Cui found a cancer-resistant mouse! This is a mouse that would never get cancer. It didn't matter what type of cancer cells were administered to it, the mouse would not get cancer. Dr. Cui took the cells of the immune system of this mouse and gave it back to mice that did have cancer and he cured them of the cancers. We currently have a clinical trial that is ongoing in humans where we are using a very similar approach to identify individuals who are cancer resistant and ask them to donate some of their white cells so that we can treat patients who have cancer.

THE IDEA IS THAT IF WE ARE USING THE WHITE CELLS OR THE IMMUNE SYSTEM OF INDIVIDUALS WHO ARE CANCER RESISTANT, THEN WE CAN GIVE THOSE WHITE BLOOD CELLS BACK TO PATIENTS WHO HAVE CANCER AND HOPEFULLY CURE THEM LIKE THE MICE.

SS: This is brand-new information to me. When I wrote *Knockout*, there were the rare aberrations showing patients who somehow survived cancer and orthodox treatment, and then there were the successes with the three kinds of cancer who did respond to chemotherapy: childhood leukemia, lymphoma, and testicular cancer, as in the case of Lance Armstrong.

BUT WHAT YOU JUST SAID IS BRAND-NEW INFORMATION... THAT *THERE ARE ACTUALLY PEOPLE WHO ARE RESISTANT TO CANCER*!

How does one tap into that good karma, to have that special gene?

DM: It is indeed good fortune not only for the individual but also for cancer advancement.

SS: This is incredible for humanity. We will all benefit from the white cells of these individuals.

DM: We have to be able to prove this in our clinical trial, but I am very enthusiastic.

SS: I thought white blood cells didn't respond well to microorganisms that cause disease, that the blood cells think the pathogen is you so they attack you, as in autoimmune diseases. Is that true?

DM: It comes back to the immune system. There are two types of immune systems: the innate immune system and the adaptive immune system. The cancer bacterial surveillance system is actually the innate immune system. Within the cells of the innate immune system there are granulocytes, monocytes, lymphocytes, dendritic cells, and natural killer cells. These are all the cells that actually will prevent cancers from developing in the first place, because when a cell becomes cancerous these immune cells will kill the cancer cell. These are the cells we are actually collecting from people who are essentially cancer resistant and giving them back to patients who have cancer.

SS: So people with a strong innate immune system are the ones who are cancer resistant? Is there a test to determine if you are one of the lucky ones to have these cells?

DM: A test called the *Cancer Killing Assay* has been developed, but we have not been able to fully utilize it because of lack of funding for this research. The idea here is to identify the genes or other factors that confer immunity against cancer and utilize this information to prevent cancer in individuals who are predisposed or to expand these specialized cells for patients with cancer.

Now the adaptive immune system is the second system: In autoimmune disease, a pathogen or toxin stimulates the adaptive immune system and this system continues to function autonomously. It's almost as if it's gone into overdrive and it continues to function without any checks and balances. Normally when a person encounters a foreign antigen, the adaptive immune system reacts to it and creates a state of tolerance so that the next time the person is exposed to it, the immune system recognizes it and destroys it without damage to the individual. In the individual with an autoimmune disease, this mechanism is abnormal and the individual's immune system continues to react to it. This is called an *immunogenic response.*

SS: Why is there so much autoimmune disease at present?

DM: Because our immune system is continuously being stimulated from immunogens, pathogens, infection, and toxins. Then it becomes automatic . . . the immune system begins to function on its own and cause damage. A disease like rheumatoid arthritis is an example of an autoimmune disease where the immune system is basically in overdrive continuously destroying joints.

SS: So keeping your immune system strong through a healthy diet and lifestyle protects you against the worst diseases and by doing so you can expect a longer life?

DM: Yes. If you ride into the future in good health, there will be a big payoff: stem cell protocols that will extend life and wipe out diseases.

SS: And right now you are having success with cancer, even in terms of using the word "cure," if the patient gets there early enough and is able to access your protocols?

DM: Yes. And also in the other areas we are exploring as well, chronic diseases like diabetes, stroke, and Parkinson's. Our research indicates that potentially these are diseases that will be treatable using patients' own stem cells with good results.

SS: What can we the patients do to be able to access these advancements?

DM: As I said earlier, I feel it is a good idea to bank and store your own stem cells while you are healthy. But more than that I want to be part of the movement that informs people about the crucial necessity of diet and lifestyle, so there is less likelihood that they ever have to see me to get treated for cancer. But if they do come, I am hopeful that the chances of success will be significantly better than what is currently offered as standard-of-care cancer treatments. I believe in what I am doing, and the progress we are making. I want to change the paradigm; cancer is not a death sentence. If we can educate people and simultaneously develop these new methods of restoring the immune system, then if cancer did occur in a patient, we could regulate his or her immune system and knock out the cancer stem cell.

SS: This is exciting progress for the future and for what is happening at present.

DM: I am extremely upbeat and hopeful that we can treat patients very, very effectively.

SS: What do you dream about?

DM: My dream is that each day when I wake up I make a difference in the lives of everyone I impact or who I meet. I want to make a positive difference in their lives, and by my own example, I can share with my family, my friends, and anyone with whom I come in contact, to set a good example of how we can live a good and healthy, long life.

SS: Thank you. A lovely way to end.

CHAPTER 14

BOMBSHELL #10:
A SKIN PATCH
MAY SLOW DOWN AGING

It is clear that the more you abuse your body by insulting it with toxic substances, the more likely one of your repair systems will undergo an early breakdown.

–David Kekich, *Life Extension Express*

A patch that uses nanotechnology to prevent aging? Sound too good to be true? It's not. You wear these patches and changes happen in your body? Yep. They help you sleep, help you with pain, help you detoxify and repair cell damage; there is one in development that may even help to prevent breast cancer. But the big one is available now: a patch that may slow down aging!

Slowing down aging is a Bombshell! This is a book about redefining aging. I am always looking for the nondrug way to accomplish the impossible. I am so enthusiastic about these patches that I have been the ambassador for this company for the past few years. I use these patches for pain, sleep, detoxification, energy, and preventing disease.

As a result of these patches, and the other self-care measures that I practice, I have not taken an over-the-counter drug in years with the exception of my stem cell breast surgery earlier this year, when I took pain medication for a couple of days. Again, I'm a believer. See what you think.

DAVID SCHMIDT

David Schmidt *is a fascinating man. He is a scientist and the founder of LifeWave, Inc. He was educated in management information systems and biology at Pace University in Pleasantville, New York. He went on to specialize in energy production technologies for both the military and commercial applications. He developed new methods for producing hydrogen and oxygen and constructed metal combustion engines. He also designed emergency oxygen systems for General Dynamics and the U.S. Navy and was invited to participate in the navy's next-generation minisub program. His background in biology helps him to explain how individual human cells operate and why we need to care for each and every cell in our bodies as a means of preventing cancer and other disease. If the human body is made up of cells reproducing, then taking care of each and every cell is crucial to life. His patches are about that, as he will explain.*

SS: Hello, David, so good to speak with you. You've had such a positive effect on the nation's health. You developed LifeWave for the military in what eventually became your energy patches: a nondrug way to maintain energy for our nation's submariners without the use of drugs or caffeine. Then you created the patch for battling the environment, a nondrug but powerful antioxidant. So tell us how your patches can help us fight the toxic assault that every living human being who is alive cannot escape.

DS: Thank you, Suzanne. The patches are about utilizing the biophysical properties of the human body.

SS: Okay, stop right there, what do you mean by biophysical?

DS: Most of us are familiar with body biochemistry but don't realize it. We're told that if we have a healthy, clean diet, free of artificial ingredients and if we drink clean, fresh water, that is going to lead to good health and all this is true because we are promoting a healthy environment and a healthy "biochemistry" in our body.

SS: Okay, that makes sense.

DS: The LifeWave patches are about utilizing the biophysical properties of the human body that most people are less familiar with. This has to do with the energy that travels through the nervous system, the bioelectrical energy, and the signaling methods the cells use in communication. As we age, the energetic systems in our bodies break down as well as the communication systems. Then the biophysical properties of the body change. It deteriorates.

SS: That's not good.

DS: Right. LifeWave is the first technology that goes after this mostly misunderstood or unknown problem and improves the biochemistry in our bodies as we age, through the biophysical properties.

The body's first line of defense against aging is its antioxidant system, which is what protects us from free-radical damage. When our bodies' antioxidant levels become decreased, these radicals can get out of control and damage healthy tissue, organs, cells, and even our DNA. It's very important as a first line of defense in antiaging to keep our antioxidant systems elevated. This is what our glutathione patches do if worn daily.

The planet is, as you always say, a "toxic soup," and people are getting very sick as a result, so we have to do everything in our power to fight the bombardment—healthy eating, good nutritious food, exercise, et cetera—but even that is not enough to ensure good health. So I created the glutathione patch, knowing that glutathione is the body's master antioxidant, to detoxify the body on a continuing basis. Antioxidants protect us from free-radical damage, so the glutathione patch is another form of "protection."

SS: In this unavoidable toxic soup it gives me comfort, like I am a step ahead, wearing my glutathione patch every day. As I've written in this book, the major factors in aging are oxidation, inflammation, and glycation, but also free-radical damage is a major cause of aging. Would your technology help manage these issues?

DS: Yes, our glutathione patch helps to manage oxidation, our Aeon patch is a very powerful anti-inflammatory product, and our carnosine patch is perhaps the most powerful method for reducing cellular glycation. But from my perspective, the real cause of aging is stress. Stress initiates in the autonomic nervous system. If your body is under a significant amount of stress and the antioxidant system fails, then elevated levels of oxidative chemicals lead to an increase in inflammation. These inflammatory markers—such as cytokines—will end up damaging the cells in the body and causing accelerated aging.

From the point of view of antiaging, we want our bodies to be in a balanced state. The human body has a tremendous communication system both inside the cells and through the nervous system. There are thousands of nerve endings and we can activate these with LifeWave technology. When we become imbalanced from stress, we begin to see an increase in oxidative chemicals in the body; and when that happens, we see inflammatory markers rise. These elevated levels of inflammatory chemicals get out of control (C-reactive proteins, fibrinogen, homocysteine, and lipid peroxides), and they will damage the DNA, the cells, the organs. We see the results of this process as aging. The good news is that when we balance the nervous system, then we can balance these chemicals and slow down and even reverse aging. Yoga, and deep breathing, is a way to reduce stress; however, now we can use technology to create stress reduction all day. Our Aeon patch is capable of balancing the autonomic nervous system for stress reduction, and this results in a very powerful antiaging effect.

SS: Before you explain your amazing Aeon patch, you mentioned lipid peroxides earlier. Please explain the importance or function of lipid peroxides. Why should we care about our levels of lipid peroxides?

DS: Every cell in the body has a membrane and it's made from fat.

SS: Right, and that fat should be made from omega-3s so that it is soft and pliable to allow water and air to flow through (hydration and oxygenation), the essence of life!

DS: Right. Lipid peroxidation is an inflammatory process that will oxidize the cell membranes.

SS: So the water and air cannot flow through?

DS: Right. When that happens, the high levels of lipid peroxide create more oxidative stress that ends up damaging the communication system in the cells. Now you no longer have maximum ability to transport nutrients to eliminate toxins, and eventually it will end in a state of disease.

SS: So you want to cut it off at the pass . . . how?

DS: One of the exciting clinical tests we performed using blood analysis demonstrated that our Aeon patch was capable of reducing levels of lipid peroxides, as well as other inflammatory chemicals. In addition, it's critically important to keep our antioxidant levels elevated. As I stated a little earlier, our first line of defense in aging is to keep our antioxidant systems elevated, which is what happens when you wear the glutathione patch daily. As we age, the energetic systems in our bodies break down and the nervous system, communication system, and the biophysical properties of the body change. Meditation has been used for thousands of years for stress reduction to help balance the nervous system. Most of us don't have time to meditate, so when the nervous system gets imbalanced into a sympathetic state, we see an increase in oxidative chemicals in the body. This then causes an increase in inflammation. The immune system deteriorates. The glutathione and Aeon patches are a sophisticated but easy way to improve health and alleviate this deterioration.

SS: How do they work?

DS: The patches emit specific wavelengths of light; this process is called *photobiomodulation*. Most people know that sunlight causes our bodies to make vitamin D. The patches do a similar thing; they emit specific wavelengths of light to trigger very specific chemical reactions, and we can use our technology to elevate antioxidants such as glutathione, instead of taking a pill.

IF WE WANT TO GET TO THE ROOT OF AGING
WE HAVE TO FIND A WAY TO DECREASE INFLAMMATION.
THAT IS HOW WE SLOW DOWN AGING.

SS: So clearly the job of the glutathione patch is to decrease inflammation from free-radical exposure. What else do you have in your arsenal? Do you have a patch that will, say, prevent cancer?

DS: I am happy to say that we have just formed a LifeWave company in Europe, and one of the new patch products in development is designed to prevent breast cancer. When women are in a precancerous state, there is an increase in the vascularity of breast tissue. It is currently believed that malignant cells create this vascularity as a method to draw blood and nutrients to the developing tumor. Our method would be to interfere in this process by elevating antioxidants such as glutathione and SOD (superoxide dismutase) to help protect normal tissue, while decreasing inflammatory chemicals such as cytokines to reduce tissue damage. In a pilot study performed by LifeWave, this method was successful at decreasing the abnormal vascularity in breast tissue in only ninety days.

SS: So you've got me thinking . . . if I can decrease inflammation by wearing an Aeon patch, and if cancer is inflammation gone crazy because the cells are multiplying out of control because of free-radical damage, it seems to me that you are on to something.

DS: We think so . . . I know you are interested in cancer therapies and how cancer begins. There was a clinical study reported in the journal *New Surgical Horizons*, and it talked about this connection between chronic inflammation, oxidative stress, and how this will lead to DNA damage and the initiation of cancer in the body.

In our clinical research, we found the Aeon patch was capable of balancing the activity in the autonomic nervous system by decreasing inflammation. (We worked with Dr. Stanislaw Burzynski, the famous cancer doctor out of Houston, Texas, also featured in this book. This is what is so great about you, Suzanne; you have this ability to bring scientists and doctors from all over the world together where they can brainstorm.) In clinical studies, we used a piece of equipment manufactured by a company called Biocom Tech and thought to look at the enervation of the heart response using a diagnostic technique called *HRV.* In simple terms, what we found was that if people were type A personalities, it helped bring them into a more relaxed state, and if they were already in a relaxed state, it brought them back into balance so their immune system would be more efficient.

SS: So if Aeon reduces inflammation in the body, it would make sense to me that it would be preventative. I know we can easily determine our inflammation levels by taking a simple blood test called the *high-sensitivity CRP test* (a test for C-reactive protein). I take this blood test every year. You want to keep your inflammation under 1.0.

So by wearing the Aeon patch, you found in your studies that it lowered people's levels of oxidative chemicals and inflammation markers and helped balance their immune systems?

DS: Yes, we found this in two separate blood studies. Then we did another clinical study using Electro Interstitial Scanning, which is a medical device in Europe, to see what would happen after thirty days of using this technology. After thirty days, there was a dramatic improvement of organ function throughout the entire body. So this showed us that the Aeon patches created an environment where the cells could repair. The patches are a new way to tap into the body's healing system to reach new levels of antiaging by promoting an environment that hasn't been able to be reached by conventional supplements.

SS: Cancer is uncontrolled cell multiplication. Too many damaged cells and you are in trouble. So if the Aeon patch repairs cells, then that would be a big advantage in prevention. So the Aeon patch instigates the body's ability to begin healing itself? Reversing cell damage and inflammation, right?

DS: Yes, the Aeon patch triggers a series of antistress factors in the body (inflammation reduction) so when people use them, they experience improved energy, a reduction in pain and inflammation, and their skin improves . . . it just looks younger.

SS: Is the Aeon patch a substitute for supplements?

DS: Supplementation is still very important, but for raising the antioxidant levels in your body and reducing inflammation, the glutathione and Aeon patches surpass supplements on many levels.

SS: Chronic inflammation affects telomeres, causing them to shorten at a faster rate than normal. I also know that people with heart disease have shorter telomeres in their heart tissues, and people with Alzheimer's seem to have a disproportionate shortening of the brain's telomeres. Once you have that kind of inflammation, can it be reversed through, of course, proper diet and lifestyle, coupled with the daily application of the Aeon patch?

DS: Absolutely; of course, it's always going to depend on how many years a person has been living in an unhealthy state and how old they are at the time, but yes, it's possible to reverse this damage and our research has shown that. Scientists have concluded that shorter life expectancies were linked to high fibrinogen (which is an inflammatory) levels and if you could keep this specific inflammatory marker decreased, then you could get a longer life span. We've shown in studies on the Aeon patches that they reduce the stress levels through the autonomic nervous system, and this has a cascading effect of reducing harmful levels of C-reactive proteins, reducing fibrinogen, reducing homocysteine, and reducing lipid peroxides.

When you are reducing the body's levels of inflammation, it gives the body a chance to recover and heal and that's exactly what we see.

SS: All this without drugs . . . You must be proud of this patch.

DS: I am, and thanks, but like you, I'm a messenger. I'm happy to do my part in bringing these products to the market. We now have over a hundred thousand customers worldwide in about a hundred countries, and the testimonials we receive from our Aeon products are extraordinary.

SS: Give me examples.

DS: I received a testimonial yesterday from a woman in England who was reaching for a tea kettle and got distracted and suffered a third-degree burn just between her wrist and elbow. She was rushed to the hospital but on the way there her husband applied the Aeon patch and our IceWave pain patches for reducing the inflammation and controlling the pain. Not only were they able to get 100 percent pain relief for that third-degree burn, but also the burn healed much more quickly. That's an extreme example.

SS: What about its effects on aging skin?

DS: I know a lot of your readers are women, and I think they will find this next fact interesting. We did a clinical study in Australia with two medical doctors and found that after ninety days of using the Aeon patch, glutathione patch, and carnosine patch, there was an average improvement in the quality of the skin of 300 percent. This means fewer wrinkles, better hydration, and improved smoothness of the skin.

SS: That's impressive. As I said before, the skin is a reflection of what is going on inside the body. So if you are creating healthy skin from the inside out, that means that your organs are getting healthier.

DS: Yes, that's true.

SS: I know you are forty-eight, but you look like you are in your twenties. A lot of it is your diet, lifestyle, and exercise regimens. But what patches do you wear daily?

DS: I am fortunate that I don't suffer any chronic pain, so I always start with my energy patches because the energy patches increase fat burning and this is a very powerful antiaging mechanism. As we age, our bodies metabolize less fat for energy. Second, I use a combination of Aeon, glutathione, and carnosine patches because these keep my antioxidant system charged and help protect me from the effects of aging. I use the Silent Night patches before bedtime, which elevate melatonin and help put you into a peaceful state of sleep. It's also great because when you wake up in the morning, you don't feel drugged. So that's my entire protocol.

SS: Where's it all going, David? How do you feel about the future?

DS: I feel great about the future. LifeWave is now at the point in Europe where our products will be used by medical doctors in hospitals and clinics to alleviate chronic pain, and in the near future we hope to help prevent breast cancer as well. Technology is going to provide many of the solutions for the future, but it has to start with a change in our awareness that in the last hundred years, mankind has created a tremendous amount of damage to our planet and now we have to have a philosophical change in the way we are conducting our business on this planet if we are going to survive. In my travels around the world, I see people who want to be part of this change. We must pull the next generation into this thinking and inspire them to make a commitment to solving these problems.

SS: How long do you think you will live?

DS: I do not see a limit, and in my mind I'm thirty years old. But conservative scientists are already saying that we can get to 150, and with telomere lengthening, when cells keep dividing, then the sky's the limit. I plan to live a long time, and my goal is to be productive and continue making contributions to mankind, while enjoying everything life has to offer. All this can happen for all of us if we are in good health.

SS: You mean healthy as in biophysically! [Laughs.] See, I got it! Thanks, David.

CHAPTER 15

BOMBSHELL #11:
YOU CAN "SWITCH OFF"
CANCER CELLS

Today, more people than ever are thinking about their "capital" in terms of time, instead of money. Put another way, each American born today gets an account with roughly thirty thousand days in it. Some of us will waste our capital with poor lifestyle decisions, thus losing time. But some of us are actively looking for ways to expand that original capital far beyond the eighty or so years we started with.

—Stanislaw Burzynski, M.D., Ph.D.

One evening I was enjoying dinner with Dr. Stanislaw Burzynski at his beautiful clinic in Houston, Texas, and I asked him the question, "Why do we get cancer?" He said simply, "We get cancer when the cancer protective genetic switches get turned off." I asked him how that happens. He then explained how the diet and lifestyle choices we all make on a daily basis affect these "switches." In knowing about them we can take control and keep these "switches" turned on. It's actually quite simple. As I've said before, you must ask yourself each day whether the choices you are making move you toward your goal of living longer with great health or move you away from it. In this interview, Dr. Burzynski will explain the switches that go a long way toward helping you become one of the ones who do NOT get cancer. I say it again and again in this book; the choices we make determine our outcomes.

STANISLAW BURZYNSKI, M.D., PH.D.

Dr. Stanislaw Burzynski *was born in Lublin, Poland, in 1943 and is an internationally recognized physician and scientist who has pioneered the development and use of biologically active peptides, known as anti-neoplastons, in diagnosing, preventing, and treating cancer and other diseases since 1967. He operates the Burzynski Clinic in Houston, Texas, and has effectively treated more than fifty types of cancer but has had the most consistent success with cancers of the brain, breast, head and neck, prostate, colon, lungs, and ovaries, as well as non-Hodgkin's lymphoma.*

Dr. Burzynski is a brave and courageous pioneer. No one has worked harder and no one has been more persecuted for his maverick approach. His successes are a threat to orthodox cancer protocols. But in speaking to his "cured" patients, I became very aware that he is on track. I believe one day Dr. Burzynski will be honored as a historic figure in the vein of Jonas Salk. To know more about his cancer protocols and testimonials, read his interview in my book Knockout. *Today, in keeping with the theme of this book, I wanted to know from him what we can do to prevent getting cancer in the first place so that we can live longer with quality and disease-free. He has the answers.*

SS: Hello, Dr. Burzynski, it is my pleasure to talk with you again. You are a scientist and a cancer doctor. Cancer, as you know so well, is a complex disease. If you had a simple message, though, what might it be about the proactive steps we can take to protect ourselves? Is there something we all can do?

SB: Thank you, Suzanne. It's always my pleasure to speak with you. We can definitely take steps to prevent cancer. It takes a long time to develop cancer, and this process involves numerous steps. Cancer is easier to control in the early stages because we see a change in the structure of the genes early on, like a mutation. This mutation would mean the gene is "switching off," and these could be the genes that protect against cancer.

SS: Is this what you call *epigenetic control*? And is there a specific test we should be taking that would allow us to see these mutations at an early phase before the genes get turned off?

SB: Epigenetic change occurs without altering the structure of the gene, which is mutation. This change typically happens before mutation. For instance, the tumor suppressor gene is switched off (silenced epigenetically) and the cell with the mutated oncogene, which stimulates cancer growth, survives instead of being killed through the action of tumor suppressors.

A simpler way of saying epigenetic control would be described as "switching off the genes that control against cancer."

SS: So epigenetics essentially looks at factors such as lifestyle and diet and how these factors affect the way the genes get expressed?

SB: Yes. It can be the factors inside your body, which enter from the food you eat and the life you live. For instance, stress and lack of sleep can silence cancer-protective genes. But were you to take nutrients seriously, like eating good-quality organic food, and take the steps to modify your behavior by learning to sleep again and managing your stress, then it is possible that the protective gene can become active again and the cancerous process that was triggered by neutralizing this gene from diet and lifestyle changes will be reversed.

SS: So it's like cutting it off at the pass. Once again, the stark reality is that the food choices we make can determine our health.

SB: Without question, and exercise is also a major component . . .

SS: People always say, "Well, I have bad genes; my mother had cancer, my father had cancer," et cetera, but I have heard and read that only 20 percent of our health is determined by our genes and 80 percent is determined by lifestyle. Do you agree?

SB: In some instances these genes are hereditary, but the changes in genes I'm talking about occur during your life, because of the way you live your life.

SS: So we are in control of not getting cancer!

SB: That is right, except for environmental factors. Maybe you lived next door to a chemical plant, or you've had radiation exposure or a virus is affecting your genome causing changes in your genes.

These things can't be blamed on genetics. So if you know you've been exposed, you deal with it by making a real attempt to live a clean, healthy life. Very few seem to grasp the importance of this.

SS: Why is there so much brain cancer?

SB: For one thing, people are living much longer and outliving the usefulness of their own brains. Silencing of tumor suppressors and mutations of oncogenes accumulate and cause brain tumors. On the other hand, in the last decade, researchers found that dementia affects approximately 40 percent of the population above the age of eighty-five, and 75 percent of these have Alzheimer's.

SS: Losing one's brain is the worst thing imaginable. How do we protect aging neurons?

SB: Well, if you've undergone general anesthesia, the chemicals used for these surgeries destroy some neurons, so every time you go under, you lose some neurons. We have an abundance of neurons, so most of the time we don't feel any difference. But if you have surgery again and again, you will start to notice.

SS: Yes, I had my stem cell surgery earlier this year, and I had brain fog for weeks afterward. I didn't like it. How do we avoid the damage?

SB: There is a process in our brain called *neurogenesis*, which is the formation of neurons. Until recently no one believed that forming new neurons was possible, but now that has been proved wrong. We have now found that every day, new neurons are being formed in our brain and at the same time old neurons are dying. It's an ongoing process, but the catch is that the brain has to put these neurons to work for this process to continue, for instance, by continuing to learn and perform intellectual activities. A functioning brain directs neurons to go into certain circuits in the brain, and then damage to the neurons of the brain can be reduced.

SS: So what can we do to make this process of producing new neurons constantly happen?

SB: You have to exercise the brain through the learning process, which stimulates the neurons to form new circuits. Once they have been incorporated in new circuits, they don't die. You have to keep your brain active.

SS: So you're saying, "use it or lose it." Amazing. Nature is perfection. Of course it makes sense; if we are old and not interested in learning anything new, we are pretty unnecessary to society. So nature has a built-in plan to get rid of us when we are useless. I guess that's why older people do a lot of crossword puzzles.

SB: Exactly. If you are active most of the time, you are using the part of the brain that stimulates the neurons. New neurons and circuits then memorize what you are learning. The bottom line is, if you want to keep your brain from deteriorating, you have to keep exercising it to keep it as sharp as possible.

SS: How else do we exercise our brain?

SB: Reading and, as you mentioned, things like doing crossword puzzles, writing memoirs, learning new languages—any activity that requires you to think. That is brain exercise.

SS: But here's where I see a problem. Our aging population is all "pilled up." They can't think through the disastrous haze of pharmaceuticals. Plus, they are eating chemicals and drinking diet soda. Older people seem to love their sugar, and generally, they don't realize that the bags of cookies and candies they get from the supermarkets are loaded with brain-killing chemicals. As a result, they may care less about learning.

SB: And that's why the percentages of demented and Alzheimer's patients are so high with older people in America; too much TV, no exercise, chemicals, bad-quality food, not reading much—it's all a horrible combination. These nonactivities are eating up the brain and deteriorating it along with the rest of the body.

In other countries where people are maintaining activity until they are quite old, you don't see much of this phenomenon. You don't see abuse of diet soda or abuse of watching too much TV. People in other countries try to stay active all their lives. Unfortunately, here in our country, the bottom line is that we are creating a population of people who are getting more and more stupid.

SS: It's sad but true.

SB: And it leads to more cancer. Memory is a very active process. During twenty-four hours, a person needs to construct completely new circuits of neurons. This is very extensive and requires involvement of numerous genes. If there is abnormal function of these genes (an inactive brain), and if this system becomes disorganized, you will end up with useless cells in your brain, which can form a brain tumor.

We talked about the genetic switches. You can keep the cancer-protective genetic switches turned on by implementing simple changes. You must have a proper diet of (preferably) organic food, and that includes adding herbs and spices that provide antioxidant protection such as turmeric, curcumin, and Indian spices. My wife and I eat at an Indian restaurant once a week, because it tastes very good and also I like to get all the important spices they use in their cooking. There were studies done on this that found significant differences between people who eat a diet high in herbs and spices versus those who don't. And there was clearly less cancer in those who used spices on a regular basis.

Exercise is important: at least one hour a day. Supplements and antioxidants are all helpful, avoiding chemicals is important, getting proper sleep is important, and managing your stress is important. If people would just do these things, the cancer rate would go way down.

And then you have to make an effort to learn. It may be difficult, but try to learn for at least one hour a day. You could learn poetry or a foreign language, or try to read a more difficult book. But those who don't try to change their lifestyle and diets will likely decline.

At the moment we are approaching the biggest paradigm shift in our approach to illnesses in the last 150 years. We are switching from categorizing the illnesses based on what we see under the microscope to categorizing the diseases based on different genomes. For instance, there is a genome for one type of breast cancer and another genome for another type of breast cancer. Of one hundred thousand different varieties of cancer, each will have different genomes. The right way to approach disease is to identify the changes and use proper molecular switches. I believe in the next ten years very few doctors will be using an optic microscope because they will be looking primarily into genomic characterization of various illnesses. This could be the answer to numerous problems like cancer (obviously), Alzheimer's, and even bacterial infections, which is important because we are running out of antibiotics due to overuse; they are just not working anymore. And infections in the future will be deadly because of this. So hopefully these new changes get here in time. We are now learning how to turn on the genes that produce antibiotics in our body.

SS: So what are they going to call this other direction?

SB: It will be called *synthetic biology*, which means proper identification of proper circuits, proper switches, and inserting them into normal cells so they can turn on the switches that are silent and direct the cell in the right way or develop it.

SS: I have a lot of friends who are developing memory problems; can't remember the end of the sentence type of thing. Will this happen in time for them?

SB: Some of them could reach the point of no return. You see, once you destroy too many neurons it's too late, especially for the neurons involved in the initial phase of memory. These are the neurons that concentrate your attention. Without these neurons you won't be able to remember simple things because you'll have lost your ability to have attention recall. On the other hand, those who have partial decline of memory may still have time to replenish them.

SS: What can they do?

SB: Sounds simple, but, make drastic changes in their diet. It's about the fuel they give their bodies. Nutrition is fuel. The brain needs proper fuel.

SS: Amen. I say this over and over. You have to give your body high-quality fuel, high octane.

Let's talk about methylation, because it is one of the factors that cause us to age. Lots of supplements have the word "methyl" or "methylation" in them, but I don't think the average person really understands what methylation means and why it's important.

SB: Methylation is one of the processes by which genes are expressed. Our cellular DNA requires constant enzymatic actions (called *methylation*), for activation, silencing, maintenance, and repair. Aging cripples youthful methylation, causing DNA damage that can manifest as cancer, organ damage, and brain cell degeneration.

SS: So methylation controls the gene activity, such as turning switches on or off?

SB: Right. Methylation is like the ignition to turn the gene "off" and "on."

SS: And we want to keep "on" our cancer-protective genes.

SB: Correct. If you remove these methyl groups, it's like removing the plastic cover from around the gene, and the gene will become active again. I am talking about methylation of the part of the gene that is responsible for the activity of the rest of the gene. Methylation is like blocking the ignition key of the gene.

SS: So methylation is *not* a good thing.

SB: Well, it depends on what you are methylating. It's bad when methylation turns "off" a gene that is important for the function of your body, like a well-working brain, but it's a good thing if methylation turns "off" the gene that is causing cancer.

SS: If the methyl group is removed, then the enzyme can reach and activate the gene?

SB: Right. Let's imagine a car with the ignition key. You want to turn on the car, so you put in the key and turn it and the car starts. If you block the keyhole, then the key can't get in and you can't start the car. Over time the gene promoter (ignition) is covered with methyl groups, which prevent enzymes from reaching it and activating it. As a result, the gene is "silenced." Increased methylation throughout life silences important groups of genes. Some of the genes that are silenced are the ones that inhibit inflammation and cancer, which helps explain why there is more cancer among the elderly.

This is actually the body's master clock.

SS: Do you mean that the defects of methylation are why we age and the number of silenced genes dictates how long we are going to live?

SB: Yes. The master clock theory unites what we know about stem cells, telomeres, and methylation. The telomere's gene in the normal cell is silenced by methylation, after approximately fifty cell divisions, allowing the cell to die. In the stem cell, the telomere's gene is not silenced and the cell lives.

SS: I like to try to simplify things, so is methylation like internal "resting"?

SB: Yes. Methylation is a chemical process like making a plastic. You put together a bunch of these methyl groups and something like a plastic is formed. What's underneath this plastic is the gene, which can't be active because it's separated from the rest of the machine. So it's *resting*. You are correct.

SS: I like to be correct! [Laughs.]

SB: This resting gene is now silenced. It's been put to sleep. Now, it's not working in your favor.

SS: So this isn't good. Here's a gene that is supposed to protect us from cancer, but it's silenced, asleep, or resting. Not doing its job.

SB: Right, but it's not damaged; it's still in good shape. Yet when it is silenced, this is the first step in the development of cancer. The gene is no longer protecting you against the development of cancer, so if you have poor eating habits and bad lifestyle habits, you don't have a gene that is turned "on" to protect you. This is methylation. If your bad habits continue, they will lead to further abnormalities because a turned "off" cancer gene is unstable. So instead of just silencing the gene, you end up with mutations, which are a permanent change in the structure of the protective gene. Now that cell is not being destroyed, and if the process continues, it will produce a number of cells that are abnormal.

SS: Okay, then that person is in trouble, possibly has cancer?

SB: Yes, and you can also see how this would affect aging. As we age, the stem cells decline, in part due to increased methylation.

SS: This means the body isn't able to renew itself as rapidly, which increases the risk of diseases and promotes aging. So how do we stop the methylation process?

SB: As I've been saying, good nutrition, improved digestion, managing stress, good lifestyle habits, daily physical exercise, and the duration of your sleep is important, seven to eight hours. Avoid chemical carcinogens, minimize free radicals with antioxidants, get sufficient exposure to sun for vitamin D intake. And restoring missing hormones is also crucial, the ones you write about, Suzanne, the bioidenticals. In other words, the choices we make every day affect the tempo of our biological clocks, which in turn affects the pace of our master clock, meaning how fast we will die. As the master clock accelerates, we are at an increased risk of cancer as well as other diseases.

SS: But you can offset disease, and lengthen your life, by changing your life and seriously utilizing your suggestions above for healthy living. So it's actually very simple: You can avoid most cancers and other serious diseases by keeping your protective genetic switches turned "on." And you do this by good diet, lifestyle, avoiding toxins, eating organic, getting sleep, managing your stress, and I imagine other factors like happiness and love in your life.

SB: Correct. I am a scientist. What I have described above is in its simplest form.

SS: That's what I want. I want my reader to walk away from this discussion with you, a great and famous cancer doctor and an innovative scientist, telling us that *we are in control of not getting cancer*!

And that control is dictated by the diet and lifestyle choices that we make. That heredity has very little to do with it, that chemicals and poor food have everything to do with it.

_____

THE BOMBSHELL! THE ANSWER TO CANCER IS SIMPLE. YOU CAN KEEP THE CANCER PROTECTIVE SWITCHES TURNED ON THROUGH DIET AND LIFESTYLE!

_____

What else will keep us alive longer? Let's talk about royal jelly and honeybees. I've heard some interesting things about them recently.

SB: Honeybees are very interesting, and through them we have made some incredible breakthroughs at the Burzynski Research Institute. Honeybees have identical genomes; you take sixty thousand honeybees and each of them is like a twin because they all have identical genomes. Why is it that some of these honeybees survive sixty times longer than others, the worker bees? The workers live only five weeks, but the queen may live two to six years. What is so different?

_____

THE DIFFERENCE IS DIET!

_____

The diet the queen consumes is only royal jelly. That's *her* diet! The workers are fed royal jelly only for three days of their life, and they live a short time.

SS: So why do you think royal jelly slows down aging?

SB: Certain flowers have molecular switches; the ones with the molecular switches turned "on" attract the honeybees.

SS: Here we go again with the switches; it even extends to flowers.

SB: It extends to all life. The flowers with the certain molecular switches that are ingredients of royal jelly have substances called *PG* (phenylacetylglutamine) and *PB* (phenylbutyrate). In fact, we decided to run experiments on these substances and a remarkable thing happened. When we injected the honeybees with PG or PB, the life span of those honeybees was almost five times longer than the honeybees who did not receive it. This is when we realized that royal jelly contains molecular switches that can activate the genes involved in lengthening aging.

SS: This is fantastic. Do you have supplements with royal jelly in them?

SB: Yes, we have supplements that contain the ingredients of royal jelly. Our theory is that by taking these ingredients, we can acquire new molecular switches that can try to reprogram the clock that protects our telomeres. If we can do that, then we can extend life.

SS: So, knowing that, who wouldn't want to take royal jelly supplements. You sell them, right?

SB: Yes, these supplements contain ingredients present in royal jelly, and you can get them on my Aminocare website.

SS: Finish this sentence for me: My dream is . . .

SB: My dream is that we put an end to cancer . . . that people take control of their life choices seriously and take preventive measures to avoid this terrible disease.

Until that happens, my dream as a doctor is to be allowed to put to use a new approach to cancer that is genomic based and actually available right now. It's frustrating to have the technology and medications available and not be allowed to use them because of bureaucratic control. Many doctors could be using these advancements and saving human lives now. It can only change if the American people get involved; if there are many of us protesting, then we could promote this change.

I dream for all doctors to have more freedom to practice medical art and use our discoveries to help people. This is why we became doctors; this is why I became a doctor. If medicine was not ruled by bureaucrats and lawyers, then we would have the freedom to move forward and win the war on cancer. If not, we'll be waiting for another forty years for orthodox medicine to catch up.

It can be done, it should be done. People should understand that bureaucrats, lawyers, and big business should be removed from controlling medicine. Doctors should be allowed to utilize protocols and medications that will help people and be able to honor our oath, "Do no harm."

SS: Well, my dream is that your dream comes true. Another great conversation, Stan. I thank you for your time.

Given that cancer is about to be the biggest killer in the world, the odds are that someone reading this book is going to get it. I've already had it, and as a result it put me on a path of good health, good diet, and good lifestyle habits, paying particular attention to prevention. Next we hear from Dr. Nicholas Gonzalez about the important work he does with cancer patients and the anticancer protocol he recommends. Once again it is very clear that we can avoid cancer, even genetic aberrations and environmental cancer, and that it is not inevitable if you know the steps to take to avoid this nasty killer. Following a preventative protocol such as Dr. Gonzalez's is not for sissies, but it seems a small thing to do to be proactive about preventing cancer or a cancer recurrence. I have chosen to do this and the by-product for me is great energy, healthier-looking skin, and a well-working body.

NICHOLAS GONZALEZ, M.D.

Dr. Nicholas Gonzalez *is a physician in private practice in New York City. With his colleague, Dr. Linda Isaacs, he treats patients with advanced cancer and other serious degenerative diseases, utilizing a nutritional-dietary approach. For more information, consult his website at www.dr-gonzalez.com.*

I do not have cancer but I did eleven years ago, so it made sense to me to use Dr. Gonzalez's protocol preventatively. Of course, he does not have to prescribe for me the supplementation that is as aggressive as that for someone with active cancer, but still it's a lot. I happily take my supplements and enzymes knowing I am keeping my body in an alkaline state with gobs of pancreatic enzymes to eat up the bad guys.

SS: Hello, Nick. Everyone is afraid of cancer; should they be?

NG: I've been in practice now nearly twenty-five years. I was researching cancer five years before that, and I've seen so many patients with advanced cancer get well. I feel it's sad that most of us still harbor some great terror about the illness. It's understandable; after all, cancer is a common problem, affecting one out of two Americans, killing one out of three. And despite all the hoopla and the media excitement, conventional cure rates really aren't changing much. For most cancers, once it has spread it's going to kill—so the fear is reasonable. But I have a much different experience with most of our patients, even those with advanced cancer, who come through smiling and well.

SS: Does everyone get well?

NG: No, not everyone gets well. There are so many factors involved with a patient's course—extent of disease, stress, family situation, amount of previous toxic therapy, even issues from childhood—all these things impact progress and prognosis. But most who do the work in our world get well, and get back to their lives. So with that kind of experience, in my mind, fear is unnecessary. Just make reasoned, thoughtful choices about treatment should you be diagnosed with the disease.

SS: I can hear my readers asking, "But how do you avoid it in the first place?"

NG: The rest of us without cancer should do the work to prevent the disease from occurring—you know, from the basics on up, no smoking, no junk food, no whites—white flour, white sugar, white bread—no chemicals, or as few as possible in the food, or in and on our bodies. Take supplements, take pancreatic enzymes, live clean and eat clean, and immediately your risk drops.

EVEN CONVENTIONAL EPIDEMIOLOGISTS NOW RECOGNIZE UP TO 80 PERCENT OF ALL CANCERS ARE PREVENTABLE, SO WE HAVE THE CHOICE TO INCREASE OR DECREASE OUR RISK. *WE*, NOT SOME UNSEEN ENEMY, ARE IN CONTROL.

Cancer tends to be frightening because most look at the disease as some wanton force, striking its helpless victims without warning, randomly, without rhyme or reason, but that's not the case at all. Good habits, good food, lower our risk substantially. So to get rid of the fear, become proactive; make the choices that minimize the chances of this ever striking your life.

SS: You once told me that cancer was manageable. Can you explain?

NG: We—my colleague, Dr. Isaacs, and I—approach cancer the way an endocrinologist approaches diabetes—as a chronic disease that can be managed for years, for decades, while patients lead normal or near-normal lives. A diabetic who sticks to the prescribed diet, who avoids the junk and sugar, who eats whole foods and takes insulin can lead a perfectly normal, productive life. You don't technically "cure" the diabetes, but patients can do fine with a disease that before the advent of insulin could kill in months.

We have patients initially diagnosed with stage IV cancer of various types who have been with us in excess of fifteen and twenty years. They may not be completely "cured." They may even have residual tumors in their bodies, but they do fine as long as they follow their prescribed diet and take the pancreatic enzymes we use to treat cancer.

SS: Do you ever cure them of cancer?

NG: Yes, we have patients, even patients with poor-prognosis cancers such as pancreatic cancer, who have been with us for years whose tumors on CT or PET scans have completely resolved. Yet even such patients may still harbor residual microscopic disease, but as long as they follow their diet and take their enzymes, they appear safe.

My mentor, the brilliant but eccentric Dr. William Kelley, first suggested forty years ago that we need to change our thinking about cancer. In those days, and even during my training, oncologists and physicians in general looked at cancer as an "all or nothing" situation. You either destroy every single cancer cell, or eventually you are going to die. We don't see this to be the case; if patients follow our therapy they can live a normal life span with their disease nicely controlled, if not always completely eradicated.

SS: So you're hopeful about the future of cancer treatment?

NG: It's been gratifying in recent years to read editorials in mainstream journals in which experts themselves are changing their minds about the disease, actually evoking the diabetes model as the correct approach to cancer, thinking of malignancy as a disease that can be managed and controlled for many, many years. That change in thinking should help lessen the pervasive fear of the disease that is everywhere. People used to be terrified of diabetes because it, like cancer, was so deadly, but though we all know diabetes can be nasty, it just isn't the life-threatening illness it was a hundred years ago. Someday I hope we look at cancer the same way, as a potentially nasty situation that can be overcome and managed nicely.

SS: As I mentioned in the introduction to your piece, I wanted to be proactive about preventing a cancer recurrence, so I asked you a while ago to design a protocol for me. Would you explain my program?

NG: Sure. I told you to eat organically, which you were already doing. Everyone should eat organically. Everyone should strive to eat whole foods, in as close to natural form as possible—fresh, locally grown produce, eggs from barnyard chickens, beef from grass-fed animals. Everyone should minimize their exposure to toxic chemicals in our food, water, air. I read an article recently that stated we in America are exposed to seventy-nine thousand synthetic chemicals, most of which have not been tested for safety. We can't completely eliminate our exposure—we all have to breathe, and when I walk down the streets of New York, I am taking in heavy metals that can be aerosolized, even pesticides that waft in on the wind currents to New York. But by eating organically, for example, we immediately reduce our exposure to many toxic chemicals. Pesticides, remember, are for the most part nerve toxins that kill insects by poisoning their nervous system. How is that a good thing, to add that to the food supply?

SS: I'm a big proponent of organic foods. It just makes sense.

NG: Organic is always best. Organic foods also tend to have higher levels of many nutrients than conventionally grown produce, as Sir Albert Howard, the great English scientist, proved eighty years ago. Fresh organic is better than canned or frozen, though I realize in a pinch sometimes we have to go with food that isn't right off the farm. But the metal of cans does leach into the food, not a good thing, and even frozen organic food is blanched to facilitate the freezing process—and with blanching comes the loss of some nutritional value. Food should also always be as untampered with as possible: no refining, no processing, no added synthetic chemicals, all of which invariably reduce the nutritional content.

SS: What else can we do?

NG: Both my office and my apartment are "green" spaces. When we had our office built in 1993, we sourced out all nontoxic materials, and instead used woods that hadn't been treated with formaldehyde and paints that had no toxic by-products or odors. We even had our office furniture built by a group of craftsmen (and craftswomen) up in Vermont, with natural woods, and natural oils for stains. In those days it was tough to find such products, but nineteen years later, the situation has changed dramatically for the better as people increasingly demand nontoxic building materials.

My apartment is the same, nontoxic—we had it painted not too long ago and purchased only low-VOC paints. There was no chemical odor, only a fresh scent, and even the painters commented how much better they liked our paints, and how much better they felt.

SS: What about water? I see it as a key to healthy cells.

NG: In my home and office, we have very state-of-the-art water filters. I know, there are all kinds of arguments about which filter is best, but we are sticking with reverse osmosis. There is no such thing as a perfect water filter, but RO comes close. People criticize reverse osmosis because it removes minerals, but it also removes the tiniest of pollutants, even viruses, and I just add a little good-quality sea salt, like Celtic Salt, to each glass of water to replenish the lost minerals. The upside of filtered water is enormous: chlorine is a carcinogen, very toxic; fluoride, which is still in many water systems, is a toxic chemical that poisons enzymes—not good. Fluoride is essentially a waste product from aluminum manufacturing that industry has convinced our politicians is a good thing, not the poison it really is.

Though we may not be able to control what's in the air outside, we certainly can control what we put on our bodies. Many preservatives and additives added to personal care products like shampoos are toxic—parabens, for example, added to many of these body care products for their antibacterial effect, are absorbed systemically and behave like estrogens in the body—not a good thing for a man, or for anyone. We recommend all our patients use natural body products, from shampoos to toenail polish—fortunately, organically based and nontoxic products are increasingly available, like your wonderful line.

SS: Thank you. I am extremely proud of Suzanne Organics, my line of certified toxic-free cosmetics. Your wife, Mary Beth, is my best customer.

NG: Yes, she is . . . So again, live as clean as possible. Eat clean. Eat whole fresh organic foods as much as possible. Avoid chemicals in the food and water, and live in a clean house. And, oh yes, exercise, good old exercise! A recent study confirmed that cancer patients receiving conventional treatment for their disease who exercised vigorously on a regular basis did better than those who didn't exercise. Traditionally, oncologists encouraged their patients not to exercise, in order to conserve their energy, but it turns out to be far better if they are active. Having said that, I do see a lot of patients who are very sick and simply can't exercise. It happens. Yet most everyone can walk every day, and twenty to thirty minutes of walking stimulates circulation—and with improved circulation, healing speeds up whatever the underlying problem. Walking also stimulates lymphatic flow, which assists the removal of toxic materials from our tissues and organs. So, exercise vigorously, regularly, and at least walk on a daily basis.

SS: What about supplementation? How important is it?

NG: Of course with supplements, you know we individualize our regimens for each patient, so it's difficult to offer general rules. However, we use pancreatic enzymes derived from a pig source to treat cancer, and in my opinion we believe that not only do these enzymes kill active cancer, but they also prevent cancer cells from forming and growing. The best supplements for cancer prevention, in my opinion, are pancreatic enzymes. For someone without cancer who wants a preventive program, like yourself, I would suggest maybe three to four capsules with meals, three times a day. With active cancer, of course, we get much more aggressive.

In terms of other supplements, we use many products, from A to zinc. Many alleged experts claim, even some of the organic raw-foods fanatics, that we should be able to get all the nutrition we need for good health from food. I've been hearing that for some forty years, and it is nonsense . . . if you want to enjoy good great health. It's simply impossible in this day and age to get sufficient nutrition from food alone—first of all, most of the soils, even those on organic farms, have been depleted of many nutrients so the food has less value than it did fifty years ago. Then, the ambient pollution in the air depletes nutrients—air pollution, for example, destroys both vitamin C and vitamin E. Our bodies are exposed to an assault of toxic chemicals we weren't designed to handle, which increases the demand for many nutrients. We all live with stress, and stress burns nutrients—I once read an article claiming that an animal exposed to extreme stress in a laboratory situation can burn up all its vitamin C in fifteen minutes. For these reasons, we need supplementation in addition to a wholesome organic diet, to help overcome the ravages of the toxic, stress-filled world in which we live.

SS: Why are enzymes so important?

NG: Dr. John Beard, the brilliant English scientist, first proposed in 1902 that pancreatic enzymes represent the body's main defense against cancer and would be useful as a cancer treatment. At the time, physiologists had already identified the many classes of pancreatic enzymes, which they acknowledged served a major digestive function, breaking down complex proteins, fats, and carbohydrates into simpler, easily absorbable molecules. But Beard claimed that above and beyond this digestive activity, the protein-digestive enzymes kill cancer cells. Subsequently, in both laboratory and human tests, he proved his point, reporting the successes of his treatment in the mainstream medical literature. He published his wonderful book *The Enzyme Treatment of Cancer* in 1911, but by the time he died in 1924, his work was forgotten. Fortunately, my mentor, Dr. Kelley, revived Beard's thesis in the 1960s with great success in his practice treating patients with advanced cancer. We've been employing high-dose enzyme therapy since we opened our practice in 1987, again with gratifying success.

SS: Are there other enzymes that are important?

NG: Of course, pancreatic enzymes represent only one class of enzymes in the body. Enzymes are a catalyst, which means they allow complex chemical reactions to occur quickly and efficiently, without much heat being produced. With enzymes, for example, reactions in our cells that might require a thousand degrees of heat—and make life impossible—occur rapidly at normal temperature. Every cell in our many tissues uses hundreds and thousands of enzymes as part of its normal metabolic machinery.

We don't tend to think of these many metabolic enzymes as nutrients, but Dr. Edward Howell was the great American researcher who spent more than fifty years of his life studying these "food enzymes" as he called them. These molecules, he claimed, could be absorbed like a vitamin or mineral and be used in the body to enhance metabolism and repair damage from injury or disease. However, these enzymes are very heat sensitive, being rendered inactive generally when the temperature hits 117 degrees Fahrenheit. So Howell proposed we should all eat, if not a completely raw-foods diet, at least some raw food to get the complement of these naturally occurring enzymes. We agree that most of us should consume some raw, but we vary the percentage of raw food in each patient's diet depending on their underlying metabolism. We prescribe diets, for example, that are largely raw but also diets that are largely cooked—cooking does destroy enzymes and some vitamins like vitamin C and folate, but it also breaks down the cells and essentially converts the food into a more or less predigested mix that doesn't require as much effort in the digestive system. Some of our patients are so inefficient from the effects of their disease or prior treatment, they initially can't tolerate too much raw food, but they do fine with cooked food. As they improve, we often increase the percentage of raw food.

SS: But this goes against the belief of some that all "raw" foods are best for you, doesn't it?

NG: For most of us, some raw food is beneficial—juicing particularly is a good way to get concentrated raw nutrition, including the food enzymes in a very enjoyable form. Fortunately, with the increased interest in juicing in the United States, there's been a host of books on the subject published.

SS: For those who haven't read *Knockout* as well as your critics, what is the benefit of coffee enemas?

NG: No part of our therapeutic regimen elicits more derisive comments from our conventional colleagues than our use of coffee enemas with our patients. Ironically, coffee enemas come right out of the mainstream academic literature, a point that seems lost on the critics. For example, many twentieth-century nursing texts recommended the enemas, as did the esteemed *Merck Manual*, a compendium of conventional orthodox wisdom. According to my conversations with a former editor of the manual, the text editors included the enemas right up until 1977 or so, when they were removed more for space considerations than anything else.

SS: That's a Bombshell. *Merck*! Any others?

NG: We have put together a nice collection of articles from the peer-reviewed medical literature discussing the positive effects of coffee enemas. One article I particularly enjoy appeared in 1922 in the *New England Journal of Medicine*, our most prominent of medical journals, discussing reversal of what today we call bipolar illness with the use of "rectal instillations," that is, enemas. A wonderful article I dug up in the Latin American medical literature dates from the early 1940s, in which a team of doctors in Uruguay reversed septic shock—almost invariably fatal in those days, and pretty fatal even today—with coffee enemas.

SS: Why do you think orthodox medicine turned away from their use?

NG: When the famed and brilliant Max Gerson started treating cancer patients with his whole-foods, raw-foods-type plant-based diet in the 1930s or so, he lost patients, not because the diet wasn't working but because it was working too fast—tumors were breaking down so quickly the patients' bodies were overloaded with dead tissue wastes, which can be deadly. Cancer cells are very abnormal and produce all kinds of proteins and enzymes that are foreign and toxic to normal tissue, so while breaking down a tumor is certainly a good thing, breaking down a tumor too fast can be overly toxic and deadly. Gerson began incorporating coffee enemas into his routine and saved his patients when they went through this toxic healing crisis. Gerson proposed that the enemas must be helping the liver, the body's main organ of detoxification, to work better.

SS: How does it work? What does it do?

NG: In terms of its physiological action, oddly enough when you drink coffee it stimulates the sympathetic or stress nervous system, so we get an energetic lift but also suppression of liver function. When you do the coffee as an enema rectally, it stimulates a completely different collection of nerves located in the lower pelvis called the *sacral parasympathetics*, and these nerves, when turned on, work through a reflex to stimulate the liver to release its toxic load. We believe that the coffee enemas enhance what scientists now refer to as *Phase I and Phase II detoxification systems*, which are responsible for neutralizing toxins whatever the source—from our diet, the environment, or our own metabolism. Coffee enemas in my experience help both these pathways work more effectively.

SS: Do you do them?

NG: Though I've never had cancer, I've done coffee enemas since I learned about them from Dr. Kelley in the summer of 1981, more than thirty years ago, and I have no intention of ever giving them up. The day I die I'm going to do my enema first, then go off and die. Patients often initially approach the enemas with some trepidation, as did I thirty years ago, but the great majority of patients report the enemas are one of the best, if not the best, part of the program because they feel so much better, whether the problem is toenail fungus or brain cancer. Coffee enemas help the liver work better, and when the liver works better, everything else in the body works better. Kelley, and Gerson before him, came to believe that an efficient liver was the key to healing, and I suspect they were both right.

SS: I know you design diets for your cancer patients according to their nutritional type based on genetics and ancestry. What diet do you recommend for cancer prevention?

NG: As you know, unlike many other alternative practitioners who use nutrition in their cancer programs, we don't have one magical "cancer diet." Kelley realized different patients need different diets, and we agree—our diets range from a largely animal fat and red meat diet to a largely raw-foods plant-based diet. We utilize ten basic diets, and dozens of variations, depending on the particular metabolic profile of the patient. Remember, humans are quite a flexible species, and our ancestors occupied a variety of ecological niches ranging from the Arctic of the Eskimos to the tropical rain forests. Each of these environments provided a unique source of food for whatever humans happened to be living there. For example, to use the extreme, the Eskimos adapted to and thrived on a diet of all fatty meat, 80 percent fat and 20 percent protein, with no fruits, veggies, nuts, seeds, or grains—there aren't any of these plant foods in the Arctic. And as long as the Eskimos stayed on a high-fat diet, they did great. As soon as our civilization crept in with white flour, white sugar, canned, processed, and refined foods, Eskimo health deteriorated tragically.

Groups living in tropical climes, on the other hand, had access to a wide variety of edible plants and adjusted to a more plant-based diet. Then you have the traditional Masai, who thrived—as Dr. George Mann of Vanderbilt reported forty years ago—on a diet of exclusively raw fermented milk, a gallon a day for an adult male, mixed with cow blood and occasional meat. So the idea that we should all be vegans, or as Atkins thought, all meat eaters, is incorrect—we're not that simple.

SS: Can you give our readers some "takeaways" on what they can do?

NG: Though it might sound complicated, I can throw out some general rules. Patients with the typical solid tumors, tumors of the breast, lung, stomach, colon, pancreas, liver, uterus, ovary, and prostate, do best with a plant-based diet—though even for these patients, some animal protein and fat is indicated, the amount varying depending on the patient. On the other hand, patients with the immune cancers like leukemia, lymphoma, multiple myeloma, and the sarcomas—connective tissue cancers we relate to immune cancers—do best with animal-product-based diets, with lots of red meat, fat, yes horror of horrors, even cholesterol, fatty fish, poultry, eggs. For these patients we also allow plant foods, the amounts and forms depending again on each patient's particular metabolism.

Balanced patients, those falling between the vegetarian and meat extreme, do best with a variety of foods, of both plant and animal origin. They do great at a buffet (organic, of course), with a variety of foods available: fruits, vegetables, nuts, seeds, whole grains, eggs, cheese, fish, poultry, and some red meat. But balanced people don't tend to get cancer, and as long as they follow a mixed diet, they should be able to avoid the disease nicely.

SS: How would a person know which diet "fits" him or her?

NG: We're frequently asked how anyone can tell what diet they need to follow without coming to see me. We wish, of course, that all doctors had the training in nutritional individuality and dietary prescription, but of course that isn't the case. Nonetheless, it really isn't that hard to tell for oneself. If the thought of fatty pot roast makes you gag, if you love fruit for lunch and don't need much else or crave salads, I promise, you are on the vegetarian side. Genetic meat eaters could care less if they never see a salad again, their idea of dessert is cheesecake and a piece of bacon, fatty food—and eating this way, they do great. Balanced people do indeed crave a variety of foods, of both plant and animal origin. So without all the fancy testing we do, it is possible to determine what kind of foods one should be eating.

SS: What other lifestyle changes need to be made to prevent cancer?

NG: Exercise, exercise, exercise—yes, I work long hours every day and on weekends, but I walk vigorously every day, from work—it's not like hiking a mountaintop but even these intense walks make me feel better and help maintain my boyish charm. Be active.

Try to minimize the stress in your life. I know, we all have stress, and none of us can get rid of it, and some stress is helpful to us physiologically—stress, to a certain degree, keeps the brain wired and active like mental exercise; we all need challenges at work and in our private lives. But too much stress, as the brilliant Hans Selye said fifty years ago, kills. New research shows it also helps bring on cancer. So do the best you can to keep stress under control (exercise helps with this, for sure).

Also, very important, get rid of negative people in your life. Gerson said he lost more patients from negative family members than from cancer itself, and at times I think he was on to something. We have patients in our practice with the worst kinds of cancer, but who enjoy each day as a gift, and these people seem to do well. Over the years, we've learned how to keep out of our office negative, angry, hostile people, who interpret every action of others as a threat or an act of revenge. You can usually get a sense of these people pretty quickly, and we don't take them as patients. We're not trying to be mean to unfortunate people with a terrible disease; we just know they won't do well—they have too many unresolved resentments and issues, often going back to childhood, and it's going to do them in. Such

unresolved issues create chronic stress, and chronic stress creates
physiological breakdown, which is the opposite of healing. When
we're in a stress mode, the sympathetic nervous system breaks down
stored tissues to provide energy for our brain and muscles so we can
think fast or react fast—but when stress is chronic, the breakdown of
tissues never ends, disease follows, and healing remains blocked.

So try to keep stress to a tolerable background noise, not the main
event every day.

SS: It seems to me from our talks that the answer to cancer is
simpler than we've been led to believe. Do you agree?

NG: It's simple in that we see patients with the worst cancers,
pancreatic, metastatic ovarian, metastatic colon, patients you've interviewed yourself, who've turned their cancer around, gotten through
the crisis, and lead happy healthy lives with a therapy involving diet,
supplements, pancreatic enzymes, and coffee enemas. It seems pretty
simple to me, but maybe I like simple answers. So yes, I think the
answer is indeed simple. Beard had it all figured one hundred years
ago, when he proposed that pancreatic enzymes are our main defense
against cancer, Kelley added the nutritional-dietary-detox components, and you have a nice approach to the disease that works most of
the time.

SS: Why don't we know about this? Why haven't we heard about
these treatments from our established cancer prevention bodies, like
the American Cancer Society? Are they doing a good job?

NG: I think the American Cancer Society is a blight on our
civilization—I've read that much of its income goes to high salaries
and maintaining the luxurious lifestyles of ACS executives. There
are wonderful articles on the Web about corruption at the ACS, and
the large donations from pesticide manufacturers and drug manufacturers. The ACS should have taken the lead with environmental
causes of cancer, but they kicked and screamed and hollered to avoid
having to face the issue, promoting such silliness as the viral cause of
cancer (which would have given a free pass to industry friends had it
proven true).

SS: Who, as you say, took the lead in discovering the connection
between environment and cancer?

NG: My dear friend the late Ernst Wynder was the first scientist
to propose way back in 1950 that cigarette smoking causes cancer.
His evidence even at that time was irrefutable, but he said one of his
biggest obstacles, along with the tobacco industry, was the American

Cancer Society. Only when the federal government announced that cigarette smoking causes lung cancer did the ACS belatedly come on board, and eventually they gave Wynder some type of award.

SS: Okay, so they were slower to recognize his important work, but playing devil's advocate, why does that make them a blight?

NG: They urge Girl Scout troops in Toledo to raise money to "fight cancer" while they give themselves ridiculously high salaries. The ACS also has traditionally hated anything that even remotely smacks of alternative.

SS: Why hasn't there been a cure after all the billions of dollars that have been raised?

NG: The billions go into drugs, and radiation, and the targeted therapies, and after sixty years of high-tech pharmaceutical inventions and interventions, we still have the same handful of cancers that respond. To date, most cancers, once no longer surgically curable, do not respond to chemotherapy, or radiation, or targeted therapies. Even the alleged miracle of antiangiogenesis is turning out to be a bust; Avastin does little for any of the cancers for which it is used, and the FDA has already rescinded its approval for its use in breast cancer.

Throwing money into the same bottomless pit doesn't make much sense to me—especially since Dr. Beard nicely presented a scientifically sensible and clinically demonstrated answer to cancer. But to the ACS and the National Cancer Institute, nutrition is silly, it's too simple, it's stupid, it can't possibly work.

SS: I've said before in this book, if it's too simple, there isn't enough money to be made . . . so it gets ignored.

NG: It's interesting when one reads medical history, they said the same thing about Dr. James Lind's citrus cure for scurvy, which he proposed in 1753. As a result, the British Admiralty refused to allow ships to recommend citrus to prevent scurvy for another forty years, and thousands of sailors died miserable unnecessary deaths. Truth is so often beautifully simple, as was Lind's suggestion and Dr. Beard's thesis about pancreatic enzymes.

SS: You have one of the best track records for managing cancer. Is it because these patients are totally compliant?

NG: One recurring complaint of my critics is that we select our patients. Of course we select our patients! First, there is absolutely no benefit for us to take on a patient who is too far gone, whom we cannot help. It's not fair to the patient. We select patients we think

cally we might be able to help, and who psychologically
asant attitude and will comply. It's a waste of everyone's
pecially the patients', if we take them on and they don't com-
rtunately, because we select our patients, compliance is very
and they generally do very well.

S: How important is God or spirituality as part of prevention?

NG: I am devoutly religious and begin each day with prayer and
Bible study. We are human beings, not laboratory rats; we are very
complicated, and we have a spiritual side that must be acknowledged
and nourished as much as our physiologic side. It's always easier to
heal patients who have a spiritual life that brings them to think about
greater things than immediate needs. Spiritual practice heals, powerfully.

SS: Do you feel hopeful about the end of cancer?

NG: When I first started out I was very idealistic, thinking this
wonderful therapy would change medicine and help change the
world—I wasn't giving myself megalomaniacal credit, it was that I
thought those who had come before me, Beard, Kelley, Weston Price,
were so brilliant. But I've come to realize scientists can be as corrupt
as anyone else. So I fear they will keep throwing billions into chemotherapy and more chemotherapy, and still more chemotherapy, and
boast about two-month improvements in average survival for some
deadly cancer as if the Second Coming were being witnessed.

But I'll keep doing what I'm doing, helping those patients I can
help in the best way I can. I have no greater aim than that.

SS: Thank you, Dr. Gonzalez. I have met with and talked to so
many of your happy patients. In fact, they are the only cancer patients I know of who are happy with their disease; it's a hard concept
to grasp, but I know it to be true. And you offer an option in a field
where options are dismal. Now you are offering your advice on prevention. There are those who will comply and those who won't. To
me it just makes sense. Thanks so much.

CHAPTER 16

BOMBSHELL #12:
YOU CAN KEEP THE ENVIRONMENT
FROM KILLING YOU

We have so polluted our environment and bodies that many folks require extreme measures in order to get well.

–Dr. Sherry A. Rogers, *Detoxify or Die*

We're going to explore *survival medicine* in this chapter. Okay, what do I mean by *survival medicine*? Over the years, I've written extensively, exhaustively, about the changing planet. We are under the greatest environmental assault in the history of humankind, and if we expect to live longer, healthier, and keep our brains intact, then having an *environmental doctor* in your coterie is now necessary and essential.

This new specialty rose out of necessity. Orthodox doctors have been caught unprepared and uninformed about the effects of toxicity on the human brain. Yet we continue to be told by mainstream medicine the "myth" that toxins are safe, that our healthy livers and kidneys keep us protected from nearly all levels of toxic accumulation. In fact, James Dillard, an assistant clinical professor at Columbia University's College of Physicians and Surgeons, said, "Most Americans have hundreds of toxins stored in their livers, and the liver is very capable of taking this kind of chemical load." Really? This is *not* true; in fact, our livers are *groaning* with toxic overload.

The liver is a magnificent organ, but if it is so impenetrable, then why is cancer about to be the biggest killer in the world, with liver cancer taking a spot in the top ten deadliest cancers? We can only ask so much of our livers and our kidneys. Toxins enter our bodies through our skin, lungs, or stomach. These intruders must eventually confront the liver, where they are detected and then usually dispatched in one of three ways: They are tucked away in the far reaches of the liver itself, sent on for elimination in the filtering system of the kidneys, or, as I wrote about in *Sexy Forever*, stored in the fat cells. It's in the fat cells that many of the long-term problems arise.

Toxins in the fat cells make and keep you fat. The more toxins you take in, the more fat is needed to store them, thus the obesity epidemic. It's not so much the volume of food, but the quality of the food that we take in that causes the problems. It's called the *toxic burden*, and burden it is. Our bodies were never designed to protect themselves against this chemical onslaught. Our systems fail to process and remove most of the chemicals once they have entered our bodies, so the toxicity starts building up inside us. According to Paula Baillie-Hamilton, a British authority on the health effects of toxic chemicals, "Every single human on the face of this earth is now permanently contaminated with these modern synthetic chemicals."

Imagine!

How did this happen?

When I was a kid there was a brand called Scotchgard. Everybody in my childhood had a can of Scotchgard in their house. It was a wondrous thing. My mother sprayed our furniture to protect it from stains. Our clothes were sprayed with it to protect against spills. It was fascinating stuff too; water would roll off it in little droplets. I loved to watch it and play with it.

But wait . . . it *was* too good to be true. How did Scotchgard end up accumulating in the body tissues of just about every human being on the planet and creating a huge health scare that continues to this day? Scotchgard is produced by the 3M Company as a stain-resistant coating for fabrics, leather, furniture, and carpets; its active ingredient, perfluorooctane sulfonic acid (PFOS), even found its way into the packaging of processed foods and fast foods. Its residues began turning up in the blood of the general population and in wildlife as early as 1976, and in 1983, a long-term study of PFOS in rats found that it stimulated the growth of cancer, particularly *liver* tumors. Amazingly, it wasn't taken off the market.

By 1999, the CDC had begun to monitor the effects of this chemical and found that it had been detected in the blood of most people everywhere from the United States to Sweden. Tests showed that it stayed in the bloodstreams of humans for up to four years. Finally, in May 2000, under pressure from the EPA, this PFOS ingredient was phased out of 3M products. But the damage had been done. And what about the effects of combining all the other chemicals we are knowingly and unknowingly accumulating? How do they react when mixed together?

Since 1950 skin melanoma is up 690 percent; prostate cancer, up 286 percent; thyroid cancer, up 258 percent; and non-Hodgkin's lymphoma, up 249 percent. Liver cancer is up 234 percent and growing; kidney and renal cancers are up 182 percent. Connect the dots.

I'm not trying to discourage you. This is, after all, a book to redefine aging, a way to live longer and healthier, without disease. Yet it seems the odds are stacked against us, and sadly, yes, the odds of escaping contamination are impossible, but—and this is the big but—there is a new specialty arising from necessity and it is called *environmental medicine*, or as I call it, *survival medicine*!

If you are not feeling well; if you are old before your time; if you are fearful of cancer and other diseases; if you suspect you are carrying a toxic burden because you have used and consumed products all your life you thought were safe; if you suspect or know you have mold, or bacteria, or gut issues that no doctor seems to know how to tackle; if you have unexplained aches, pains, painful joints, headaches, constipation, or colon problems—then environmental medicine could be your answer.

The job of the environmental doctor is to rid you of chemicals, molds, toxins, and contaminants.

ENVIRONMENTAL MEDICINE WORKS TO GET THE TOXINS OUT OF YOU BEFORE THEY CAN LEAD TO CANCER OR OTHER TERRIBLE DEBILITATING DISEASES.

This is a Bombshell!
Doctors who specialize in environmental medicine are in a rapidly expanding field. In addition to Dr. William Rea, whom you'll hear

from here, two others I've found are Dr. Rick Sponaugle, founder and medical director of Florida Detox and Wellness Institute, and Dr. Robin Bernhoft of Brentwood, California, in the L.A. area. These doctors have dedicated their lives to the detoxification of environmental toxins, including mold. (For more information on Dr. Sponaugle and a bonus chapter, go to my website, www.suzannesomers.com, and click on my blog.) As I vet more environmental medicine doctors, I will list them in my blog. Most antiaging doctors specialize in detoxification. Dr. Rea and the others I mention take the "last resort" patients, those so sensitive to chemicals that their lives are threatened.

But right now, I introduce you to Dr. Bill Rea, one of the original pioneers in environmental medicine. The doors at his Dallas, Texas, clinic have been open for thirty-five years, and more than thirty thousand patients have come to him from all over the world when no other medical protocols have worked.

WILLIAM REA, M.D.

Dr. William Rea *founded the Environmental Health Center in Dallas, Texas, where he offers an innovative, nontoxic approach to solving human health problems that are related to environmental pollutant exposure, including chemical and electromagnetic sensitivity. The center is considered by many people to be pioneering, and Dr. Rea is a recognized world authority on the manipulation of the patient's environment. As I said above, Dr. Rea has treated more than thirty thousand environmentally sensitive patients with his innovative techniques.*

SS: Hello, Dr. Rea. You are an environmental doctor located in Dallas, Texas. What is your definition of environmental medicine?

WR: Thank you, Suzanne. Environmental medicine understands that a toxic accumulation gathers in the human body from the air we breathe, the water we drink, bacteria, viruses, chemicals, mold toxins, and exposure from electromagnetic fields such as cell phones and technology. We environmental doctors determine what the individual toxic load is in each patient and work to detoxify these harmful toxins and get them out of the body.

SS: I find it very hopeful that you *can* clean the body of toxins.

WR: We can tell what is or is not in the blood, but it's more difficult in the tissues. To determine the amount of toxins in the tissues requires biopsies. We have breath analysis that can determine the amounts of over a thousand chemicals in the body. In the years I've been doing this, we have patients who have been treated with our protocols and appear to have none to very few toxins left in them after they change their lives and their environments.

SS: Lucky people. But even though you are able to clean out a patient using time, diligence, and patience, do you feel that we are constantly being reintoxicated?

WR: Unfortunately, you are going to have to breathe and drink water and eat food, and even if it is organic, you are still going to get some exposure. It's frustrating. That's why these changes we make have to become a way of life.

SS: I just came back from New York and I laughed to myself that you never see a bug in a hotel anymore, and you can't open a window.

WR: You could take aluminum foil with you, which is nearly 100 percent impervious to most toxic chemicals. You put it over the mattress and therefore "wall off" the toxins; you can even put the aluminum around the floors. Now these are for extreme cases. If you go to my website, you will see that for some people who have such a toxic load, they are virtually horribly allergic to everything. It makes their lives miserable.

SS: Are you joking? Aluminum on your bed and on the floors? Is it that bad out there?

WR: This is in extreme cases, but, yes, it's awful. You can get a breath analysis of a thousand chemicals and every time, a new one crops up. It can drive you crazy.

SS: But isn't our government keeping us safe?

WR: Suzanne, you've been around long enough to know that answer.

SS: Sorry, just playing devil's advocate.

WR: The human race is the most resilient on this planet, along with the cockroaches; otherwise we wouldn't have seven billion people. On the other hand, that doesn't mean we have seven billion *functioning* people. And how many people have good brain function? How many have good energy? Aches, pains, joints—you can go down the list—heart disease, cancer, and more; these are all usually environmentally induced.

SS: But when you talk about it, people get overwhelmed.

WR: I know, their eyes glaze over. So what we focus on are the informed people who really want to know about it, and those who want to be well.

SS: Who comes to your clinic?

WR: I get everybody's failures . . . people from all over the world, from all continents, who have their backs up against the wall. They've tried every protocol and they have failed, and now they are nonfunctional.

SS: Is there an age range?

WR: Not really; we usually see from twenty- to fifty-year-olds. But it can be any age, even kids and teenagers. The older ones also come, but they are generally not as informed and usually have a tendency to go to what they understand in orthodox medicine.

SS: So you treat those who have been on the planet long enough for their toxic burden to have reached critical mass?

WR: Yes, exactly; they have maxed out. There are four or five areas of the brain in addition to the GI tract (which is where you get the food sensitivities), and if those areas get off a little where the olfactory tract goes right up into the brain, it's like a sensor and a computer and then these toxins in the brain are devastating.

We found with people coming to us from Mexico City, where they are breathing in all those toxins, that unfortunately these toxins come right up through people's olfactory tract, and as a result they are getting Alzheimer's, Parkinson's, multiple sclerosis, and nonspecific neuropathy. Mexico City is number one in the world for pollution, although Shanghai is coming up on them. Some experts also found these toxins in kids from Mexico City who were in accidents, as well as finding them in wild dogs running around Mexico City. So every living thing in that area is breathing in these poisons, and the kids and animals have less resistance to them.

SS: My granddaughter has severe food intolerances. She is allergic, it seems, to just about everything.

WR: Well, that's how I got into this specialty; my oldest son almost died from food intolerances. He was allergic to about thirty of the most common foods—milk, beef, wheat, dairy, eggs, you name it. The intolerance causes terrible yeast infections, migraines, vomiting, diarrhea, and stomach issues. This is all classic; it's called *neurovascular injury*, which is nerve and blood vessel injury caused by breathing and eating these foods. Maybe children are not getting it at home, but they are getting exposed at school. Some kids are more receptive than others. I went to my grandkids' school and the smell of natural gas knocked me over. It was from their stoves in the kitchen. Something had gone wrong with their ventilation system and they hadn't gotten around to fixing it, but if a kid is sensitive, this is a big problem. Then there are the cleaning solutions they use at school; none of the schools are using organics, plus they spray for bugs, and in addition, most people use toxic chemicals in their homes to clean so it is quite pervasive.

SS: I often laugh at a commercial about a woman who lives in her apartment and friends come over and she gets embarrassed because she has a dog and her apartment smells. But the next time they come over, she has sprayed the entire apartment with a freshener (chemical) spray and now she is happy and her friends are smiling.

WR: Yeah, except now she's going to get sick and so will her dog. It shows the ignorance. No one understands the slow but sure damage we are doing to ourselves, our families, and our pets.

SS: Yes, but we've been led to believe these agents are not harmful.

WR: I had a state trooper from Georgia come to my clinic and he had uncontrollable heart irregularities, kinds that were killing him. In fact, they had to resuscitate him a couple of times before he got here. We traced it down to a Christmas tree deodorizer hanging in his car. He almost died, and he was twenty-seven years old.

Everybody has their own toxic burden. Some people can clear it better than others because their detox systems work better. What we look for in our patients is, What are the environmental triggers for each individual?

SS: Didn't you start your career as a cardiovascular surgeon?

WR: Yes, but then it started melding. At one point I had twenty heart patients in the hospital, and at the same time I had twenty environmental patients in the hospital. And finally I realized that no one was taking care of the environmental patients and that I knew how. I also think having my son so sick from being affected by pesticides was a sign to me that this was the direction I needed to take.

Everyone in our family was affected; in fact, at one point we had six rotary diets in the house. "Rotary" is when you don't eat the same food except for every four days.

SS: How did you turn your son's health around?

WR: Well, number one, I cleaned up his environment. I now grow organic foods and use safe water. No pesticides, no formaldehyde, no natural gas exposures. I used an intradermal neutralization technique we use now in my clinic for neutralizing foods, and also molds and chemicals. Then I put him on a high-nutrient program. I made an immune modulator out of his own blood, which he still takes. He's forty-seven now, rides his bicycle to and from work each day, and does just super. This has been going on for over twenty years.

SS: Is he able to eat most everything now or is he still allergic?

WR: He still has to be a little bit careful, but he takes his food shots and that allows him to eat almost anything. He still can't eat red watermelon. Strange, he can eat yellow watermelon, but not red. That's how subtle the environmental overload can be.

SS: What's a food shot?

WR: It's a shot where we neutralize the patients and desensitize them for molds. We have injections for that and also we have injections that neutralize chemicals.

SS: So if a patient came to you not knowing what's wrong, but he or she did not feel well, walk me through the steps of how you would treat this patient.

WR: Well, first we would take a good history and physical, not only an environmental history but also a medical history. You have to remember that almost all patients who come to me have already been to at least fourteen doctors. We review those records to see which direction it takes us. If necessary, we have apartments at Marriott that are environmentally clean, very simple but environmentally clean. Usually the patients stay there. So they are getting the treatment the minute they walk in, because we are reducing the total body pollutant load. We put them on safe water, and then if they can tolerate food, we feed them organic—only with a rotary diet.

Then we test them for molds and the different foods, and for chemicals. We give them a skin test, and of course we have a whole nutrition department. We try our best to keep the expense down as much as possible for them.

We might build a new booster shot for them; we see what their gamma globulins look like, because they are often deficient. We also might give them oxygen therapy.

SS: How long does a patient stay?

WR: Well, again, it depends on the contamination in their house . . . at this point we've modified around thirty thousand houses or built new ones. We try to have them have someone clean up their bedroom while they are in the clinic. By living at the hotel apartments while the patients are under treatment, they see the difference in how they feel. Then we have them go home to see if they can tolerate the bedroom at home. If they can't, then we most likely have to have them put in a hardwood floor or ceramics.

SS: Are there some houses that are just not salvageable?

WR: Yes, some of them are unsalvageable. You just can't do anything with them because they are so contaminated. Those people have to move. Most of them don't have to. I'd say 90–95 percent don't have to move. Some do have to change out the gas for electric heat, though.

SS: I'm one of those 5 percent. We, sadly, had to move out of our beautiful house recently because the mold was so pervasive. We had an unfinished basement and lived near the ocean, and there was water sitting underneath the house and coming up through all the air-conditioning ducts. It got inside the walls, behind the marble in the bathroom, everywhere. I never thought it would happen to me. But then again, two years before that our house burned down and I never thought something like that would happen to me. That's life. Are carpets a big culprit?

WR: They are, but the number one offenders in the house or buildings are natural gas and pesticides. Number three is formaldehyde and that comes from Sheetrock and carpets. Solvents are a big issue, toluene or xylene, things like that. If formaldehyde is the issue, then we recommend steam cleaning the carpets and covering the Sheetrock and in many cases to go with a hardwood or tile floor.

SS: What about organic carpets?

WR: No, organic can be contaminated also. The fiber may be organic, but the glue may not be. Organic mattresses are okay, but I find that they stink. But that's my opinion. We tell people to buy organic clothes and then wash them about six times to get the odor out. Even though it's a natural odor, a lot of people can't tolerate it. We all have individual senses of susceptibility. For some people it is so intense we help them build their own mattresses with springs and washable mats that they can layer to their comfort. It's a lot.

SS: I have an organic mattress and it smells perfectly fine. I guess there are different manufacturers with differing products. What about pets living in a house with mold?

WR: They should be outside. If not a lot of pets get sick, it's an indicator. If your pet gets sick or dies, it's a signal to get out of the environment. Kind of like the canary in the coal mine.

SS: Is it Sheetrock or what they call drywall that is mold food?

WR: It is. Insulation is mold food; corners are also mold food, because it can accumulate there. All you need to create mold is sweating or leaking pipes. Have one good hard rain and if it creates a leak, you are going to have problems. It's a fight all the time. For my severest patients, we eliminate Sheetrock altogether and use porcelain. It is free of formaldehyde and mold-free.

SS: Is porcelain considerably more expensive?

WR: It was common right after World War II. The feds built a whole lot of porcelain houses, but then that stopped and they went to Sheetrock. Porcelain is fused on steel. It never needs repairs, so amortized over the years it's actually cheaper.

We have glass walls in our waiting room, and then put Sheetrock behind it. This keeps the synthetic toxins out, along with the mycotoxins. We also use composite tiles as toxic-free options, ceramic tile that's put down with old-fashioned grout as there are few chemicals in it. Porcelain tile is also an option, and it's beautiful. We are always trying to find options for people that are not too costly. People need to be educated about buildings; I wrote a book about that.

SS: What's it called?

WR: *Optimum Environments for Optimum Living and Creativity.* I also wrote *Energy and Brain Function.*

SS: My assistant has been sick for four months. She's been vomiting, can't keep food down; her doctor said she had IBS. So he put her on an antidepressant.

I encouraged her to take the food intolerance allergy stool test and it turns out she has a parasite and an "off the charts" gluten intolerance. I mention this because if this is how the majority of people are being treated by their orthodox doctors today, it is terrible. He put her on an antidepressant to calm her down. What kind of medicine is that? This means people are getting care that is actually detrimental to their health.

WR: Yes. It's the philosophy of "wait until the disease gets worse and then we might be able to diagnose you." We should be preventing illness by getting the mold toxins, getting the chemicals, and creating nutrient programs before all this ever happens. I see this all the time with teenagers who come here incapacitated and on our program get better real fast.

SS: And then do they have to come back regularly or do you teach them how to detoxify themselves?

WR: We make sure before they leave us that they understand "cause and effect." We teach them that the body is a wonderful sensor, but it's been underdeveloped and ignored. We've got a supercomputer in our brain that can analyze these things, but it gets masked over and ignored. So once we teach our patients and their families this concept, so that they truly understand it, they can understand what needs to be done in their environment. I have some patients who check in about once every twenty years. I'd like to see them more often, but they are from Singapore, Japan, England, and Spain, so it's not easy to drop by. But they learn how to manipulate them-selves and keep their environments pristine.

SS: Do the green builders get it?

WR: They don't, and you would expect that they would. But the Bau-biologists, they are German, and some do understand how to build a toxic-free house.

SS: How can people check for chemicals in their home?

WR: We have kits now that measure indoor air. One is called an "Indoor Air Analysis Kit," and there's an "Outdoor Air Analysis Kit."

SS: After the patients get their kit, they can start eliminating toxins from their houses. Will these kits analyze if there is mold?

WR: Yes. Mold is serious. How does nature disintegrate things? We rot. Right? And our homes and bodies are broken down into dirt for lack of a better explanation. What we are doing is trying to live in harmony with nature, but we are also fighting nature when the negative aspects get into excess. Molds can lead to Parkinson's dis-ease, multiple sclerosis, Alzheimer's disease, arteriosclerosis, and so on, and so many other horrible conditions.

SS: Can molds lead to death?

WR: Yes, molds can. That's why we have to keep fighting. I've been treating molds since I was a thoracic surgeon. I knew about this as a surgeon because we had all these things like coccidioidomycosis, blastomycosis, and even some other pulmonary cardiac diseases—all were caused by molds. Aspergillosis can be caused by mold in the lungs. Environmental illnesses will alter brain function, they will alter heart function, they will alter intestinal function, and they will spark food intolerances and food sensitivities, which can be devastat-ing and even deadly.

SS: So, it's rethinking your house and what you have in it, as well as what you clean it with, and rethinking your food and your water.

WR: Drink from glass bottles, not plastic. Install reverse osmosis fil-ters. And your sinks should be made of ceramics and steel. Your water should be double filtered. You have to understand that public water supplies are contaminated, fluoride is a disaster, and so is chlorine. Ozone aids the water. A lot of cities in Europe use ozone in the water.

SS: Do we need to return to more natural ways of living in our everyday lives?

WR: Yes, natural living using modern technology. Like water; you need to filter it, and modern technology makes that possible. Learn to steam things to kill them, like bugs. Pesticides will surely eventually do you in, as will gas and mold. But decreasing toxins can be done. We can live and be healthy, if we understand how to manipulate our own personal toxic load. And then each of us has to take responsibility for implementing changes. It is possible to decrease toxin loads; we can neutralize toxins and teach you what nutrition your individual body requires. We see individual miracles in our clinic every day. It's very rewarding work.

SS: And what do people say to you after they've finished your program?

WR: Most of them say they've never felt better in their lives.

SS: It's almost like you've turned a light on in them.

WR: We have. That's what's happening.

PART III

PUTTING IT ALL TOGETHER

When you have to make a choice and don't make it, that is in itself a choice.

–William James

CHAPTER 17

THE BOMBSHELL AGE REVERSAL PLAN

I often read that I am considered controversial in my approach to my health. I thought I would dispel that notion by describing my plan, what I do on a daily basis to combat the toxic, stressful world we have inherited. I try to live a healthy life physically and spiritually. I have love in my life and that is a tremendous advantage. Also, I treasure my family and have gratitude for all I am so blessed with. So what do I do that people consider so "odd"?

Here it is.

I start each day by checking in with myself . . . how am I feeling?

Today's assessment:

Emotionally: great.

Physically: energetic, happy.

I slept eight hours last night, deeply, soundly, such a blessing. No sleeping pills for me; instead, I give myself assistance by taking melatonin before I go to bed plus three chewable GABAs to turn off the "noise." You know that noise, all those "lists" of projects and activities that need attending to, those "to-dos" for tomorrow, as well as the always difficult task of turning off the mind from continuing to review what you did today. I also wear a LifeWave sleep patch between my big and second toes. It has the magical effect of shrinking the time the melatonin naturally starts to pour and the effect is a long, dreamy drugless sleep.

I take sleep seriously. It's our bodies' replenishing time. Like a race-car, got to cool down, rest the machine. Sleep is the "tune-up." Remember when you were a child? Did it ever enter your mind that when you went to bed at night you wouldn't sleep? Of course not! In fact, before your mom even got through a bedtime story, you were conked out. When did that change? Oh right, adulthood with all its stress, lists, exhaustion, and hormone imbalance.

Sleep is when all the healing hormone work happens. It's when the organs and glands are given a rest to replenish and reenergize. But most people push and push themselves, even take pride in it, until they push so hard that the internal self starts to collapse. Sleep is perhaps the most important overlooked source of health in anyone's antiaging arsenal.

What else do I do? I always take a nightly, long, hot bath before going to bed. Relaxes me, calms me down, destresses. No small thing, that. And there is something I love about sliding between clean sheets all fresh and shiny. I rub my organic skin creams all over (wild orange and vanilla). It's like superfood for my skin, and they are a new concept: creams that not only soften skin but also provide nutrition that ends up in your bloodstream.

Then of course, without fail, before bed I always rub on my hormone creams: estradiol, estriol, and testosterone; progesterone if it's the second half of the month. I take my vital hormones every day in different amounts to create a natural rhythm of nature. My hormone amounts are determined by lab work, individualized just for me.

Somewhere in the middle of the night I usually wake up, probably because I drink a lot of water right before bedtime when taking my vitamins and enzymes. This momentary awakening works positively for me because in nature human growth hormone (HGH) pours in in the middle of the night while we are sleeping. I have a deficiency, determined by my IGF-1 (insulin-like growth factor) levels. Most people my age are deficient in HGH, seeing as how our bodies stop producing it in our late thirties. Again, we are living longer than nature planned due to technology, and so the new thinking in extending life is to reproduce an optimal quality of life replicating our healthiest prime. We were never healthier or stronger than when our bodies were making a full complement of hormones, and HGH is one of them. HGH gets a bad rap, mainly because of how it's used by some athletes who routinely use a hundred times more than natural physiologic levels. The proper way to replace anything is to mimic nature.

Nature never made HGH in increments one hundred times more than our bodies could produce. So I take only what my body is missing and no more than that.

As always, I try to replicate as closely as I can the rhythm and routine of nature. If nature pours human growth hormone in the middle of the night, who am I to question? HGH builds lean muscle, strong bones, and a strong heart. Plus it is part of the "hormonal song." All hormones work together. When one is off, they all get off.

My daily routine is part of my *plan* for aging well. I believe visualizing my own end point is an essential component of living a long, healthy life.

If you make simple changes on a daily basis, you can turn around the decline and destruction resulting from today's modern assault. My daily routine is about restoring those parts of me that are declining to be sure the luster and shine of all that is golden about aging becomes my reality.

We once thought about the golden years as two little old people with silver hair sitting together happily looking out to the sunset in their rocking chairs. That would be lovely if that was the present template of aging. Sadly, that picture of happy little old people no longer exists. Instead, the golden years are now usually spent in the nursing home, conveniently drugged to a foggy haze in order to become easier to warehouse. This present desperate end results in isolation and loneliness, with people cut off from family and loved ones except for excruciating visiting days from family members who are forced to make awkward small talk with their once vibrant loved ones who can no longer think due to the overdrugging from pharmaceuticals and a lifetime of exposure to toxins.

What a crappy way to end a beautiful life. But it's what we now expect.

Don't accept this as your end point. Refuse to accept the scenario of a helpless, sick ending. Instead, choose to be the new face of aging: productive, healthy, energetic, sexual, and vibrant. Make changes in how you are living your life at present. It's not difficult, not crazy expensive, and not overwhelming. So far, it's little more than rubbing on a few creams, taking a nightly warm bath, avoiding toxins, taking supplements, and eating good food. You can do it, too.

Back to my routine: Every morning I rub on my prescribed hormones, including DHEA cream, a vital antiaging hormone. Then, because I have a sensitive stomach, I take glutamine powder to heal the lining of my gut. I also take a packet of minerals in a glass of water to replace what has been depleted from our food and soil.

As I said, I have a sensitive stomach, and I don't think I'm alone, so I take great care to keep my GI tract in balance and healthy. Gut disturbances are a relatively new phenomenon that has happened not only to me but to so many as we age because we did not realize that processed, refined, chemicalized fake foods, which we get from having to eat in restaurants so often, have wreaked havoc on our guts. People accept bloating, constipation, heartburn, acid reflux, yeast, and its overgrowth as normal. There is nothing normal about it.

I also take a packet of super vitamin C in a glass of water. In addition, I take a spoonful of fiber in a glass of water to keep my system regular. I take daily vitamins, determined by a blood test that indicate my exact deficiencies, and I add in my pancreatic enzymes with each meal and before I go to bed. In addition, I wear my nanotechnology patches during the day for energy; if I have any pain, I wear a pain patch. And every day I wear my glutathione detoxification patch to help with the toxic assault none of us can avoid.

Perhaps my routine sounds like a lot of steps, but remember your end point. What do you visualize? I've told you what my picture looks like, and these simple but vital steps are what are necessary to get me there. You have to make your own choices. You can do some of it, or all of it—whatever best suits your lifestyle and needs. But to do nothing likely means that your end point will be the present awful template.

Finally, I exercise. You've got to exercise; it's a must! Think of that Maserati . . . even if it was brand-new, if you never drove it (exercised it), it would run stiff. It would sputter and choke. It would be rusty. The parts would not be lubricated. Well, the body works the same way.

To keep fit and limber and ensure my joints are lubricated, I do yoga three to four times a week (stretching keeps us all flexible), I do some cardio every day for twenty minutes until I get my heart rate up, and I do weight training in my bedroom every other day, for about twenty minutes.

There you have it. This is the daily plan I have adopted, personalized to my individual needs in order to live long with quality.

Adding to my plan of action are the things already mentioned in this book such as my stem cell breast regrowth, new hormones for sexuality, cell rejuvenation, and nanotechnology advances, some of which are available to use now, such as my nondrug patches. I believe all these proactive health endeavors will allow me to access the near future—when those advances described by Ray Kurzweil with nanobots and biotechnology are available, and the reprogramming of genetic switches that Dr. Burzynski spoke about effectively helps to eliminate disease. The future is exciting indeed!

So what do you feel comfortable doing? What might you want to test out with the help of your antiaging doctor? Here are some ideas to consider.

18 AGE-REVERSING IDEAS TO CONSIDER

1. Take melatonin nightly to naturally sleep the required eight hours.
2. Consider GABA (the chewable kind) nightly to turn off the "noise" in your mind.
3. Be mindful of overworking, so as to eliminate unnecessary stress.
4. Work with your doctor to replace the minor and major hormones if a deficiency exists—for example, estrogen, progesterone, testosterone, DHEA, and HGH; thyroid adrenals, cortisol, or insulin levels.
5. Take a long, relaxing nightly hot bath, add Epsom salts two times a week and soak for twenty minutes.
6. Use organic cosmetics to moisturize and soften but also to provide superfood for your skin.
7. Drink plenty of water, eight glasses a day preferably.
8. Take daily vitamins determined by a blood test.
9. Eliminate toxins from your life and home.
10. Consume organic food.
11. Follow an anti-inflammatory diet (see the next section for more details).
12. Take a spoonful of glutamine powder to heal the lining of your gut, if applicable.
13. Take a daily packet of minerals to replace what is now missing in your food.
14. Take vitamin C daily.
15. Take a spoonful of natural fiber daily.

16. Exercise regularly.
17. Use nanotechnology nondrug patches for pain, sleep, energy, and body detoxification.
18. Avoid pharmaceutical drugs unless absolutely necessary.

It's a little bit of effort, a moderate expense layout, but vital to combat the destructive forces working against all of us in today's toxic, chemicalized world. This is where you step on board and buy your ticket to your positive end point. Along the way you get to enjoy a great, and I mean *great*, quality of life. It's worth it!

GO ALKALINE:
EAT AN ANTI-INFLAMMATORY DIET

Inflammation is also associated with high levels of acidity. Cancer loves acid, and for those who suffer from chronic yeast infections, yeast also loves an acidic environment. (By the way, the best way to heal the gut from chronic yeast and yeast infections told to me by Dr. Gonzalez is Candex by Pure Essence Labs, two tablets morning and night. Really works.) Your health is very sensitive to the tiniest change in your pH levels. Being too acidic can lead to disease. Being too alkaline is rare, but can cause problems as well. Ideally your pH should be around 7.0. The lower you go on the pH scale, the more acidic you are. Using pH indicator strips to test your urine (a good brand is Cardinal Health) is an excellent way to keep a check on yourself. If your pH strips say 5.0 or 5.5, you are way too acidic.

Some foods are acid causing, so if your pH is low, then you might try avoiding meat and poultry, eggs, cheese, grains, legumes, and most nuts until you get back in balance. Another good way to bring your alkaline levels into the 7.0 range is by taking a teaspoon daily of Bio-Terrain Alkaline pH balancer available at the Tahoma Clinic (www.tahomaclinic.com).

Most people are too acidic. The best way to avoid colds and flu and other serious conditions is to keep your body slightly alkaline; vegetables and fruits help to alkalize your system, and supplementing with four alkaline minerals—calcium, magnesium, potassium, and sodium—will also bring you into balance. A teaspoon of baking soda in water daily can also help alkalize.

What else can you do to enjoy Bombshell health? You can remember your telomeres and how important they are to longevity.

KEEPING TELOMERES HEALTHY

EATING QUALITY FOOD IS THE BEST
DEFENSE AGAINST DISEASE
AND ACCELERATED AGING.

That sentence says it all. TA-65 appears to be a miracle supplement. But if it is not affordable, there are foods that are great "alkalinizers," and also telomere friendly!

Here are the best of the best.

ALMONDS
A true superfood, an amazing source of protein and fiber as well as minerals, including calcium, magnesium, iron, potassium, and zinc. They are also high in vitamin E and contain monounsaturated fats, which help to keep arteries supple. Raw, unsalted is best. Sorry salted fans.

APPLES
This old standby contains the phytonutrient quercetin, which prevents oxidation (damage) of LDL cholesterol and thereby lowers the risk of damage to arteries, and in turn the risk of heart disease. Apples also contain pectin, a soluble fiber that seems to be effective in lowering levels of blood cholesterol.

AVOCADOS
These provide more heart-healthy monounsaturated fat, fiber, vitamin E, folic acid, and potassium than any other fruit. They are the number one source of beta-sitosterol, a substance that can prevent macular degeneration and reduce total cholesterol, and lutein, an antioxidant that prevents cataracts and lowers the risk of prostate cancer.

BEANS

Rich in calcium, iron, folic acid, B vitamins, zinc, potassium, and magnesium, beans are a Bombshell of a food. They contain large amounts of both soluble and insoluble fiber. Soluble fiber helps reduce cholesterol levels, insoluble helps regulate bowel movements.

BEETS

Low in calories and loaded with nutrients, especially high levels of carotenoids and flavonoids. What's not to love?

BLUEBERRIES

The U.S. Department of Agriculture lists blueberries as an excellent fruit source of antioxidants. Studies indicate their role in fighting memory loss, high cholesterol, diabetes, and strokes. Blueberries improve blood flow, keeping your brain and heart healthier. They also contain pterostilbene, shown to be effective in reducing LDL (bad guys) cholesterol. A half-cup serving has as much antioxidant power as five servings of other fruits and vegetables.

BROCCOLI

This cruciferous vegetable is a powerhouse of antioxidants such as indole-3-carbinol (I3C), di-indolymethane (DIM), and sulforaphane that detoxifies cancer-causing chemicals. Cruciferous vegetables also contain compounds called glucosinolates that have antidiabetic and antimicrobial properties.

CABBAGE

Rich in isothiocyanates and other cancer-preventing nutrients, high in fiber, and with the ability to stimulate the immune system and kill bacteria and viruses, cabbage is not just an ingredient for coleslaw! It inhibits the growth of cancerous cells, protects against tumors, helps control hormone levels, improves blood flow, and stimulates your sex drive. It also inhibits the growth of polyps in the colon, and consuming large amounts boosts estrogen metabolism, reducing cancer risk. Studies show eating cabbage just once a week reduces the risk of colon cancer by 60 percent.

GARLIC

Many clinical trials show garlic as a cancer fighter—preventing colon, breast, skin, prostate, stomach, and esophagus cancers. It keeps your immune system vigilant by maintaining healthy function and numbers of natural killer cells, which are your first line of defense.

GRAPEFRUIT
Eating one grapefruit a day for thirty days can significantly reduce cholesterol by as much as 15 percent and triglycerides by 17 percent; and if you eat the fruit and the skin, you get more fiber and more antioxidants. Grapefruit also helps fight heart disease. But it should not be eaten if you're still on a statin.

KALE
This green veggie regulates estrogen and is cancer protective for bowel, breast, bladder, prostate, and lung cancers. It also protects against heart disease and regulates blood pressure. It's also a good source of calcium, which protects against osteoporosis, arthritis, and bone loss.

MEAT
This protein source supplies needed iron, B_{12}, carnosine, taurine, glutamate, choline, and zinc. Eat only organic and grass fed.

OLIVE OIL
Provides important monounsaturated fats that can help prevent heart attacks and allow for pliable cell membranes.

ORANGES
These tasty citrus fruits have hesperidin, an important flavonoid that can lower rates of heart attack. They are also a rich source of pectin, which lowers cholesterol, as well as potassium and folic acid, which lower homocysteine.

SEA VEGETABLES
The consumption of these vegetables may account for the low rates of cancer in Japan. They contain a high level of iodine. Nori is exceptionally high in protein and vitamins A and K, iodine, and potassium. Dark sea vegetables like arame, wakame, hijiki, and kelp contain alginate, which works in the GI tract to reduce the reabsorption of heavy metals.

SWEET POTATO
I like baked baby yams the best. They are like candy and loaded with protein, fiber, and beta-carotene for your arteries, as well as potassium, which controls your blood pressure.

TEA
Drink it black, green, and now white. All contain numerous and powerful unique polyphenols that may inhibit breast, digestive, and lung cancers. The polyphenols in green tea are wonderful antioxidants and function via unique mechanisms to protect against common ailments. A study showed people who drank two or more cups daily also had higher bone density than those who didn't.

TOMATOES
Lycopene, found in tomatoes, reduces the risk of prostate, lung, and stomach cancers. Also, they contain potassium and vitamin C, all of which are essential for the immune system. Tomatoes are also good for the skin.

WILD SALMON
This is the perfect food. But it has to be wild as it is loaded with omega-3 oils. Wild salmon has been shown to protect against many cancers and autoimmune diseases, such as rheumatoid arthritis and asthma. The more omega-3 oils you have in your system, the longer the length of your telomeres. Also, wild salmon is generally found to be low in heavy metals like mercury, which can be a big problem in other fish like swordfish and large tuna.

The more daily servings you eat on average of these foods, the less likely you are to develop a chronic disease. Research shows that people who consume at least seven to ten servings a day get the most benefit. To do that, animal protein can no longer be the predominant portion on the plate. It's hard to eat a large portion of protein at each meal and expect to get enough vegetables and fruit.

Ready to do even more? Then turn the page and find out in the next chapter, "Advanced Age Reversal," how to knock down the other age promoters we discussed earlier.

CHAPTER 18

ADVANCED AGE REVERSAL

Based on new findings about the *mechanisms of aging*, the universal dream of a longer life is now a scientific reality. But what if you want to go deeper than making just a few changes and you want to dive into a more advanced age-reversing program? I asked Bill Faloon of Life Extension to provide a plan to counterattack the eighteen most common things that age us. Consult with an antiaging physician to see which of these might be issues for you, so that you can tailor your plan of attack to your individual needs.

The phenomenon known as "aging" is the result of pathological changes that are somewhat controllable using existing technologies. By prolonging our healthy life span, we put ourselves in a position to take advantage of future medical breakthroughs that could result in dramatic extensions of the human life span.

This chapter reveals what do about the eighteen controllable causes of age-related disease; follow these simple steps to correct them.

AGING FACTOR 1: CHRONIC INFLAMMATION
SOLUTION: COMPREHENSIVE ANTI-INFLAMMATORY REGIMEN

An array of *clinically proven* nutrients and hormones has been shown to effectively *target* the mechanisms behind inflammation. The agents listed below operate in multiple ways to neutralize pro-inflammatory processes.

NUTRIENT	TYPICAL DAILY DOSE	SUGGESTED PRODUCTS
Fish oil	1,400 mg EPA and 1,000 mg DHA	Super Omega-3 EPA/DHA with Sesame Lignans and Olive Fruit Extract
Curcumin*	400–800 mg	Super Bio-Curcumin®
Bromelain	500–1,000 mg	(enteric-coated tablets)
DHEA (dehydroepiandrosterone)	15–50 mg	(micronized for optimal absorption)

* 400 mg of enhanced bioavailable curcumin (BCM-95®) equates to 2,500 mg of standard curcumin supplements.

The most commonly used *blood test* for inflammation is known as *high-sensitivity C-reactive protein*, or hs-CRP. Any doctor should be able to provide this test for you, or you can order it directly by logging on to www.suzannesomers.com. CRP levels in men should ideally be below 0.55 mg/L while women should be below 1.50 mg/L.

In addition to the nutrients and hormones described in this section, those with persistently high levels of C-reactive protein should seek to reduce their fasting blood glucose levels to below 85 mg/dL of blood.

Carrying excess fat pounds, especially in the belly, is a common cause of systemic inflammation. There are nutrients that impede the absorption of carbohydrates and thus facilitate weight loss along with reductions in fasting blood sugar. (You will read in Aging Factor 16 about natural ways to reduce belly fat and lower blood glucose.)

Those with stubbornly high blood sugar levels may need to take a standardized *green coffee bean extract* (350 mg three times daily) that has been shown to naturally block the overproduction and release of glucose into the bloodstream.

High LDL (bad cholesterol) can also spark systemic inflammatory fires. Your LDL levels should ideally be kept below 80–100 mg/dL. The presence of inflammatory factors in the blood is why blood testing is so important when designing an individualized program to neutralize your Aging Factors. To inquire about low-cost compre-

hensive blood testing in your area, log on to www.suzannesomers
.com and click through to Life Extension.

AGING FACTOR 2: GLYCATION
SOLUTION: FACILITATE GLUCOSE METABOLISM AND INHIBIT GLYCATION

Numerous studies have shown that the nutrients listed below *suppress* dangerous glycation reactions in the body.

NUTRIENT	TYPICAL DAILY DOSE	SUGGESTED PRODUCTS
Carnosine	1,000 mg	Mitochondrial Energy Optimizer with BioPQQ™
Pyridoxal-5'-phosphate (active form of vitamin B_6)	100 mg	
Benfotiamine (a form of vitamin B_1)	150 mg	
Chromium	500 mcg	Optimized Chromium with Crominex® 3+

AGING FACTOR 3: METHYLATION

The DNA within every cell of your body requires constant enzymatic reactions called *methylation* for maintenance and repair. Aging *cripples* youthful methylation metabolism. The resulting DNA damage can manifest as cancer, liver damage, and brain cell degeneration.

SOLUTION: METHYL DONORS

Low-cost nutrients can safely *restore* methylation activity to youthful levels.

Taken together, the following nutrients are referred to as "methyl donors." They induce so-called remethylation reactions—boosting levels of methylation activity and restoring healthy cellular function and repair.

Nutrient	Typical Daily Dose	Suggested Products
L-methylfolate (active form of folic acid)	1,000 mcg	Optimized Folate
Pyridoxal-5'-phosphate (active form of vitamin B_6)	100 mg	
Vitamin B_{12}	1,000 mcg	
TMG (trimethylglycine)	500–1,000 mg	
S-adenosylmethionine (SAMe)	200–400 mg	

AGING FACTOR 4: MITOCHONDRIAL DYSFUNCTION

Over 350 studies published in 2010 alone show how mitochondrial *degradation* leads to the onset of virtually every degenerative disease. Mitochondrial dysfunction can result in congestive heart failure, muscle weakness, fatigue, and neurological disease. The good news is that researchers have found that age-related mitochondrial decline may be *reversed*.

SOLUTION: MITOCHONDRIAL SUPPORT

To energize and restore aging mitochondria, the following four nutrients should be taken each day.

Nutrient	Typical Daily Dose	Suggested Products
CoQ_{10}, as ubiquinol	100–200 mg	Super Ubiquinol CoQ_{10} with Enhanced Mitochondrial Support™
Pyrroloquinoline quinone (PQQ)	10 mg	Mitochondrial Energy Optimizer with BioPQQ™
Acetyl-L-carnitine arginate	675 mg	
R-lipoic acid	150 mg	

AGING FACTOR 5: HORMONE IMBALANCE
SOLUTION: BIOIDENTICAL HORMONE REPLACEMENT WITH NUTRIENT SUPPORT

The most effective way to bring your sex hormones into balance is by *restoring* them to youthful levels with bioidentical hormone replacement therapy. There's no fixed dosage for these hormones. You and your doctor tailor the amount that's right for you through careful monitoring of your blood test results.

HOW TO SUPPORT HORMONE BALANCE

Nutrient or Intervention	Typical Daily Dose	Suggested Products
FOR WOMEN (no prescription needed)		
DHEA*	15–25 mg	(micronized for optimal absorption)
Pregnenolone*	50–100 mg	
Natural progesterone cream	Follow label directions	
Broccoli extract	400–800 mg	Triple Action Cruciferous Vegetable Extract
Indole-3-carbinol (I3C)	80–160 mg	
Apigenin	25–50 mg	
Calcium D-glucarate	200–400 mg	
Vitamin D$_3$	5,000 IU	
FOR WOMEN (requires prescription)		
Bioidentical hormone replacement	Based on individual blood test results	

(continued)

Nutrient or Intervention	Typical Daily Dose	Suggested Products
FOR MEN (NO PRESCRIPTION NEEDED)		
DHEA*	25–100 mg	(micronized for optimal absorption)
Pregnenolone*	50–100 mg	
Saw palmetto extract	320 mg	Ultra Natural Prostate Formula
Stinging nettle root extract	240 mg	
Lignan extract	20 mg	
Vitamin D_3	5,000 IU	
Broccoli extract	400–800 mg	Triple Action Cruciferous Vegetable Extract
Indole-3-carbinol (I3C)	80–160 mg	
Apigenin	25–50 mg	
FOR MEN (REQUIRES PRESCRIPTION)		
Bioidentical hormone replacement	Based on individual blood test results	

* Consult with your physician before taking DHEA or pregnenolone. Do not use DHEA or pregnenolone if you are at risk for or have been diagnosed as having any type of hormonal cancer, such as prostate or breast cancer.

Those taking bioidentical hormones should consider taking nutrients shown to help aging men and women safely utilize their hormones, protect against hormone-dependent cancers, and eliminate potentially carcinogenic compounds found in our diet and environment.

Estrogen imbalance poses a major threat to both women *and* men. Clinical studies reveal that too much or too little estrogen puts men at greater risk for heart disease, atherosclerosis, stroke, prostate cancer, and osteoporosis. Compounds found in *cruciferous vegetables* help our bodies regulate estrogen metabolites, neutralizing dangerous ones.

The chart in this section describes bioidentical hormones you can obtain right now and the nutrients you should take with them. Fortunately, many of these nutrients are available in special multiformulas, so you don't have to take a lot of pills.

AGING FACTOR 6: EXCESS CALCIFICATION

Aging *disrupts* calcium transport, resulting in excess calcium infiltration into the soft tissue cells of the brain, heart valves, and middle arterial wall (causing arteriosclerosis). Many age-related disorders are related to excessive calcification, including memory loss, aortic valve stenosis, atherosclerosis, vision problems, even dementia.

Gradual calcium buildup in your coronary arteries can constrict blood flow, causing chest pains and putting you at greater risk for a heart attack.

These deadly age-related processes can be halted and possibly *reversed* using two low-cost nutrients.

SOLUTION: VITAMINS K AND D

Lining our blood vessels is a *protein* that regulates whether or not circulating blood calcium *infiltrates* (calcifies) our arteries. This protein requires *vitamin K_2* to function. When one is deficient in vitamin K_2, vascular calcification occurs. When sufficient K_2 is present, this protein functions to shield against arterial calcification.

Vitamins D and K work *together* to help remove calcium from circulation in the blood, trigger bone formation, and maintain bone strength. Vitamin D helps your bones absorb calcium. Vitamin K ensures that calcium is deposited in your bones and stays out of your arteries. Together they work to prevent excess calcium from depositing in your brain, arteries, and other soft tissues.

NUTRIENT	TYPICAL DAILY DOSE	SUGGESTED PRODUCTS
Vitamin D	5,000 IU (and sometimes higher)	
Vitamin K_1*	1,000 mcg	Super K with Advanced K_2 Complex
Vitamin K_2 as MK-4	1,000 mcg	
Vitamin K_2 as MK-7	100 mcg	

* If you're taking anticoagulant drugs like Coumadin (warfarin), talk to your doctor before starting on a vitamin K regimen.

AGING FACTOR 7: DIGESTIVE ENZYME DEFICIT

Digestive enzymes are essential to the body's absorption and full utilization of food. They speed the chemical reactions that break down food in the digestive tract. Raw foods also provide enzymes that naturally break down food for proper absorption. The capacity of the living organism to make enzymes diminishes with age. One reason we pack on the fat pounds, feel sluggish, and grow more vulnerable to infectious disease as we grow old may surprise you. It's a connection I never made until I started talking to antiaging experts.

Our aging bodies no longer produce sufficient amounts of the active chemical compounds we need to extract essential nutrients from the foods we eat.

Meeting the full range of our nutritional requirements can create a high demand for these *digestive enzymes*. Their gradual loss accounts for many health problems that plague aging adults, from impaired immunity to digestive distress and nutritional deficiencies.

SOLUTION: TAILORED ENZYMATIC AND NUTRITIONAL SUPPORT

NUTRIENT	TYPICAL DAILY DOSE	SUGGESTED PRODUCTS
A complete high-potency digestive enzyme blend	Per label instructions	Enhanced Super Digestive Enzymes with Probiotics
Prebiotic fiber blend	About 6 grams	Agave Digestive-Immune Support

Another way to restore digestive enzyme balance is to ensure you have enough beneficial bacteria in your gut. Supplements that supply these living bacteria are called *probiotics*.

You also need to ensure that "good" bacteria are getting enough of the nutrients they need to thrive. Dietary deficiency of these nutrients—known as *prebiotics*—is another reason we don't have the robust digestive enzyme balance of our younger days.

So your digestive support strategy is threefold:

1. Replenish youthful levels of digestive enzymes.
2. Repopulate your gut with beneficial bacteria using probiotics.
3. Nourish beneficial bacteria so they can thrive with prebiotics.

One final word of caution, and something else that might surprise you: High-quality digestive enzyme supplements can cause you to gain weight if you're not careful.

They work so well in helping your body break down food efficiently that you don't get that "full" feeling as quickly. So you may wind up eating more than you should, *even though you know you shouldn't*.

AGING FACTOR 8: FATTY ACID IMBALANCE

Aging *distorts* the metabolism of *essential* fatty acids, throwing their delicate proportion and interplay off balance. The resulting *fatty acid imbalance* may manifest as anything from irregular heartbeat and skin disorders to heart disease, high blood pressure, and stroke.

SOLUTION: FATTY ACID INTERVENTION

NUTRIENT	TYPICAL DAILY DOSE	SUGGESTED PRODUCTS
Fish oil	1,400 mg EPA and 1,000 mg DHA	Super Omega-3 EPA/ DHA with Sesame Lignans and Olive Fruit Extract
Gamma-linolenic acid	300–600 mg	Mega GLA with Sesame Lignans
Lecithin granules	10 grams	

AGING FACTOR 9: DNA MUTATION

We are continuously exposed to synthetic *and* natural carcinogens in our food supply, in everyday household products, and in our environment. Cooking any food at high temperatures (above 250 degrees Fahrenheit) also generates toxic cancer-causing agents. These environmental and dietary compounds *mutate* cellular DNA.

Aging cells gradually lose their ability to repair DNA from these constant assaults. The resulting DNA damage can cause normally functioning cells to proliferate out of control, turning them into cancer cells.

These processes can be halted and reversed with a number of plant-based compounds that break down carcinogens, prevent cells from becoming cancerous, and *disable* mutated cells.

SOLUTION: TARGETED DNA PROTECTION AND REPAIR

NUTRIENT	TYPICAL DAILY DOSE	SUGGESTED PRODUCTS
Chlorophyllin	100–300 mg	Chlorophyllin
Curcumin*	400–800 mg daily	Super Bio-Curcumin®
Broccoli extract	400–800 mg	Triple Action Cruciferous Vegetable Extract
Watercress extract	50–100 mg	
Rosemary extract	50–100 mg	
Apigenin	25–50 mg	

* 400 mg of enhanced bioavailable curcumin (BCM-95®) equates to 2,500 mg of standard curcumin supplements.

AGING FACTOR 10: IMMUNE DYSFUNCTION

As the aging *immune system* loses its ability to attack bacteria, viruses, and cancer cells, it instead generates excessive levels of *inflammatory* chemicals that turn on its host and create autoimmune diseases such as rheumatoid syndrome.

SOLUTION: SUPERCHARGE YOUR IMMUNE SYSTEM

You can restore your immune system using a few safe, low-cost compounds that target age-related immune conditions. They enhance different parts of your immune system at the same time to optimize your defenses against infectious disease, including pneumonia, the flu, and other highly infectious diseases.

NUTRIENT	TYPICAL DAILY DOSE	SUGGESTED PRODUCTS
Vitamin D	5,000–8,000 IU	
DHEA	15–50 mg	(micronized for optimal absorption)
Beta 1,3/1,6 glucan	100–600 mg	Immune Protect Formula
Probiotic	333 million colony forming units (CFU)	
High-potency multinutrient formula	Two tablets	Life Extension™ Two-Per-Day tablets
Lactoferrin	300 mg	

AGING FACTOR 11: ENZYME IMBALANCE

Youthful functions within your cells depend on multiple *enzymatic* reactions occurring with precise timing. Aging causes enzyme imbalances in the brain and liver. The result can manifest as neurological diseases such as Parkinson's or persistent memory loss. Impaired liver function results in toxic damage to every cell in the body.

SOLUTION: RESTORE YOUTHFUL ENZYME COFACTORS

NUTRIENT	TYPICAL DAILY DOSE	SUGGESTED PRODUCTS
L-methylfolate	1,000 mcg	Optimized Folate
S-adenosylmethionine (SAMe)	200–400 mg	
High-potency multinutrient formula	Two tablets	Life Extension™ Two-Per-Day tablets

AGING FACTOR 12: LOSS OF MITOCHONDRIA

The increasing weakness and fatigue we inevitably experience as we get older isn't only the result of a steady age-related decline in the amount of energy our mitochondria can produce. The *number* of healthy mitochondria throughout our bodies declines sharply as well.

SOLUTION: STIMULATE GROWTH OF NEW MITOCHONDRIA

Mitochondrial biogenesis is the scientific term for the process of growing *fresh* mitochondria. The most recent research indicates that the following nutrients listed can trigger mitochondrial biogenesis and *increase* mitochondrial energy output.

NUTRIENT	TYPICAL DAILY DOSE	SUGGESTED PRODUCTS
Pyrroloquinoline quinone (PQQ)	10–20 mg	PQQ Caps with BioPQQ™
CoQ_{10}	100–200 mg	Super Ubiquinol CoQ_{10} with Enhanced Mitochondrial Support™
R-lipoic acid	300–600 mg	
Trans-resveratrol	250 mg	Optimized Resveratrol with Synergistic Grape-Berry Actives
Acetyl-L-carnitine	1,000–2,000 mg	

AGING FACTOR 13: EXCITOTOXICITY

Excitotoxicity is the pathological process by which nerve cells are damaged and killed by excessive stimulation by neurotransmitters such as glutamate. The result is brain cell damage and destruction leading to neurological disorders. Excitotoxicity contributes to lasting brain damage that arises from events like stroke and traumatic brain injury.

SOLUTION: COMPOUNDS THAT PROTECT AGAINST GLUTAMATE INJURY

There are nutrients that can protect brain cells and neurons from excitotoxicity injury and *regenerate* damaged cells.

NUTRIENT	TYPICAL DAILY DOSE	SUGGESTED PRODUCTS
Vinpocetine	15–30 mg	
Methylcobalamin	1 mg	
Magnesium threonate	1,000–2,000 mg	
Blueberry extract	500–2,000 mg	
Melatonin	1–10 mg before bed	Enhanced Natural Sleep®
Carnosine	1,000 mg	

AGING FACTOR 14: CIRCULATORY DEFICIT

Delivery of nutrient- and oxygen-rich blood to the brain, heart, and extremities is impaired as a part of normal aging. Major strokes and ministrokes are common problems associated with circulatory deficit to the brain. The skin of all aged people shows the effects of lack of nutrient-rich blood to the upper layers. An underlying cause of circulatory deficits is *endothelial dysfunction*, which destroys the inner lining of blood vessels and decimates their ability to efficiently transport blood.

SOLUTION: MULTIMODAL SUPPORT FOR HEALTHY CIRCULATION

With all the mainstream medical and media attention focus on cholesterol and high blood pressure for heart health, a major issue facing most maturing people has been overlooked: *healthy circulation*.

Anywhere from two-thirds to three-fourths of Americans are concerned about circulatory issues by some estimates. Ruptured blood vessels, embolism, stroke, and varicose veins affect many people. Many resort to blood-thinning medications with potentially dangerous side effects. Most have been kept in the dark about low-cost, *natural* alternatives.

One of the most exciting is a brand-new, cutting-edge, high-potency *tomato extract*. This tomato extract is specially processed in such a way that provides benefits you cannot obtain by consuming cooked tomato products. In human clinical trials, it's proven to be completely safe with no side effects. Just three grams improves blood flow within ninety minutes and lasts for more than *twelve hours!*

It's already been approved in Europe for clinical use. It works by helping improve the balance of clotting factors—platelets—in your bloodstream. Even more exciting, it worked for 97 percent of test subjects, which means it will most likely work for you, without the risk of hemorrhaging, organ damage, and other side effects associated with blood-thinning drugs.

To protect against endothelial dysfunction, a critically important nutrient is *pomegranate*. In human clinical studies, those who drank pomegranate juice along with taking their standard therapy are able to *reverse* markers of circulatory deficit. In one study, circulation to the brain increased by 30 percent after one year in the pomegranate group, compared to *reduced* circulation to the brain in the placebo group not getting pomegranate. Both groups continued with their standard therapies.

NUTRIENT	TYPICAL DAILY DOSE	SUGGESTED PRODUCTS
Tomato extract	3 grams	Fruit Flow®
Pomegranate extract	500 mg	Full-Spectrum Pomegranate™
Fish oil	1,400 mg EPA and 1,000 mg DHA	Super Omega-3 EPA/ DHA with Sesame Lignans and Olive Fruit Extract
Sweet orange extract	600 mg	European Leg Solution Featuring Certified Diosmin
Vinpocetine	10–30 mg	

AGING FACTOR 15: LOSS OF YOUTHFUL GENE EXPRESSION

In response to normal aging and environmental toxins, changes occur in *genes* required to sustain youthful cellular function. What happens is that genes that maintain cellular health slowly "turn off," while genes that make us vulnerable to degenerative pathologies become overexpressed (turned on). As cells lose their youthful gene expression profile, we succumb to a plethora of discomforts, diseases, and eventual death.

SOLUTION: ACTIVATE YOUR LONGEVITY GENES

Longevity researchers have known for seventy-five years that consuming far fewer calories while meeting all nutritional needs can greatly increase life span in some species. More recently, geneticists discovered why: caloric restriction activates genes that slow cell aging.

In 2003, remarkable news arrived from the scientific community that a compound found in red grapes and other plants called *resveratrol* extended the life span of certain cells by as much as 70 percent. Even more exciting were findings in 2006 from a team of Harvard researchers showing that resveratrol "switches on" many of the same genes as caloric restriction!

Today this remarkable compound has attained celebrity status, with nationally known doctors endorsing its use. Medical researchers have found it combats not only aging but also the *diseases of aging*.

Further research into the area of *youthful gene expression* has brought to light a new class of compounds like resveratrol that enables aging cells to reverse course and function as though they were young again. These compounds work in *synergy* with resveratrol, mutually complementing and reinforcing its rejuvenating biological effects.

The following box describes four nutrients that help promote more youthful gene expression. Many of them can be found in multi-ingredient formulations, so you only need to take a few pills each day to obtain these potencies.

NUTRIENT	TYPICAL DAILY DOSE	SUGGESTED PRODUCTS
Trans-resveratrol	250 mg	CR Mimetic Longevity Formula
Fisetin	48 mg	
Trans-pterostilbene	3–100 mg	
Vitamin D	5,000 IU	

AGING FACTOR 16: LOSS OF INSULIN SENSITIVITY

In youth, we efficiently utilize ingested carbohydrates to produce cellular energy with a minimal amount converted to body fat storage. Aging reduces cellular sensitivity to insulin, which results in most people suffering chronically high blood glucose and insulin. This not only contributes to common age-related disorders but also unfavorably influences gene expression patterns.

Even if a blood test shows fasting glucose levels are normal, too many of us suffer from constant exposure to excess glucose throughout our normal days. In the presence of excess glucose, healthy tissue comes under an incredibly destructive free-radical assault. The ensuing cellular destruction has been linked to everything from blood vessel damage and stroke to cancer.

The bottom line is that most of us are playing with fire when it comes to excess blood sugar. Without knowing it, we place ourselves under a lifelong assault from excess glucose that wreaks havoc on our bodies long before we or our doctors recognize it. This is why some experts call glucose *the silent killer*. Even modest spikes in blood sugar (fasting glucose above 85 mg/dL) have been linked to increased risk of heart attack.

SOLUTION: RESTORE YOUTHFUL GLUCOSE CONTROL

The good news is that forward-thinking researchers have identified a number of safe, completely natural substances that work in different ways to keep our after-meal blood sugar levels in check.

The most recently discovered of these is *green coffee bean extract*. I'm going to go into a bit of detail here because it really is exciting.

It works by blocking the destructive elevation in blood sugar that occurs after meals. Researchers have identified the active compound in raw coffee beans that combats excess blood sugar as *chlorogenic acid*. It brings blood sugar under control by both reducing the release of stored glucose into our bloodstreams *and* stopping the creation of excess glucose within our bodies.

In a recent clinical trial, just 350 mg three times a day of green coffee bean extract produced a remarkable 35 percent reduction in after-meal glucose spike. After twelve weeks, study participants shed on average almost eleven pounds, with fat loss accounting for 92 percent of the weight.

Nutrient	Typical Daily Dose	Suggested Products
Green coffee bean extract	350–1,050 mg	
Chromium	500 mcg	
Green tea phytosome	300 mg	Optimized Irvingia with Phase 3™ Calorie Control Complex
Irvingia gabonensis extract	300 mg	
Cinnamon	175–350 mg	CinSulin® with InSea™ and Crominex® 3+ (chromium)
R-lipoic acid	150–300 mg	

AGING FACTOR 17: LOSS OF BONE DENSITY

Aging gradually weakens bones through decalcification and trace mineral loss. A compromised skeletal system negatively affects immune strength, blood cell production, nervous system function, insulin sensitivity, energy metabolism, and weight management.

SOLUTION: BROAD-SPECTRUM BONE SUPPORT

Ninety-nine percent of the calcium in our bodies resides in our teeth and bones. It stands to reason that if our bones and teeth store so much calcium, we would need to obtain additional calcium to preserve their strength. The real controversy is why mainstream doctors remain unenlightened about the need of maturing people to take the *right* kind of calcium supplement—and the proper nutrients to support it.

Ideal forms of calcium to look for on labels are *dicalcium malate, calcium bis-glycinate,* or *calcium citrate.* They're easily tolerated by the body, highly absorbable, and supportive of bone mineral density—the key measure of a calcium supplement's value.

A daily dose of at least 1,000 mg is recommended for female adults. Women can take up to 1,200 mg. You won't get any additional benefit from high doses. (Men only need around 800 mg a day of supplemental calcium.)

Your body can't readily absorb calcium without *vitamin D_3*. This vitamin also ensures calcium deposits properly in bone tissue. There are receptors for vitamin D_3 in more than thirty different tissue types throughout the body. D_3 binds with them to promote immune function, reduce inflammation, reduce hardening of the arteries, enhance heart function, improve brain and nerve tissue performance, and even prevent cancer.

It's a good idea to have your vitamin D blood levels checked to make sure you're getting enough. The current evidence suggests that your readings for *25-hydroxyvitamin-D* should be between 50 and 80 ng/mL in blood for optimal health. Experts suggest taking at least 2,000 IU per day, with most people requiring 5,000 IU per day, to achieve blood levels in a healthy range.

NUTRIENT	TYPICAL DAILY DOSE	SUGGESTED PRODUCTS
Calcium	1,200 mg	Bone Restore
Vitamin D	1,000 IU	
Magnesium	340 mg	
Zinc	2 mg	
Manganese	1 mg	
Silicon	5 mg	
Boron	3 mg	
Vitamin K_1	1,000 mcg	Super K with Advanced K_2 Complex
Vitamin K_2 as MK-4*	1,000 mcg	
Vitamin K_2 as MK-7	100 mcg	

* If you're taking anticoagulant drugs like Coumadin (warfarin), talk to your doctor before starting on a vitamin K_2 regimen.

AGING FACTOR 18: OXIDATIVE STRESS

Free radicals are fiery unstable molecules that have been implicated in most diseases associated with aging.

At the molecular level, the continuous chemical reactions keeping your heart beating, your blood moving, and your brain working look like controlled infernos. The constant exchange of electrons wheeling inside the tiny energy-producing powerhouses in your cells called the *mitochondria* throws off enormous quantities of energy.

The problem is that as we get older, the cellular structures that once kept these fires under control begin to degrade, including the mitochondria themselves. Aging causes our cells to lose control over these reactions and renders them more vulnerable to destruction.

SOLUTION: QUENCH THE RAGING FIRES WITHIN

Antioxidants have become popular supplements to protect against free-radical-induced cell damage, but few people take the proper combination of antioxidant supplements to adequately compensate for age-induced loss of endogenous antioxidants such as SOD, glutathione, and catalase.

NUTRIENT	TYPICAL DAILY DOSE	SUGGESTED PRODUCTS
Superoxide dismutase/ Gliadin complex (GliSODin®)	500 mg	Endothelial Defense™ with GliSODin® and Full Spectrum Pomegranate
Pomegranate extract	500 mg	
Green tea extract	725 mg	
Grapeseed extract	150 mg	
S-adenosylmethionine (SAMe)	200–400 mg	
Astaxanthin	5–6 mg	
R-lipoic acid	300–600 mg	

(continued)

NUTRIENT	TYPICAL DAILY DOSE	SUGGESTED PRODUCTS
High-potency multinutrient formula	Two tablets	Life Extension™ Two-Per-Day tablets
Gamma-tocopherol/ sesame	200 mg gamma-tocopherol with 20 mg of standardized sesame lignans	

ONE FINAL NOTE

Children can benefit by taking vitamin supplements, but it is the *aging human* whose body is depleted of the endogenous antioxidants, hormones, enzymatic repair systems, and other biological chemicals needed to sustain life. What is optional in childhood becomes *mandatory* as humans enter middle age and become vulnerable to a host of degenerative diseases that await them if they fail to protect themselves.

The encouraging news is that supplements like fish oil, vitamin D, lipoic acid, curcumin, coQ_{10}, resveratrol, DHEA, vitamin K, and SAMe function to circumvent multiple aging factors that conspire to rob us of our youthful health. This means that you don't have to take gobs of pills to counteract the multiple mechanisms of aging described in this chapter.

To find out about low-cost sources where you can obtain these nutrients in concentrated multi-ingredient formulas, log on to www.suzannesomers.com and click through to Life Extension or call 1-888-884-3666 any time of the day or night.

THE WRAP-UP

Thank you for reading this book. I hope at this point you have been encouraged to take your health into your own hands, and form a *plan* enabling you to live longer and healthier.

ONLY YOU CAN DO IT!

I've tried to expose you to the best and the brightest, those who have dedicated their lives and professions to making life an exciting, healthy, and long-lasting experience. You now know what's coming in Ray Kurzweil's future: advancements that will make the present paradigm of aging and the current approach to health obsolete. You've been introduced to nanotechnology and the most cutting-edge advancements in medicine and health that are accessible now. You now know you can regrow body parts with one's own autologous stem cells, as I have been able to do with my breast.

You have learned that there are unavoidable toxic forces that are damaging our health and in many cases killing us. You know that there is a new specialty called *environmental medicine* that understands the toxic planet and how to deal with it; you also know you

can detoxify and clean your blood regularly to remove these dangerous toxins; and you know that there are supplements available that
not only lessen the intensity of the toxic assault but also actually kill
free radicals to protect you.

You know why you age, and how to stop it, and you now know
there is a new supplement that is being hailed as the Holy Grail,
the enzyme that actually lengthens telomeres, which allows for longer life and reverse aging. Imagine, we can now turn back the clock
without surgery or drugs. You now know that cancer is manageable,
and that there are steps *you* can take to prevent cancer by keeping
the "cancer-protective genetic switches" turned "on." You now know
there may actually be cancer-resistant human beings and that their
white blood cells could be the ones to save your life or that of a loved
one. You now know that there is a natural answer to regressing prostate cancer that will change men's lives. And you now know that
there are patches that repair, give energy, and prevent disease.

You know that hormones are the juice of youth, and that restoration of these vital hormones prevents deterioration. You know there
are hormones to make you sexy, hormones to help you sleep, hormones to invigorate your energy, and hormones that protect your
brain. You know there is a new kind of medicine and a new kind of
doctor who understands that it's a different world and we have to
treat our bodies differently as a result.

I want this book to be life changing for you. It was for me. You
can utilize some of the information, all of it, or none of it. But more
than anything, this book is meant to put your health and *how you
age* where it belongs, in your hands. If the present paradigm of aging
is not attractive to you then *do something about it, now*! It's not too
soon; in fact, the sooner the better. But anytime you start, you will
be better off than never having done anything at all.

MAKE YOUR PLAN

What's your plan going to be? Change your eating habits, change
your sleep habits. Manage your stress, eliminate the toxins from your
home and your food, and be grateful for the love in your life. It's all
part of aging well.

SEE YOUR END POINT

What does it look like? How old are you? What do you look like? Are you in good health? Are you happy? Do you have energy? Are you having sex? Are your bones strong? Is your brain working?

It's your life. You can redefine aging. It's all up to you. See it. See exactly what you want. Visualize it. And then go get it.

And one more thing. Think good thoughts. Each cell in the human body is important and every cell communicates with all the other fifty trillion or so cells that make up *who we are*. So every day talk to just one cell and feed it something positive: "I am happy" or "I am well." The job of that one cell is then to communicate to all the other cells alerting them that "We are happy." It works.

This quote hangs on the wall of the Palm Greens restaurant, a small organic eatery down the hill from my home where I go in the mornings to get my "green smoothie." It says:

> We are what we think. All that we are arises with our thoughts.
> With our thoughts, we make the world.
>
> —Buddha

Thank you,

FOREVER HEALTH—RESOURCE SITE FOR QUALIFIED DOCTORS

I have always included a resource guide at the back of my books directing my readers to qualified doctors specializing in bioidentical hormone replacement and antiaging medicine. Initially, and astonishingly, in my book *The Sexy Years*, the resource section of qualified doctors was only a total of eleven doctors. By *Ageless* it grew to over a hundred, and then by *Breakthrough*, the list grew so large it had to be put on my website. Now we are in the thousands, and it shows the power of patients being informed about their bodies and how they function. Women read the books and realized they could feel good again. And to my great surprise, they brought their husbands along and they started feeling good also: The result is happier couples, more stable marriages, and healthier people. This has been the thrill of my life.

But no one, especially the doctors, was ready for the huge onslaught. The doctors' practices became at times overwhelmed—front desks that couldn't handle the load, secretaries having meltdowns. Something had to be done. It had to be simplified not only for the patients so they weren't hanging on the phone forever trying to get an appointment, but also for the doctors so their front offices were not overrun and unmanageable.

The answer is *Forever Health*, a newly created source for qualified antiaging doctors.

The resource guide will direct patients where to go in their area to find a qualified specialist in this type of medicine. Under the Forever

Health guidance program, patients will be able to be in contact with their doctor whenever they want.

The patient will not be a number. Even with thousands of patients already under a doctor's care, the new patient will feel that he or she is the doctor's only patient. Patients can get their appointments made easily and not be left in cyberspace because they can't get through to anyone.

How can this be done?

Forever Health has come up with a software system that will make it very easy for patients to find the help they need. These doctors will have been trained in the specialty of bioidentical hormones and antiaging medicine. Everything you read about in any of my books will be common knowledge to all of them.

Up until now, all the doctors have been taught different protocols and most have elected to specialize in only one. Forever Health doctors will be able to offer various protocols as a result of standardized training under the guidance of a medical advisory board. Forever Health takes patients right to each doctor's website. They can read all about the physician and find out what he or she has available, what that doctor offers, and then individuals can decide which doctor is the right "fit" for them.

Then people can click on and make an appointment. The doctor's calendar will open and the person clicks on when he or she wants an appointment. Then it's set. The doctor can electronically send out all the forms and paperwork the patient needs to fill out. Once the patient fills out the forms and sends them back, the lab requests can be sent out as well. For patients, everything is taken care of . . . when they walk in the door of their new doctor's office, the doctor has everything he or she needs electronically and now the doctor has the information to sit down and spend quality time with individual patients. I was so impressed with the system—which trained the doctors, modernized the mechanics of making orders, and made the patient visit more meaningful—I decided to join forces with them.

It doesn't matter where you live, there will be a doctor in your town; if not, Forever Health will direct you to the qualified doctors nearest you.

The goal of Forever Health is to offer a nationwide, validated, turn-key approach to superb quality health care. Each clinician will be held to the highest standard. Forever Health and its advisory board will be doing research at all times. They will continue raising the level of excellence to ensure the doctors on this roster continue to be updated and aware of the latest advancements.

To access Forever Health, go to www.foreverhealth.com.

SUGGESTED READING

Balch, Phyllis A. *Prescription for Nutritional Healing*, 5th ed. New York: Avery, 2010.

Blaylock, Russell L., M.D. *Excitotoxins: The Taste That Kills*. Albuquerque, N.Mex.: Health Press, 1997.

———. *Health and Nutrition Secrets That Can Save Your Life*, rev. edn. Albuquerque, N.Mex.: Health Press, 2006.

———. *Natural Strategies for Cancer Patients*. London: Kensington, 2003.

———. *Nuclear Sunrise* (e-booklet).

Brownlee, Shannon. *Overtreated: Why Too Much Medicine Is Making Us Sicker and Poorer*. New York: Bloomsbury, 2008.

Campbell, T. Colin, and Thomas M. Campbell. *The China Study: The Most Comprehensive Study of Nutrition Ever Conducted and the Startling Implications for Diet, Weight Loss and Long-Term Health*. Dallas, Tex.: BenBella Books, 2004.

Canton, James, Ph.D. *The Extreme Future: The Top Trends That Will Shape the World for the Next 5, 10, and 20 Years*. New York: Dutton, 2006.

Critser, Greg. *Generation Rx: How Prescription Drugs Are Altering American Lives, Minds, and Bodies*. Boston: Houghton Mifflin Harcourt, 2005.

Dayton, Martin. *The Case for Intravenous EDTA Chelation Therapy*, 1999.

Elias, Thomas. *The Burzynski Breakthrough: The Most Promising Treatment . . . and the Government's Campaign to Squelch It*. Lexikos Publishing, 2000.

Faloon, William. *Pharmocracy*. Mount Jackson, Va.: Praktikos Books, 2011.

Fitzgerald, Randall. *The Hundred-Year Lie*. New York: Dutton, 2006.

Fossel, Michael, M.D., Ph.D., Greta Blackburn, and Dave Woynarowski, M.D. *The Immortality Edge*. Hoboken, N.J.: John Wiley & Sons, 2011.

Fox, Cynthia. *Cell of Cells: The Global Race to Capture and Control the Stem Cell*. New York: W.W. Norton, 2007.

Galitzer, Michael. *Clinical Bioenergetics* (pamphlet).

Goldberg, Burton, W. Lee Cowden, and Ferre Akbarpour. *Longevity*. Alternative Medicine.com Books, 2001.

Graveline, Duane, M.D. *Lipitor, Thief of Memory*. Self-published, 2006.

Greene, Robert A., M.D., and Leah Feldon. *Perfect Balance: Dr. Robert Greene's Breakthrough Program for Finding the Lifelong Hormonal Health You Deserve*. New York: Clarkson Potter, 2005.

Haltiwanger, Steve. *Winning in the New World: With Help from the Power of Anti-Aging Peptides and Hormones*, audiobook. Intec Publishing, 2002.

Hertoghe, Thierry, M.D. *The Hormone Solution*. New York: Three Rivers Press, 2002.

Hinohara, Shigeaki. *Living Long, Living Good*.

Hotze, Steven F., and Kelly Griffin. *Hormones, Health, and Happiness: A Natural Medical Formula for Rediscovering Youth*. Houston, Tex.: Forrest Publishing, 2005.

Kekich, David A. *Life Extension Express*. BookSurge.com, 2009.

Kurzweil, Ray. *The Singularity Is Near*. New York: Viking Penguin, 2005.

Kurzweil, Ray, and Terry Grossman, M.D. *Fantastic Voyage*. New York: Plume, 2005.

———. *Transcend*. New York: Rodale, 2009.

Life, Jeffry S., M.D., Ph.D. *The Life Plan*.

Lipton, Bruce H., Ph.D. *The Biology of Belief*. Carlsbad, Calif.: Hay House, 2008.

Mahmud, Khalid, M.D. *Keeping aBreast: Ways to Stop Breast Cancer*. Bloomington, Ind.: AuthorHouse, 2005.

McLeod, Donald M., and Philip A. White. *Doctors' Secrets: The Road to Longevity*, 2001.

Mercola, Joseph. *Take Control of Your Health*, 2007.

Miller, Philip Lee, M.D., and the Life Extension Foundation with Monica Reinagel. *Life Extension Revolution: The New Science of Growing Older Without Aging*. New York: Bantam Books, 2006.

Morgentaler, Abraham, M.D. *Testosterone for Life: Recharge Your Vitality, Sex Drive, Muscle Mass, and Overall Health*. New York: McGraw-Hill, 2008.

Moritz, Andreas, and John Hornecker. *Simple Steps to Total Health*. Enter-chi.com, 2006.

Morrison, Jeffrey A., M.D. *Cleanse Your Body, Clear Your Mind*. New York: Hudson Street Press, 2011.

Moss, Ralph W. *Alternative Medicine Online: A Guide to Natural Remedies on the Internet*, 1997.

Moss, Ralph W., and Theron G. Randolph. *An Alternative Approach to Allergies: The New Field of Clinical Ecology Unravels the Environmental Causes of Mental and Physical Ills*. New York: Harper & Row, 1989.

Niehans, Paul. *Introduction to Cellular Therapy*. New York: Pageant Books, 1960.

Owens, Paula. *The Power of 4: Your Ultimate Guide Guaranteed to Change Your Body and Transform Your Life*, 2008.

Plasker, Eric. *The 100 Year Lifestyle: Dr. Plasker's Breakthrough Solution for Living Your Best Life*. Avon, Mass.: Adams Media, 2007.

Ragnar, Peter. *The LifeWave Experience to a New You! The Official Handbook.* Asheville, N.C.: Roaring Lion Publishing, 2007.

Rea, William J., M.D. *Energy and Brain Function.*

————. *Optimum Environments for Optimum Living and Creativity*, 2002.

Rogers, Sherry A., M.D. *Detoxify or Die.* Hampton, Va.: Prestige, 2002.

Rothenberg, Ron, M.D., Kathleen Becker, and Kris Hart. *Forever Ageless.* Encinitas, Calif.: HealthSpan Institute, 2007.

Rowe, John Wallis, and Robert L. Kahn. *Successful Aging.* New York: Dell, 1999.

Segala, Melanie, ed. *Disease Prevention and Treatment.* Hollywood, Fla.: Life Extension, 2003.

Sinatra, Stephen T., M.D., F.A.C.C., C.B.T. *A Cardiologist's Guide to Optimum Health.* New York: Lincoln-Bradley, 1996.

————. *CoenzymeQ$_{10}$ and the Heart.* Keats Publishing, 1999.

————. *The CoenzymeQ$_{10}$ Phenomenon.* Keats Publishing, 1998.

————. *Heartbreak & Heart Disease: A Mind/Body Prescription for Healing the Heart.* Keats Publishing, 1996.

————. *Lose to Win: A Cardiologist's Guide to Weight Loss and Nutritional Healing.* New York: Lincoln-Bradley, 1992.

————. *Lower Your Blood Pressure in Eight Weeks: A Revolutionary Program for a Longer, Healthier Life.* New York: Ballantine Books, 2003.

————. *Optimum Health: A Natural Lifesaving Prescription for Your Body and Mind.* New York: Bantam Books, 1996.

————. *The Sinatra Solution: New Hope for Preventing and Treating Heart Disease.* North Bergen, N.J.: Basic Health Publications, 2005.

Sinatra, Stephen, and Connie Bennett. *Sugar Shock! How Sweets and Simple Carbs Can Derail Your Life—and How You Can Get Back on Track.* New York: Berkeley, 2006.

Sinatra, Stephen, and James Roberts. *Reverse Heart Disease Now.* New York: John Wiley & Sons, 2007.

Sinatra, Stephen, Graham Simpson, and Jorge Suarez-Menendez. *Spa Medicine: Your Getaway to the Ageless Zone.* North Bergen, N.J.: Basic Health Publications, 2004.

Sinatra, Stephen, and Jan Sinatra. *L-Carnitine and the Heart.* Keats Publishing, 1999.

Sinatra, Stephen, Jan Sinatra, and Roberta Jo Lieberman. *Heart Sense for Women: Your Plan for Natural Prevention and Treatment.* New York: Plume, 2000.

Small, Gary, M.D., and Gigi Vorgan. *The Longevity Bible: 8 Essential Strategies for Keeping Your Mind Sharp and Your Body Young.* New York: Hyperion, 2007.

Starr, Mark, M.D. *Hypothyroidism Type 2.* Irvine, Calif.: New Voice Publications, 2005.

Sutherland, Caroline. *The Body Knows . . . How to Stay Young: Healthy-Aging Secrets from a Medical Intuitive.* Carlsbad, Calif.: Hay House, 2008.

Thomas, John. *Young Again: How to Reverse the Aging Process.* Medford, N.J.: Plexus Press, 2002.

Thompson, Robert, and Kathleen Barnes. *The Calcium Lie: What Your Doctor Doesn't Know Could Kill You.* In Truth Press, 2008.

Van Zyl, Bernard. *Stem Cells Saved My Life: How to Be Next*. Bloomington, Ind.: AuthorHouse, 2006.

Wallach, Joel D., and Ma Lan. *Dead Doctors Don't Lie*. Franklin, Tenn.: Legacy Communications, 1999.

Watson, Brenda. *The H.O.P.E. Formula*. Palm Harbor, Fla.: ReNew Life Press, 2007.

———. *The Road to Perfect Health*. Sherman Oaks, Calif.: Health Point Press, 2011.

Watson, Brenda, and Leonard Smith, M.D. *Gut Prescriptions: Natural Solutions to Your Digestive Problems*. Palm Harbor, Fla.: ReNew Life Press, 2006.

Wright, Jonathan V., M.D. *Dr. Wright's Book of Nutritional Therapy: Real-Life Lessons in Medicine Without Drugs*. Emmaus, Pa.: Rodale, 1979.

———. *Maximize Your Vitality and Potency*. Petaluma, Calif.: Smart Publications, 1999.

Wright, Jonathan V., M.D., and Alan R. Gaby, M.D. *Natural Medicine, Optimal Wellness*. Ridgefield, Conn.: Vital Health Publishing, 2006.

Wright, Jonathan V., M.D., and Lane Lenard. *D-Mannose and Bladder Infection: The Natural Alternative to Antibiotics*. Auburn, Wash.: Dragon Art, 2001.

———. *Why Stomach Acid Is Good for You*. New York: M. Evans and Company, 2001.

———. *Xylitol: Dental and Upper Respiratory Health*. Auburn, Wash.: Dragon Art, 2003.

Wright, Jonathan V., M.D., and John Morgenthaler. *Natural Hormone Replacement for Women over 45*. Petaluma, Calif.: Smart Publications, 1997.

Wright, Jonathan V., M.D., and John Neustadt. *Thriving Through Dialysis*. Auburn, Wash.: Dragon Art, 2005.

Wright, Jonathan V., M.D., et al. *The Natural Pharmacy*. New York: Three Rivers Press, 1999.

Young, Simon. *Designer Evolution: A Transhumanist Manifesto*. Amherst, N.Y.: Prometheus, 2005.

INDEX

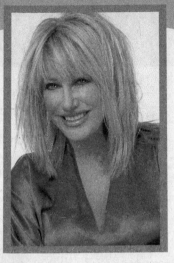
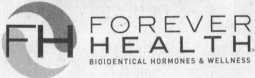